SAUNDERS

POCKET
REFERENCE
for
NURSES

SAUNDERS

POCKET

REFERENCE
for

NURSES
SECOND EDITION

KATHLEEN MELONAKOS, RN, MA
Nurse Consultant
Palo Alto, California

SHERYL A. MICHELSON, RN, MS
Nurse Educator, Operating Room Region
Stanford Health Services
Stanford, California

W.B. SAUNDERS COMPANY
A Division of Harcourt Brace & Company
PHILADELPHIA, LONDON, TORONTO, MONTREAL, SYDNEY, TOKYO

W. B. SAUNDERS COMPANY
A Division of Harcourt Brace & Company

The Curtis Center
Independence Square West
Philadelphia, PA 19106

Library of Congress Cataloging-in-Publication Data

Melonakos, Kathleen.
    Saunders pocket reference for nurses / Kathleen
Melonakos — 2nd ed.
      p.   cm.
    Includes bibliographical references.
    ISBN 0-7216-4459-7
    1. Nursing—Handbooks, manuals, etc. I. Michelson,
Sheryl A.
II. Title. III. Title: Pocket reference for nurses.
    [DNLM: 1. Nursing Care—handbooks. 2. Nursing
Process—handbooks.
WY 39 M528s 1995]
RT51.M45   1995
610.73—dc20
DNLM/DLC
                                        94-20443

SAUNDERS POCKET REFERENCE FOR NURSES ISBN 0–7216–4459–7

Printed in the United States of America

Last digit is the print
number: 9   8   7   6   5   4   3   2   1

To all healers—
"Healing occurs in relationships."

Dr. Peter Koestenbaum

CONTRIBUTORS

Amy Andolina, RN, MS
Nutrition Support Consultant
Lucille Packard Children's Hospital
Palo Alto, California
*Intravenous Therapy, Parenteral Nutrition,
and Blood Transfusion*

Sandra Bardas, Pharm. D
Clinical Pharmacist
Stanford Health Services
Palo Alto, California
Drug Administration

Brenda Bouvier, RN, MS, CIC
Manager, Infection Prevention
Stanford Health Services
Palo Alto, California
Infectious Disease and Infection Prevention

Kathleen A. Coryell, RN, MSPH
Epidemiologist, Infection Prevention
Stanford Health Services
Palo Alto, California
Infectious Disease and Infection Prevention

Ann Coulston, RD, MS
Senior Research Dietician
Stanford Health Services
Palo Alto, California
Nutrition and Medical Nutrition Therapy

Lorraine Hultquist, RN, EdD
Director of Nursing Education
Evergreen Valley College
San Jose, California
Selected Nursing Diagnoses and Nursing Interventions

Nancy Merritt, RN, BA, CEN
Clinical Nurse III, Emergency Department
El Camino Hospital
Mountain View, California
Emergency Assessment and Intervention

Sheryl Michelson, RNC, MS
Nurse Educator, Perioperative Services
Stanford Health Services
Palo Alto, California
The Client Undergoing Surgery

Pamela Schreiber, RN, MS
Clinical Nurse Specialist, Pain Management
Stanford Health Services
Palo Alto, California
Selected Nursing Diagnoses and Nursing Interventions

REVIEWERS & CONSULTANTS

CHARLENE DENDY-GRAVES, RN, BS
Nurse Manager for Partial and Outpatient
Psychiatric/Chemical Dependency Services
Sierra Gateway Hospital
Clovis, California

KATHY DOHERTY, RN, MS
Oncology Clinical Nurse Specialist
Stanford Health Services
Palo Alto, California

LORI HART
Clinical Instructor
Department of Diagnostic Radiology
Stanford Health Services
Palo Alto, California

LORRAINE HULTQUIST, RN, EdD
Director of Nursing Education
Evergreen Valley College
San Jose, California

KATHRYN LaGRANGE, RN, MS, CCRN
Clinical Nurse Specialist
Critical Care
Stanford Health Services
Palo Alto, California

NANCY MERRITT, RN, BA, CEN
Clinical Nurse III, Emergency Department
El Camino Hospital
Mountain View, California

PREFACE

Purpose

As a student nurse, new graduate, medical-surgical nurse, and psychiatric nurse, I noted that physicians often used pocket manuals, and recognized that nurses could well benefit from a general, eclectic pocket reference of their own. A portable volume containing the most essential information for nurses on the job was needed. I set about, with the help of friends and colleagues (many at Stanford University Medical Center) to distill the most important facts and figures that nurses constantly use when caring for adult clients with various types of medical diagnoses.

In the first edition, my colleagues and I focused on nursing responsibilities such as assessment, lab evaluation, nursing diagnoses, fluid and electrolyte balance, drug administration, and nutrition. We also included information on cancer, heart disease, surgery, psychiatry, and emergency situations. The experienced editors at Saunders helped us refine the work, and the **Saunders Pocket Reference for Nurses** (or "**PRN**") became a reality in 1990. Its immediate success showed us that we had filled a professional need.

For the second edition, Sheryl Michelson, with her wide knowledge base, joined me as co-author and co-editor. Together we endeavored to retain the nursing centered focus and organization of the first edition while reflecting changes in the evolving health care environment. Again with the help of expert colleagues, we made additions and revisions according to advances in medicine, nursing, and health care technology, including computer charting, pulse oximetry, increasingly varied IV pumps and controllers, new drugs, new diagnostic procedures, increased outpatient and laser surgery, the expanded use of endoscopy, new cancer treatments, new infection control practices, and current CPR recommendations. Throughout the book, we again emphasize the nursing process, nursing diagnosis, and client education.

Audience

Students who must grasp and apply enormous amounts of data will find this book extremely helpful. New graduates who want to ease their transition from student to clinician can use this manual as an aid. Experienced practitioners will benefit from the up-to-the-minute information and easy accessibility, as they are usually pressed for time. Advanced practice nurses such as nurse practitioners and clinical nurse specialists need reminders, too, as they cannot be expected to retain in memory the vast quantities of information and facts that are necessary to the complex provision of health care today. Psychiatric nurses may also want to refer to the **PRN** "as needed," to better meet the needs of their clients. This book will serve as a valuable resource for home health nurses as well, as practice in that and other nonhospital settings continues to expand.

Organization and Content

Clinical assessment, as the primary step in the nursing process, is referred to throughout the book, but is the primary focus of the first three chapters. Chapter 1 covers major areas of clinical assessment, along with anatomical charts and new documentation practices. Chapter 2 describes assessment of and interventions for some of the most commonly encountered and urgent nursing diagnoses, such as pain, anxiety, nausea, vomiting, and sleeplessness. Chapter 3 includes extensive laboratory data, such as the "normal" reference chart, with increased and decreased value indications. Assisting the physician to diagnose disease is a primary nursing function; therefore, Chapter 4 provides the indications, preparation, and posttest treatments in chart form for many frequently ordered diagnostic procedures.

Chapters 5, 6, 7, 8, 9, and 12 deal with areas of concern in almost all client care situations: fluid and electrolyte balance, intravenous therapy, drug administration, nutrition and diets, infection control, and psychosocial considerations, respectively. Chapter 10 covers both general perioperative care and care in specific types of surgeries, while Chapter 11 deals with general care of the cancer client. For quick and easy location, content on emergency management is placed last, with nursing implications provided for handling critical medical conditions such as myocardial infarction. Full CPR guidelines, current as of 1992, are outlined, with clear illustrations in Chapter 13.

We designed the format of this book to provide the easiest possible access to information. For instance, we frequently use concise charts or tables to allow for quick comparison. The main topics are numbered and listed at the beginning of each chapter. Sections, tables and figures are numbered and follow in sequence. Convenient cross-referencing is utilized throughout the book to save space and avoid repetition. The extensive index will also make it easy to find specific topics.

This manual is not intended to take the place of policy or procedure manuals, as protocols vary in different clinical settings. Specific hospital policy must be followed in every case. *Every nurse is responsible for knowing and following his or her own institution's policy at all times.* This book only provides guidelines for common practice.

Acknowledgements

I want especially to thank my co-author, Sheryl Michelson of Stanford, for her tireless energy and abilities in helping prepare the second edition. She cheerfully met deadlines even while carrying a tremendous workload as a nurse educator and mother of two small children. I really appreciate that we could work well together. I also want to thank my husband, Brian, who has supported me in countless ways and made my publishing efforts possible. My mother, Mary Kimball, has inspired me and helped me as well. Also, I am grateful to the friends and colleagues with whom Sheryl and I worked who either contributed or reviewed chapters. These experts are listed at the beginning of this book. Finally, let me thank Thomas Eoyang, Editor-in-Chief at W.B. Saunders, and Cass Stamato, his faithful assistant, who encouraged me and gave helpful guidelines for completing the task. It is my hope again to aid nurses in helping people.

KATHLEEN MELONAKOS

For many years now I have wanted to author a book. Perhaps my desire came from the influence of my two gifted parents; my father, Edward Michelson PhD, an accomplished writer of textbooks and journal articles, and my mother, Carole Black, who was the publisher of scientific journals. I was fortunate that Kathleen offered me the opportunity to join her as a co-author of the second edition of the **PRN.** I have grown a great deal from working with Kathleen. Our relationship allowed us to "mentor" each other and I value her friendship as well as her professional expertise. I would also like to thank my husband, Chuck, and our daughters, Samantha and Julia, who so patiently supported me through countless hours of writing, proofing, and phone calls.

SHERYL MICHELSON

CONTENTS

CLINICAL ASSESSMENT

The most fundamental skill required in nursing is the ability to assess, prevent, and solve problems. In order for problems to be prevented or solved, they must first be identified, which calls for sharp assessment skills.

As a nurse, evaluate yourself often in your ability to pinpoint and implement solutions to problems and potential problems. Develop your own personal method for doing client histories and physicals based upon your institutional policies, skill level, time, and client population. Expertise with the vital signs and neurologic assessments is essential, as crucial decisions must be made from these data. As the member of the health care team who spends the most time with the client, your assessment skills are vital.

1-1 THE NURSING PROCESS

While physicians focus on diagnosing and treating disease, nurses focus on client response to illness, and its effect on daily functioning. The nursing process is the problem-solving method nurses use to assist clients in meeting basic needs (Figure 1-1). Nursing diagnosis, a key element of the process, helps to identify which problems can be solved by nursing care and which require the health team's collaborative efforts. Then a plan of care can be formulated and implemented. When doing nursing care plans, goals should be directed at strengthening client coping mechanisms and increasing abilities to perform activities of daily living.

Assess Identify unmet client needs based on objective and subjective data:

1. The client, his family/significant others
2. Laboratory data, the medical record
3. The physical examination

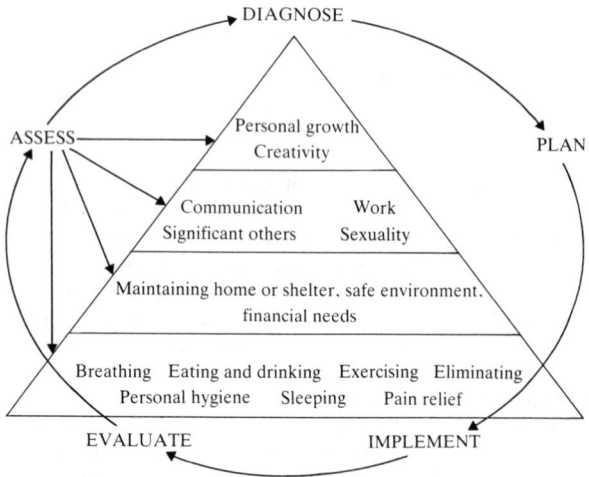

Figure 1–1. Meeting basic needs with the nursing process.

4. Nursing history, subsequent client interviews
5. Members of the health team

Diagnose   Analyze data and formulate nursing diagnosis or diagnoses. See NANDA Approved Nursing Diagnostic Categories, Appendix A, and Chapter 2. List problems separately on the medical record.

Plan   Give the most urgent and critical problems the highest priority. Establish short-term, intermediate, and long-term goals (outcomes) together with client. List nursing orders and expected outcomes with time limits in the nursing care plan.

Implement   Put the plan into action. Coordinate the activities of client, health care team, and family members. Record responses.

Evaluate   Compare client behavioral outcomes with the expected outcomes. Determine the extent to which goals are achieved. Identify alterations needed in the nursing care plan.

1-2   THE HEALTH HISTORY

Obtaining the nursing history and physical assessment are the first steps in establishing nurse-client rapport, determining the nursing diagnoses, and formulating a plan of care. Facilitate meaningful nurse-client communication in the initial and subsequent interviews by doing the following:

- Provide a quiet, private atmosphere.

- Introduce yourself and state your purpose.

- If the client is unable to give a history, ask if family or a significant other may be present. List the person giving the information at the beginning of the assessment form.

- Be relaxed and unhurried, sitting with client if possible.

- Adjust length of interview to the needs of the client. Adapt accordingly if the client is elderly or sensory impaired, i.e., sit close enough so your voice may be heard clearly or make sure hearing aid is adjusted properly. Do not overtire the client. Structure the interview using a mutual planning approach to stay within time limits and remain goal-centered.

- Convey interest in the client.
- Maintain eye contact.
- Speak slowly and clearly.
- Ask open-ended rather than leading questions.
- Avoid getting unnecessarily personal, or explain why you need the information.
- Observe nonverbal as well as verbal responses.

I. Source of Information and Reliability of Informant

II. Identifying Information
  A. Complete name, address, and phone number
  B. Age, date, and place of birth
  C. Sex
  D. Ethnic origin
  E. First/major language spoken
  F. Marital status/significant other(s)
  G. Occupation

III. Chief Complaint (Why medical care is being sought, in the client's own words)

IV. History of Present Illness
  A. Time and date of onset
  B. Sudden or gradual
  C. Location in the body
  D. Mild, moderate, or severe
  E. Aggravating or alleviating factors
  F. Associated symptoms (i.e., shortness of breath)
  G. Frequency since it began

V. Past Medical History
  A. Hospitalizations: time, duration, and diagnosis
  B. Operations
  C. Childhood illnesses and immunizations
  D. Injuries
  E. Illnesses or chronic conditions, especially infectious diseases, i.e., TB, HIV, Hepatitis
  F. Blood transfusions
  G. Foreign travel (dates and places)

    H. Allergies to foods, drugs, or other items such as iodine, tape, or latex (describe reactions to allergens)

VI. **Present Medication** (Names, dosages, routes, and frequency of all medications presently being taken or taken recently [include over-the-counter medication, birth-control pills, transdermal drug delivery systems, illicit or street drugs])

VII. **Family History**
    A. Age and health status of parents, grandparents, aunts, uncles, siblings
    B. Age and health status of spouse, children
    C. Familial illnesses: (i.e., cancer, diabetes mellitus, heart disease, hypertension, seizure disorder, renal disease, arthritis, alcoholism, mental health problems, anemia)

VIII. **Social History**
    A. Residence
    B. Work environment
    C. Hobbies
    D. Social relationships
    E. Recent stressful life events (see Table 12-5, Social Readjustment Rating Scale)
    F. Financial effects of illness or hospitalization
    G. Religious/cultural/lifestyle patterns

IX. **Health Habits**
    A. Use of alcohol, tobacco, caffeine, and/or drugs
    B. Nutrition
    C. Exercise pattern
    D. Bowel/bladder habits
    E. Sleep habits
    F. Sexual habits

X. **Review of Systems**
    A. General—height, weight, fever, chills, sweats
    B. Body systems—pain, discomfort, and/or alteration in functioning
      1. Neurologic
      2. Eyes, ears, nose, and throat
      3. Respiratory
      4. Cardiovascular
      5. Integumentary (skin, hair, and nails)
      6. Gastrointestinal
      7. Urinary

8. Reproductive
9. Musculoskeletal
10. Endocrine

1-3 GENERAL PHYSICAL ASSESSMENT

While the medical examination is for the purpose of diagnosing disease, the nursing examination is to determine lack of functioning due to illness, or alert the physician to a change in client status. Nursing goals will be directed toward restoring the functional capacity of the client as much as possible.

- Gather the following equipment:

  stethoscope (with bell and diaphragm end pieces)
  blood-pressure cuff
  thermometer
  pocket flashlight
  otoscope and ophthalmoscope
  tongue blades
  reflex hammer
  tuning fork
  client gown
  tape measure/ruler

- Before starting the examination, wash your hands in the presence of the client.

- Measure height and weight.

- Follow principles of good communication as described for taking the nursing history.

The following list is meant to serve as a reminder of general assessment principles. For detailed descriptions of the mechanics of examination consult an assessment text. See Sections 1-4, 1-5, 1-6, 1-7, and 1-8 for more detailed vital signs, neurologic, respiratory, cardiovascular, and gastrointestinal exams, respectively.

General appearance Overall assessment of the well-being of the client; evidence of weight loss or weight gain, ascites, edema, jaundice, agitation or depression, systemic toxicity, nutritional deficiency

Vital signs   Temperature, pulse, respirations, blood pressure in both arms, sitting, standing and lying down. See Section 1-4 for detailed exam.

Skin   Color, turgor, temperature, moisture, hair distribution, lesions, striae, scars

Nervous system   Current mental status as reflected by words and behavior; level of consciousness, orientation, pupil reaction. See Section 1-5 for detailed exam.

Head   Hair, skull, scalp, contour, masses, lesions, evidence of trauma

Eyes   Visual fields, visual acuity, external ocular movements, pupils, cornea, sclera, optic disk, lens opacity, conjunctiva, use of glasses, contact lenses

Ears   Auditory acuity (Weber or Rinne, whispered voice or ticking watch), canals, eardrums, mastoid process (with tuning fork), hearing aid or other device

Nose   Exterior, mucosa, septum, turbinates, discharge, bleeding, polyps, sinus tenderness, evidence of surgery, injury

Mouth and throat   Breath odor, dental hygiene, color and integrity of lips, gums, hard palate, tongue and pharynx, sputum production and characteristics, dentures, loose teeth

Neck   Nuchal rigidity, postural alignment, range of motion, thyroid enlargement or tenderness

Chest   Thorax (shape and symmetry), respiratory movement, anterior–posterior diameters (should be shorter than bilateral diameters), rib or sternal tenderness, lesions, scars

Breasts   Contour, symmetry, nipple retraction, masses, tenderness; teach breast self-exam

Lungs   *Percuss:* dullness—consolidation, atelectasis, or effusion; hyperresonance—pneumothorax or chronic obstructive pulmonary disease

Palpate: Tactile fremitus is normally felt most strongly over the bronchi and diminishes as the hands approach the lung bases as client says "ninety-nine."

Auscultate: Resonance, breath and voice sounds, rales and rhonchi, friction rub (rubbing or grating sound coincident with respirations); see Section 1-6 for detailed exam.

Cardiovascular system

Inspection: Check for edema, petechiae, ecchymosis, dilated veins, cyanosis, vascular irregularities, scars, spider angiomata, and areas of numbness or tingling. Check nails for clubbing and capillary refill (color should return immediately when nails are pressed until they blanch).

Palpation: Check peripheral pulses for symmetry, quality, and regularity (carotid, brachial, radial, ulnar, femoral, popliteal, dorsalis pedis, posterior tibialis). Palpate over precordium for point of maximum impulse, thrills, lifts, heaves, or tenderness.

Auscultation: Rate, rhythm, character of S1 and S2, extra heart sounds, opening snap, bruits, clicks, friction rub (see Section 1-7 and Figure 1-5)

Lymph nodes   Palpate for enlargement: head, neck, axillary, brachial, breast, inguinal, popliteal

Abdomen

Inspection: Check for scars, striae, symmetry, bulging, herniations, visible peristalsis, and pulsations.

Auscultation: Check for bowel sounds, rubs, and bruits before palpating or percussing, as manual stimulation may increase peristalsis. See Section 1-8 for detailed exam.

Palpation: Check all four quadrants to confirm positive findings, and check organ size and tenderness.

Percussion: Check for liver, kidney, and spleen size, distended bladder, shifting dullness, and masses.

Back   Curvature, symmetry, mobility, tenderness over spine, pelvis, kidneys (costovertebral-angle tenderness)

Extremities   Range of motion of shoulders, hips, ankles, feet; crepitus, joint pain, swelling, fluid, muscle development (see Table 2-7, Range-of-Motion Exercises, and Table 2-8, Passive Range-of-Motion Exercises). Check for Homan's sign by dorsiflexing the foot with leg extended (if pain is elicited, thrombophlebitis may be present). Check for calf tenderness.

Genitalia   Inspect and palpate external structures for pain, swelling, inflammation, bulging, growths, discharge, bleeding, scars, and foul odor. Perform or assist physician with a speculum and bimanual examination. Teach males testicular self-exam. Collect ordered specimens and return to laboratory.

Urine   Examine urine color, concentration, odor, and quantity.

Rectum   Inspect for hemorrhoids, fissures, and tenderness. Observe stool color and consistency. Hemoccult test for occult blood.

Large muscle/nerve function

Motor status: gait, involuntary movements

Coordination: finger to nose, Romberg test

Deep tendon reflexes: biceps, triceps, brachioradialis, patellar, achilles tendon. See Section 1-5 for detailed exam.

Also identify and document IV lines, NG tubes, Foley catheters, oxygen sources, ventilators, cardiac monitors, pulse oximeters, dialysis graphs, tracheostomies, colostomies, chest tubes, gastrostomy tubes, prostheses, pacemakers (date inserted, type), and transdermal or other drug delivery systems.

1-4   VITAL SIGNS ASSESSMENT

Many major therapeutic decisions are based on the vital signs. Accuracy and expertise in interpreting results are essential.

I. Temperature
   A. Oral

- Take temperature orally if client is awake, oriented, and cooperative

- Wait 15 min if client has just smoked or swallowed liquids

- Place the thermometer under client's tongue and instruct client to keep lips closed; leave in place 5 to 8 min if using a glass thermometer

- Electronic thermometers with disposable probe covers are easy to use and carry less risk of cross-contamination than glass thermometers. Accurate readings depend on correct placement of the device.

- Do not take oral temperatures on any of the following:
   a. Confused, disoriented, or comatose clients

    b. Clients with NG tubes

    c. Clients receiving oxygen

    d. Clients with endotracheal tubes

    e. Clients on seizure precautions

    f. Clients with wired jaws or facial fractures

- Normal oral temperature is 97.7 to 99.5°F (36.5 to 37.5°C)

B. Tympanic: Tympanic thermometers are accurate, timesaving, comfortable for the client, and less likely to spread infection, as the ear harbors fewer pathogens than the mouth or rectum. The sensor probe is placed in the external opening of the ear and detects infrared radiation from the eardrum. In some models you can choose whether the core temperature or oral or rectal equivalent readings should be displayed.

- Before you start, explain procedure to client, as many have never heard of taking temperatures this way.

- Accurate readings depend on correct technique. Follow the manufacturer's instructions.

- Core tympanic readings are frequently one degree higher than oral readings with electronic thermometers (oral readings are often affected by mouth-breathing, drinking, gum chewing, smoking, and eating).

- Take two tympanic readings and record the second one if the unit has been re-charging for several hours (Baird et al. 1992).

C. Rectal

- Take rectal temperatures only if oral or tympanic temperatures are contraindicated.

- Do not take rectal temperatures on clients who have had peritoneal or rectal surgery, neurosurgery, or cardiac disease.

- After lubricating, insert the thermometer 1 1/2 in into rectum.

- Leave glass thermometer in place 2 to 3 min; stay with client.

- Normal rectal temperature is approximately 1°F or 0.28 to 0.56°C higher than oral temperature: 98.7 to 100.5°F (37.5 to 38.5°C)

D. Axillary

- Take axillary temperature only if the other methods are not possible, as it is an unreliable method.

- Wait 15 min if client has just finished washing the axilla.

- Leave glass thermometer in place for 5 to 8 min.

- Normal axillary temperature is approximately 0.5°F or 0.28°C lower than oral temperature: 97.2 to 99.0°F (36.1 to 37.1°C)

E. Temperature variations

- Normal temperature fluctuates with the time of day. Both oral and rectal temperatures are usually 1 to 2 degrees F lower in the early morning. Other influences are environmental temperature, age (infants and children usually have higher temperatures than adults), exercise, and time of ovulation in women.

F. Elevated body temperature

- Pyrexia (fever) is a prime indicator that disease is present.

- Symptoms associated with pyrexia are tachycardia, tachypnea, anorexia, headache, malaise, flushing, chills, diaphoresis, and occasional delirium (hyperpyrexia). A fever may be intermittent (temperature reaches normal between fluctuations), remittent (temperature does not reach normal between fluctuations), or continued (minimal fluctuations).

- Obtain temperature at frequent intervals when elevation exists. In severe cases a rectal probe for continuous monitoring may be necessary.

- **Interpretation**
  a. Normal pyrexia: One to two days after surgery (general anesthesia), myocardial infarc-

tion, or a cerebrovascular accident, a slight elevation in temperature is not abnormal.

b. Abnormal pyrexia: The most common cause is infection. Suspect pulmonary, wound, urinary, or abdominal or systemic infection, especially postoperatively. Other causes are cerebral edema, cerebrovascular accident, myocardial infarction, brain trauma, neurosurgery, or brain tumors.

- Always report temperatures above 99.5°F (oral) and check with physician before administering antipyretics.

- The elderly do not necessarily show accurate temperature-sensitive responses. They may be afebrile even with a severe infection.

G. Hypothermia

1. Medically induced hypothermia: Body temperature may be intentionally lowered to reduce oxygen requirements in clients undergoing cardiac, neurologic, vascular, or gastrointestinal surgery.

2. Accidental exposure: Temperatures below 93.2°F or 34°C usually result in death. Hypothermia from accidental exposure is a medical emergency (see Emergency Assessment and Intervention, Chapter 13). Frequent or continuous monitoring of temperature is necessary.

II. Pulse

A. Measurement

- Evaluate radial pulse using your first, second, and third fingers on client's radial artery.

- Evaluate rate, rhythm, and amplitude.

- Obtain pulse rate per minute by counting beats for 30 sec and multiplying by 2.

- Count for a full minute and take apical pulse if irregularities are noted.

- Normal pulse rate for the average adult is 60–80 beats per min (60–90 for over age 65, and as low as 40 for some athletes).

- Check pulse whenever condition of client changes.

B. Interpretation
1. Abnormal pulse rates
   a) Tachycardia: Rate greater than 100 beats per min; causes include anxiety, anger, fear, pain, surprise, exercise, fever, anemia, shock, congestive heart failure, hypoxia, decreased blood pressure, pulmonary embolus, drugs, decreased blood volume, and thyrotoxicosis.

   b) Bradycardia: Rate less than 60 beats per min; causes include drug use, increased blood pressure, athletic conditioning, Valsalva maneuver, carotid sinus massage, sinus-node ischemia, increased intracranial pressure, increased intraocular pressure, hypothyroidism, hyperkalemia, Stokes-Adams disease, neurogenic shock.

2. Pulse rhythm
   a) Normal dysrhythmias: There are two normal dysrhythmias: 1) in young adults and children the pulse rate speeds up at the end of inspiration and slows down with expiration, and 2) occasional premature beats are normal.

   b) Abnormal dysrhythmias: When irregularities are noted in a radial pulse, auscultate with a stethoscope (see Figure 1-5) over apex of for a full minute while palpating radial pulse. *Pulse deficit* exists if the apical rate differs from the radial rate. See also Section 1-7 and Table 13-1, Recognition of Life-Threatening Dysrhythmias.

3. Abnormal heart sounds

- Quiet or muffled heart sounds, which may be caused by a thick chest wall, severe overload, or cardiac tamponade

- Gallops: "extra" heart sounds (best heard over the apex) that are a cardinal sign of congestive heart failure

- Snaps and clicks: high-pitched sounds usually associated with murmurs, caused by rapid displacement of a valve from high pressure due to stenosis

- Murmurs: high- or low-pitched sounds caused by turbulent blood flow through a valve, due to congenital or acquired defects

- Friction rub: a sound like two pieces of leather rubbing together, associated with pericarditis

4. **Pulse amplitude:** Use the following three-point scale to indicate the pulse amplitude (measurement of force or strength): 3+ = bounding pulse; 2+ = normal pulse; 1+ = weak, thready pulse; 0 = absent pulse. A bounding pulse implies a widened pulse pressure (difference between systolic and diastolic pressures). A weak, thready pulse implies narrowed pulse pressure.

5. **Pulse points:** Obtain peripheral pulses on clients having angiography, or cardiac or vascular surgery. Peripheral pulses include radial, ulnar, brachial, femoral, popliteal, dorsalis pedis, and posterior tibialis. Other pulse points include temporal, carotid, and external maxillary (see Figure 13-14).

III. Respirations
A. Measurement

- Assess respirations for rate and quality.

- Count rate for 30 sec and multiply by 2. Evaluate for a full minute if respiratory or cardiac problems are present.

- Normal respiratory rate in the average adult is 16–20 breaths per minute. Rate varies with age, exercise, and environmental conditions. There are normally three deep breaths per minute.

B. Interpretation of abnormal respiratory patterns

1. **Tachypnea:** rapid and shallow; associated with fever, pneumonia, respiratory alkalosis, salicylate poisoning

∕∿∿∿

2. **Bradypnea:** slowed but regular; associated with use of opiates and alcohol, tumors, metabolic disorders, conditions affecting the medulla oblongata

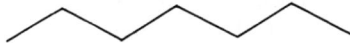

3. **Hyperventilation** or **Kussmaul's:** increased rate and depth; associated with renal failure and diabetic ketoacidosis

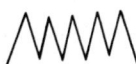

4. **Apnea:** periodic absence of breathing; caused by mechanical obstruction or conditions affecting the respiratory center

5. **Cheyne-Stokes:** periods of apnea followed by breaths of increasing depth; caused by increased intracranial pressure, severe congestive heart failure, renal failure, meningitis, drug overdose, cerebral anoxia

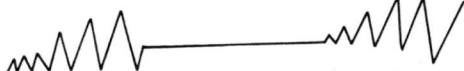

6. **Biot's:** fast, uniformly deep respirations marked by abrupt pauses associated with head injury

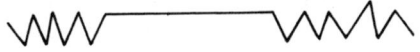

7. **Ataxic breathing:** completely chaotic and irregular respiratory pattern associated with severe brain-stem damage

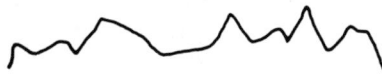

IV. Blood Pressure

A. Measurement

- Client's position (sitting, standing, lying down) may affect blood pressure. Generally, client should be sitting upright. Document if BP's are taken in other positions.

- Use appropriate cuff size: 12–14 cm for average adult arm; 18–20 cm for obese arm; pediatric cuff for infants, children, and adults with thin arms. Cuff should overlap at least 1″ when applied.

- Apply cuff 2 cm above antecubital space.

- Place center of bladder over brachial artery.

- Release inflated cuff slowly.

- If it is necessary to recheck blood pressure, allow the cuff to completely deflate before reinflating.

- Client should not speak while reading is being taken, or BP may increase.

- When doing initial client assessment, check BP in both arms. Normal difference is usually 5 mm Hg or less.

- Normal blood pressure in the average adult is 100/60 to 140/90 mm Hg (may be higher in the elderly).

B. Interpretation

1. **Hypertension:** blood pressure consistently higher than 140/90 mm Hg; causes include fever, anemia, anxiety, atherosclerosis, aortic insufficiency, coarctation of the aorta, polycythemia, renal disease, thyrotoxicosis, beriberi, Cushing's syndrome, hyperparathyroidism, CNS lesions, burns

2. **Hypotension:** systolic pressure less than 90 mm Hg; causes include shock, hemorrhage, fever, infection, anemia, cancer, Addison's disease, hypovolemia, metabolic acidosis, wasting diseases, heat exhaustion

V. Electronic Monitors

A. Automated Vital Signs Monitors:
Automated vital signs monitors may be used on the medical-surgical unit for clients who need continuous monitoring of pulse rate, systolic and diastolic pressures, and mean arterial pressures at preset intervals. These might include clients who are in chronic congestive heart failure, those who are receiving intravenous drugs such as dopamine or nitroglycerin, or those who have undergone certain diagnostic tests such as cardiac catheterization.

- Always take vital signs manually first and compare with the reading on the monitor. If results differ, call the central supply department or the manufacturer's representative.

- Set monitor for appropriate data interval. Be familiar with the particular monitor your hospital supplies. Typical intervals are 1, 2, 3, 4, 5, 10, 15, 20, 30, 45, 60, and 90 min.

- You will be able to retrieve stored data on most monitors. This includes the last data obtained, the time elapsed, and the data from the previous 99 min.

- False readings may be obtained if the tubing becomes kinked, a leak develops in the tubing or cuff, the client moves his arm too much, the cuff is too small or too big, the cuff is positioned above or below the heart level, the client has convulsions or the shivers, or if there is inadequate circulation to the limb being used to monitor vital signs.

B. Pulse Oximeters:
Pulse oximeters measure the arterial blood oxygen saturation (SaO_2) to detect the presence of hypoxemia before visible signs (such as dusky skin color or dusky nail beds) develop. It is a noninvasive device that utilizes a sensor attached to the client's finger, toe, nose, or earlobe.

- Determine if allergies to adhesive are present and also the client's hemoglobin level.

- Use a sensor appropriate for the client's weight and size, taking into account the client's adequacy of circulation in the extremity selected (follow manufacturer's instructions).

- Before applying the sensor, clean the site selected with an alcohol swab, and remove blue or black nail polish or acrylic nails.

- Ensure that the alignment of the light-emitting diodes (LEDs) and photodetector is accurate.

- Ensure adequate functioning of the alarm system.

- Inspect an adhesive finger or toe sensor site every 4 hr and a spring-tension sensor every 2 hr.

- Immobilize the sensor site, and protect it from external light sources.

- Take frequent readings, verify that hemoglobin level is normal, and document all nursing assessments.

1-5 NEUROLOGIC ASSESSMENT

The reason for performing the neurologic exam will determine the extent and thoroughness, i.e., the approach to the client brought to the emergency room with a head injury will be different from that for the conscious ambulatory client who presents with a headache.

History

Obtain a history as for a general client (see Section 1-2), but be particularly aware of mental status and functioning. Whether the client is a reliable source will be evident from his/her general appearance and behavior, sensorium, mood and affect, thought content, and intellectual capacity. If necessary, obtain the history from a person who has firsthand knowledge of the client's problems and complaints.

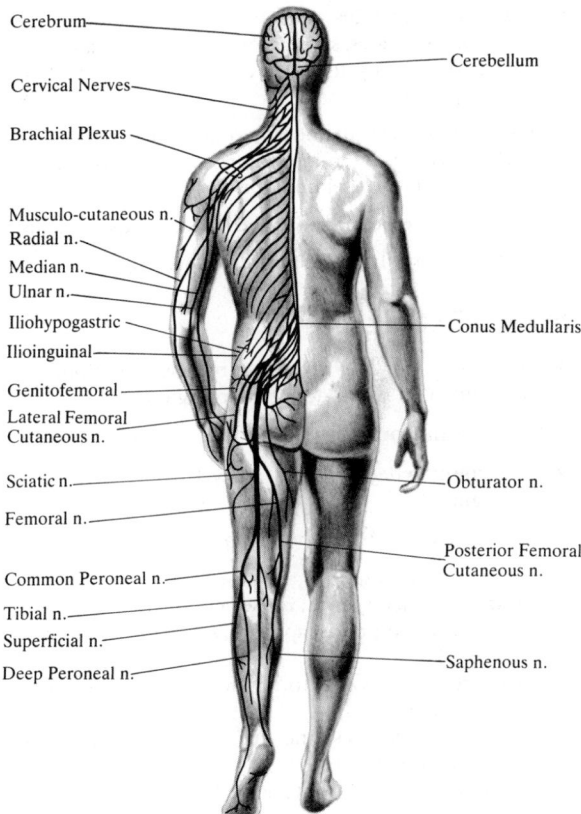

Cerebrum

Cerebellum

Cervical Nerves

Brachial Plexus

Musculo-cutaneous n.
Radial n.
Median n.
Ulnar n.
Iliohypogastric
Ilioinguinal

Conus Medullaris

Genitofemoral
Lateral Femoral
Cutaneous n.

Sciatic n.

Obturator n.

Femoral n.

Posterior Femoral
Cutaneous n.

Common Peroneal n.

Tibial n.
Superficial n.
Deep Peroneal n.

Saphenous n.

Figure 1–2. The brain and spinal nerves.

In some cases, the clinician must proceed with objective data only. Ask about

- Past illnesses
- Present problems
- Complaints, especially chronicity, remittency, exacerbating or alleviating factors, duration

- Motor abnormalities, sensory problems, auditory and visual disturbances, symptoms, such as smell and taste disorders, relating to other cranial nerves, problems with expression

- Problems related to the autonomic nervous system, such as urinary retention or incontinence, motor dysfunctions, and sexual function

- History of medication, drug, and alcohol use or abuse

- Exposure to solvents, chemicals, carcinogens

Physical Exam

Items 1–4 deal with gross neurologic function, and should be included when doing neurologic checks.

1. Level of consciousness (single most important factor):

- Determine whether client is awake by calling his or her name.

- Describe client behavioral response:

    Alert (awake, responds appropriately)
    Lethargic (sleepy, but arouses easily)
    Obtunded (responds appropriately, but difficult to arouse)
    Stuporous (responds to painful stimuli, never completely alert)
    Semicomatose (responds to painful stimuli, reflex movements only)
    Comatose (no response, no reflex)

2. Orientation: person, place, time (disorientation to time occurs first, to people last)

- If client is awake but fails any of these, he/she is said to be disoriented. Give client a simple verbal command, i.e., "squeeze my hand" to determine response to verbal stimuli.

3. Pupils

- Assess pupil size and consensual reactivity. Pupils are normally 2–3 mm in diameter and equal in size and shape.

- Normal pupil size:

Pupil size
mm

- 1
- 2
- 3
- 4
- 5
- 6
- 7
- 8
- 9

- Check for reaction to light and accommodation by covering one eye and bringing object quickly from far to near. Room lighting may affect pupil size. Normally, the lens thickens and the pupil constricts (PERLA). Use this notation: BR = brisk reaction; SR = sluggish reaction; NR = no reaction.

- **Interpretation of abnormal pupil changes:**

  Aniscoria: Congenital inequality of the pupil diameter occurs in 10% of the population. It is not pathologic.

  Fixed or irregularly shaped pupils may be found in people who are blind, have cataracts, or an eye prosthesis.

  Slowness to react to light is abnormal.

  Pinpoint pupils may be caused by myotic medications, localized pons involvement, or narcotics use.

  Dilated pupils may be caused by brain injury, third-cranial-nerve compression, anoxia (as in cardiac arrest), atropine or scopolamine use, and barbituate use.

4. **Unconsciousness:** The comatose client must be assessed carefully and frequently; monitoring changes from the baseline is key.

- **Response to painful stimuli:** Use the trapezius pinch, the sternal rub, calf pressure, interdigital compression, or supraorbital compression. One of two responses will be elicited:

  Purposeful movement: There is a clear attempt to push away the painful stimulus.

  Nonpurposeful response: There is no response at all, or only a generalized body movement.

- **Brain-stem postures:** Serious brain damage is signified by the following brain-stem postures:

  Decorticate rigidity: Flexed elbows are close to the body and wrists are flexed over the chest. Plantar flexion of the feet. A memory aid: in decorication the arms move toward the *core.*

  Decerebrate rigidity: Ankles and toes are flexed. Elbows are extended and at the side with wrists flexed. A more ominous sign than decorticate rigidity. Indicates brain stem functioning only.

- **Respirations:** Check for abnormal breathing patterns, such as Cheyne-Stokes, Biot's, central neurogenic hyperventilation, or ataxic breathing (see Section 1-4). Generally, these occur as the coma deepens from the thalamus to the brain stem and indicate brain damage.

- **Glasgow coma scale:** Use this when doing neurologic checks to evaluate improvement or decline in client's condition. Make a flowchart and add up the score every 15 min. The highest score is 14; the lowest 3. A client with a score below 8 should be in an ICU or neurological specialty unit.

		10:00	10:15	10:30, etc.
Eyes				
Open spontaneously	4			
Open to verbal command	3			
Open to pain	2			
No response	1			

		10:00	**10:15**	**10:30, etc.**

Best motor response

Obeys verbal command	6
Localizes pain from painful stimulus	5
Flexion–withdrawal	4
Decorticate posture	3
Decerebrate posture	2
No response	1

Best verbal response

Oriented and converses	5
Disoriented and converses	4
Inappropriate words	3
Incomprehensible sounds	2
No response	1

Total

5. Sensation: Assess sensation over the four extremities and trunk, with client's eyes closed.

- **Light touch:** Have client indicate when he/she feels the piece of cotton by saying "touch."

- **Pain:** Use a safety pin alternating the sharp and dull end.

- **Temperature:** Apply test tubes of cold and warm water or warm and cold alcohol swabs to the skin and ask client to identify sensation.

- **Proprioception:** Move the big toe and ask the client which way it was moved.

6. Reflexes

- **Deep tendon:** Note the grade of each reflex and the symmetry from side to side as you assess with the reflex hammer: 1) biceps, 2) triceps, 3) brachioradialis, 4) patellar, 5) Achilles tendon. Grades: 0 = no response; 1+ = diminished or below normal; 2+ = normal; 3+ = brisker than normal; 4+ = very brisk, hyperactive, or clonus.

- **Pathologic reflexes**

  Clonus: A 4+ deep tendon reflex. This may signify upper-motor-neuron disease.

Babinsky: If dorsiflexion and fanning of the toes occurs when the sole of the foot is stroked from the heel up to the ball, it could indicate pyramidal tract lesions.

Oculocephalic eye movements: In unconscious patients the eyeballs remain in midposition when head is turned from right to left.

- **Cranial nerves:** Use Table 1-1 as a reminder of cranial nerve function. The critical nerve functions to assess are nerves IX (glossopharyngeal) and X (vagus), which control the cough and gag reflexes. If these nerves are impaired, client could be at risk for silent and continuous aspiration.

TABLE 1–1. CRANIAL NERVES

NERVE		TYPE	FUNCTIONS
I	Olfactory	Sensory	Smell
II	Optic	Sensory	Vision
III	Oculomotor	Motor	Eye movement
IV	Trochlear	Motor	Eye movement
V	Trigeminal	Motor	Chewing movements
		Sensory	Sensations of face, scalp, teeth
VI	Abducens	Motor	Eye movement
VII	Facial	Motor	Facial expressions
		Sensory	Taste; salivary and lacrimal glands
VIII	Acoustic	Sensory	Hearing; sense of balance
IX	Glossopharyngeal	Motor	Secretion of saliva; swallowing movement
		Sensory	Sensations of throat, taste
X	Vagus	Motor	Swallowing; voice production; slowing of heartbeat; and acceleration of peristalsis
		Sensory	Sensations of throat, larynx, and viscera
XI	Spinal accessory	Motor	Shoulder movements; neck rotation
XII	Hypoglossal	Motor	Tongue movements

- To check cough reflex, tell client to give you the best, biggest cough they can, then stand aside (they will not want to cough on you)

- For the gag reflex, assess by placing a long tongue blade down the back of the throat to touch the uvula. The client should retch. If the uvula only moves up on one side, client is at risk and may need special feeding, or at some point a tracheostomy.

7. Signs of increased intracranial pressure

Early Client needs more stimulation to display the same responses, loses details in test of orientation, forgetful, restless, suddenly quiet after severe restlessness, increased tone (resistance) on passive movement, subtle weakness, pronator drift, sluggish pupil reaction, Cheyne-Stokes breathing

Late Unarousable, dense motor weakness, then posturing, then no response, one "blown" pupil, then both pupils dilated and fixed, Cushing's triad: increased systolic BP, profoundly slow pulse, abnormal respirations

Laboratory Values

Look for abnormal values and worsening trends, i.e., cerebrospinal fluid for blood, cell count, differential, color, culture, glucose, cytology, and VDRL.

Diagnostic Studies

Evaluate abnormal reports of x-rays, scans, EEGs, lumbar puncture, angiography, EMG, myogram, evoked potentials, magnetic-resonance imaging (MRI), positron emission tomography (PET) scan.

1-6 RESPIRATORY ASSESSMENT

While doing the thorough nursing history, physical exam, and vital signs assessment of the respiratory client outlined in Sections 1-2, 1-3, and 1-4, pay particular attention to the respiratory system and the following areas of concern.

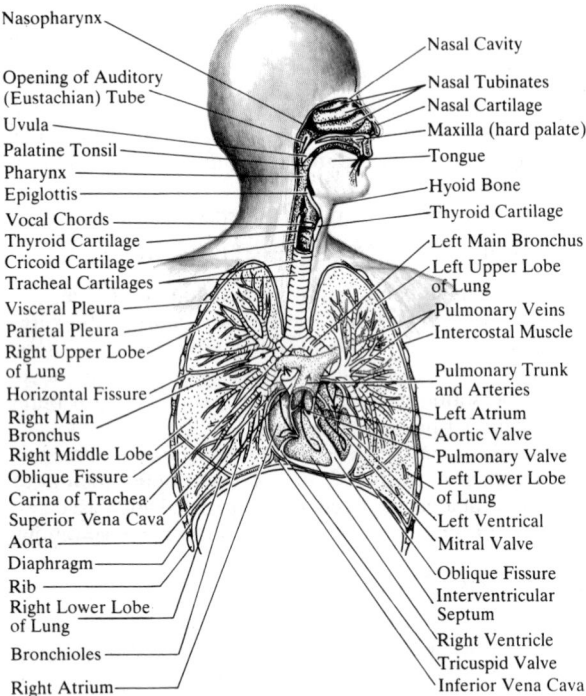

Nasopharynx

Opening of Auditory (Eustachian) Tube

Uvula

Palatine Tonsil

Pharynx

Epiglottis

Vocal Chords

Thyroid Cartilage

Cricoid Cartilage

Tracheal Cartilages

Visceral Pleura

Parietal Pleura

Right Upper Lobe of Lung

Horizontal Fissure

Right Main Bronchus

Right Middle Lobe

Oblique Fissure

Carina of Trachea

Superior Vena Cava

Aorta

Diaphragm

Rib

Right Lower Lobe of Lung

Bronchioles

Right Atrium

Nasal Cavity

Nasal Tubinates

Nasal Cartilage

Maxilla (hard palate)

Tongue

Hyoid Bone

Thyroid Cartilage

Left Main Bronchus

Left Upper Lobe of Lung

Pulmonary Veins

Intercostal Muscle

Pulmonary Trunk and Arteries

Left Atrium

Aortic Valve

Pulmonary Valve

Left Lower Lobe of Lung

Left Ventrical

Mitral Valve

Oblique Fissure

Interventricular Septum

Right Ventricle

Tricuspid Valve

Inferior Vena Cava

Figure 1–3. The organs of respiration and the heart.

History

CHIEF COMPLAINT AND HISTORY OF PRESENT ILLNESS

- Are there episodes of shortness of breath? When do they occur?

- Evaluate presence of cough: is it productive, hacking, paroxysmal, brassy (with a harsh buzzing sound), habitual, nervous?

TYPE OF SPUTUM	CHARACTERISTICS	MAY INDICATE
Mucoid	Thin, clear	Early bronchitis
Mucopurulent	Thick, viscous, greenish color, frothy	Pneumonia, later bronchitis, TB
Purulent	Thick, viscous, yellowish, offensive smell	Lung abscess, advanced TB, bronchiectasis, pneumonia
Nummular	Mucopurulent with small semisolid masses that sink in water	Advanced TB
Rusty	Mucopurulent, rust-tinged, viscous	Pneumonia
Prune juice	Dark brown, offensive smelling	Late pneumonia or gangrene of lung
Hemoptysis	Bright red and frothy	Cancer, TB, pneumonia, pulmonary embolism, mitral stenosis, or aneurysm rupturing into bronchial tubes

- What is the amount and type of sputum?
- Is there pain on inspiration?

PAST MEDICAL HISTORY

- Past history of respiratory disease
- Therapy used and effectiveness

HEALTH HABITS

- Smoking: how much and for how long?
- Is there exposure to secondary smoke, solvents, or gases?
- Exercise pattern: Is client on breathing exercises?

Physical Exam

INSPECTION

- Check chest symmetry upon inspiration.

- Look for barrel-, funnel-, or pigeon-shaped chest, spinal deformities, or other abnormalities.

- Check skin for mottling, scars, irregularities, and odor.

- Evaluate respiratory pattern, including rate and rhythm (see Section 1-4). Look for pursed-lip breathing, nasal flaring, chest breathing versus abdominal breathing, retractions, splinting because of pain, or use of accessory muscles.

PALPATION

- Gently palpate all over thorax for any tender areas.

- Check for equal chest expansion by placing your hands on either side of the chest at the lung bases and ask client to inhale deeply; hands should move equally upward and slightly outward.

- Assess tactile fremitus by palpating for vibrations on the chest wall when client says "ninety-nine." Decreased fremitus could indicate pneumothorax or pleural effusion. Increased fremitus could indicate consolidation (i.e., atelectasis, pneumonia).

PERCUSSION

- See Lungs in Section 1-3.

AUSCULTATION

- Have client cough to clear upper airway. Instruct client to breathe deeply through the mouth.

- Start at the trachea and move stethoscope in a zig-zag pattern auscultating the anterior, the posterior, and lateral parts of the thorax.

ADVENTITIOUS BREATH SOUNDS	CHARACTERISTICS	MAY INDICATE
Crackles	Sound like fizzing seltzer; may be fine, medium or coarse, wet or crackling	"Wet"—pulmonary edema, "dry"—pulmonary fibrosis
Rhonchi	Bubbling or rumbling sounds	Chronic bronchitis or any disorder with retained pulmonary secretions
Wheezing	Musical sounds, varied pitch, whistling, creaking	Asthma, chronic bronchitis, or any disorder reducing the caliber of airways
Pleural friction rub	Like a squeaky, groaning leather shoe, grating sound	Pleurisy, pulmonary embolus, TB, lung cancer

Laboratory Values

- Check CBC, electrolytes, hematocrit, hemoglobin.
- Check arterial blood gases: pH, pO_2, pCO_2 and HCO_3 for normal limits. (Table 3-5, Arterial Blood Gases)
- Pulse oximetry permits continuous monitoring of arterial oxygen saturation; it is often used for clients with chronic respiratory problems, sleep apnea, or those undergoing pulmonary function tests.

Diagnostic Studies

- Identify abnormal reports of x-rays, ECG, biopsies, fluid aspirations, lung scans, pulmonary function studies, bronchoscopy, TB tests, etc.

1-7 CARDIOVASCULAR ASSESSMENT

In order to diagnose heart disease, the physician, assisted by the nurse, will thoroughly explore the client's medical history, present symptoms, and physical status through examination, laboratory studies, and diagnostic studies. Of particular importance will be the cause of the heart ailment (valvular, structural, infection, etc.); damages or structural changes that have occurred; physiologic alterations that have occurred, such as reduction in cardiac reserve; and limitations that must be placed on the client in light of cardiac function/reserve.

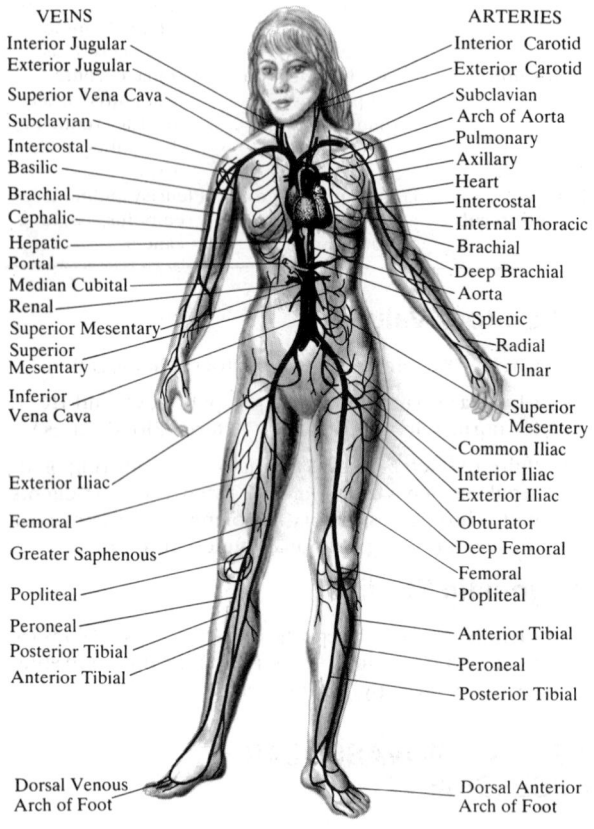

VEINS	ARTERIES
Interior Jugular	Interior Carotid
Exterior Jugular	Exterior Carotid
Superior Vena Cava	Subclavian
Subclavian	Arch of Aorta
Intercostal	Pulmonary
Basilic	Axillary
Brachial	Heart
Cephalic	Intercostal
Hepatic	Internal Thoracic
Portal	Brachial
Median Cubital	Deep Brachial
Renal	Aorta
Superior Mesentary	Splenic
Superior Mesentary	Radial
	Ulnar
Inferior Vena Cava	Superior Mesentery
	Common Iliac
	Interior Iliac
Exterior Iliac	Exterior Iliac
Femoral	Obturator
Greater Saphenous	Deep Femoral
	Femoral
Popliteal	Popliteal
Peroneal	
Posterior Tibial	Anterior Tibial
Anterior Tibial	Peroneal
	Posterior Tibial
Dorsal Venous Arch of Foot	Dorsal Anterior Arch of Foot

Figure 1–4. Major blood vessels.

Do a thorough nursing history, physical exam, and vital signs assessment of the cardiac client such as the ones outlined in Sections 1-2, 1-3, and 1-4. Pay particular attention to the cardiovascular system and to the following areas.

History

CHIEF COMPLAINT AND HISTORY OF PRESENT ILLNESS

- Is there progressive weakness, shortness of breath, syncope, diaphoresis, nausea, vomiting? What are the circumstances of occurrence?
- Find out the who, what, why, where, and how of any pain the client is having (see Pain, Section 2-3).

PAST MEDICAL HISTORY

- History of heart disease? What type?
- What therapy was used and was it effective?
- See Table 1-2 if client has a pacemaker.

PRESENT MEDICATION

- Is client on nitroglycerin, digitalis, diuretics, antihypertensives, potassium supplements?

FAMILY HISTORY

- Family history of heart disease, diabetes, stroke, thromboembolism

SOCIAL HISTORY

- Stress level of occupation, stress of commuting
- Type A behavior?
- Marital/family status: number of marriages, separations, divorces, children, health of spouse
- Recent stressful life events (see Table 12-5, Social Readjustment Rating Scale)

HEALTH HABITS

- Smoking, drinking, caffeine intake: how much per day and for how long?

- Nutrition: have client describe typical eating patterns, including salt intake, fatty foods, cholesterol.

- Activity: Is client on an exercise program or cardiac rehabilitation program?

TABLE 1–2. IF YOUR CLIENT HAS A CARDIAC PACEMAKER

Assessment Find Out:	• When pacemaker was put in (lithium batteries last between 7–10 years)
	• Date of most recent checkup, as pacemakers should be evaluated every 3 months for proper functioning
	• Why pacemaker was put in. The following are among the rate or rhythm disturbances that can warrant a permanent pacemaker: bradyarrhythmia, various forms of tachyarrhythmia, sick sinus syndrome, Stokes-Adams syndrome, permanent heart block resulting from surgical trauma or an MI
	• The client's set pacemaker rate, programming, manufacturer and model numbers. If rate is programmed, mark it in big letters on the front of the client's chart so staff is aware of pacemaker and rate.
	• Client's knowledge about his/her pacemaker.
Client Teaching:	Make sure the client knows:
	• How to take his apical or carotid pulse daily. If he is gradually losing beats, the battery may be getting weak and he should mention this to the doctor who will judge when the battery needs replacing.
	• The signs and symptoms of pacemaker failure: syncope, hypotension, bradycardia, pallor, cyanosis, shortness of breath, chest muscle spasm. Signs of pacemaker displacement: hiccups, fainting, dizziness.

**TABLE 1–2. IF YOUR CLIENT HAS A
CARDIAC PACEMAKER** *Continued*

	Unusual fatigue, dizziness, jugular vein distention, oliguria, diminished peripheral pulses, or altered mental status may also indicate improper functioning.
	• About movement restrictions during the first 6 weeks after insertion—contact sports or vigorous activity of the arms and shoulder may dislodge the electrode. Contact sports must be avoided long term.
	• That clients shouldn't wear tight bra straps or heavy shoulder purses or anything that could put pressure on the pulse generator.
	• To notify the doctor if the incision ever starts becoming tender, red or swollen.
	• About possible electrical hazards, i.e., microwave ovens over 10 years old, electrical devices held close to pacemaker that may interfere with signals, etc.
	• The importance of regular visits to the doctor or pacemaker clinic for periodic checks and programming the pacemaker's rate or impulse strength.
	• About the telephone transmitter monitoring system and how to use it if available.
Nursing Interventions	• Consult with physician if client is having electrosurgery, diathermy, radiation therapy, or MRI. The pacemaker will need to be reprogrammed during the procedure, or the procedure may be contraindicated.
	• If malfunction occurs, reduce client's cardiac demands at once, by having him rest in bed with the side rails up. Keep call light within reach. Take vital signs q 15 min, obtain a 12 lead ECG, and begin telemetry monitoring if possible. Inform the physician. Start IV, keep atropine available at bedside and O_2 if needed. Collect any old and current ECG's, prepare for chest X-ray, and probable transfer to OR or ICU.

Physical Exam

- In your thorough vital signs assessment (see Section 1-4), particularly assess

  1. Pulse rate

  2. Pulse amplitude

  3. Pulse deficit

  4. Peripheral pulses

  5. Apical pulse and listen for abnormal heart sounds (see Section 1-4 and Figure 1-5).

  6. Use both the bell and diaphragm of the stethoscope when auscultating; the bell is for low-pitched sounds, while the diaphragm is for higher-pitched sounds. The room must be quiet.

- In doing a complete physical exam (see Section 1-3), complete the following, in addition to the steps listed above:

  1. Inspect cardiac area for pulsations or other abnormalities.

  2. Neck veins should only distend as client lowers head to the supine position, not while sitting.

  3. Percuss the outline of the heart: cardiomegaly is present if the apex is percussed past the midclavicular line.

  4. Palpate for thrills or murmurs over each of the four heart-valve areas (aortic, pulmonic, tricuspid, and mitral).

  5. Use 1 +, 2 +, 3 +, or 4 + scale to describe severity of pitting edema.

Laboratory Values

- CBC: especially white blood count, hemoglobin, and hematocrit for infectious or anemic trends

- Electrolytes: particularly potassium if the client is on diuretics or potassium supplements

- Blood gases: pH, pO_2, and HCO_3 for normal limits

How to locate the auscultation points

The five auscultation locations are shown superimposed over the heart.

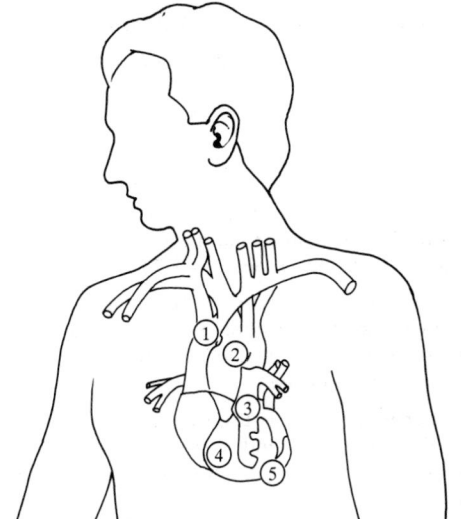

A good auscultation sequence begins with the aortic point, as follows:

1 Auscultation area—2nd right intercostal space.

2. Pulmonic area—2nd left intercostal space.

3. Erb's point—3rd left intercostal space.

4. Tricuspid area—5th left intercostal space close to the sternum.

5. Mitral area—5th left intercostal space just medial to the midclavicular line.

You may prefer another sequence, and that's all right as long as you use it consistently.

Figure 1-5. How to locate the auscultation points.

- Cardiac enzymes: trends in elevation of CPK, LDH, SGOT, isoenzyme studies, HBD

- Coagulation studies: prothrombin time for oral coagulants, partial thromboplastin time for heparin therapy

- Lipid profile: serum cholesterol, triglyceride, and lipoprotein levels to indicate risk for coronary artery disease, atherosclerosis, other lipid diseases

- Urinalysis: particularly note specific gravity and presence of protein.

- Blood urea nitrogen (BUN): kidney function

- Serum drug levels: digitalis, lidocaine, procainamide, quinidine

ECG

- Assist with obtaining accurate ECG readings, reassure client that obtaining readings is routine (see Electrographic Procedures, Section 4-7)

- Systematically evaluate ECGs; help identify acute changes or life-threatening dysrhythmias. (See Table 13-1, Recognition of Life-Threatening Dysrhythmias, for a brief summary.)

- Holter monitoring is used for a continuous ECG recording for an extended time, usually 24 hr. Client must wear the compact Holter monitor during usual activities.

Diagnostic Procedures

- Evaluate outcomes of angiography, scans, stress testing, pulmonary function tests, x-ray studies, fluoroscopy, echocardiograms, plethysmography (a noninvasive procedure that detects deep vein thrombosis in the lower extremities), etc.

1-8 GASTROINTESTINAL ASSESSMENT

More Americans are hospitalized with gastrointestinal (GI) disorders than any other group of disorders.

Do a thorough nursing history, physical exam, and vital signs assessment such as the ones outlined in Sections 1-2, 1-3, and 1-4. Pay particular attention to the gastrointestinal system and the following points.

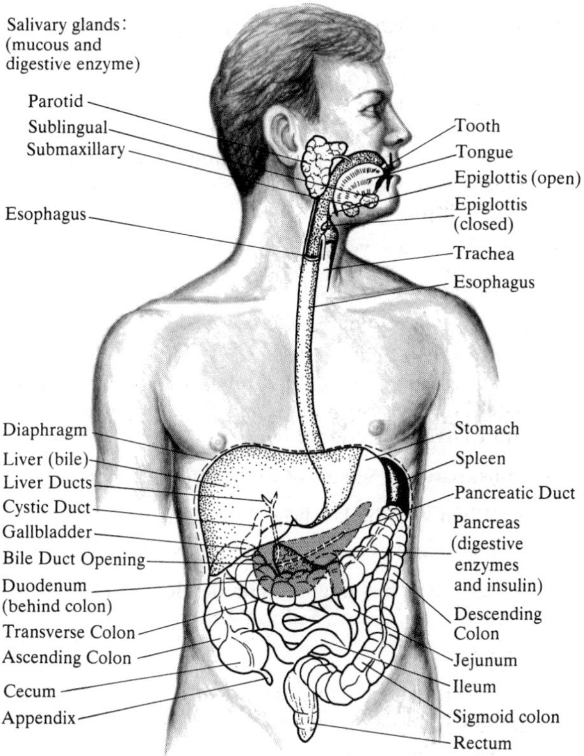

Salivary glands:
(mucous and
digestive enzyme)

Parotid
Sublingual
Submaxillary

Esophagus

Diaphragm
Liver (bile)
Liver Ducts
Cystic Duct
Gallbladder
Bile Duct Opening
Duodenum
(behind colon)
Transverse Colon
Ascending Colon
Cecum
Appendix

Tooth
Tongue
Epiglottis (open)
Epiglottis
(closed)
Trachea
Esophagus

Stomach
Spleen
Pancreatic Duct
Pancreas
(digestive
enzymes
and insulin)
Descending
Colon
Jejunum
Ileum
Sigmoid colon
Rectum

Figure 1–6. The organs of digestion.

History

CHIEF COMPLAINT AND HISTORY OF PRESENT ILLNESS

- Pain is a common symptom of GI disease. The chief mechanisms causing abdominal pain are obstruction, peritoneal irritation and/or irritation, vascular insufficiency, ulceration, altered bowel motility, nerve injury, referred pain from an extraabdominal site, and emotional stress.

- Do a thorough assessment of any discomfort the client is having. Use the who, what, where, why, and how mnemonic (outlined in Pain, Section 2-3) to obtain the character, location, precipitating factors, time and duration, severity, and possible causes of pain. Be aware that referred pain is common with GI problems, which can make diagnosis difficult (See Figure 2-1, Areas of Referred Pain).

- Is there nausea, vomiting, diarrhea?

  1. Before or after meals?

  2. Other precipitating factors, i.e., emotional stress, medications, specific foods, treatments, exercise, etc.?

  3. Describe frequency, amount, color, odor, and consistency. (See also Nausea and Vomiting, Section 2-5 and Diarrhea, Section 2-6).

- Constipation? (See also Constipation, Section 2-7.)

  1. When was the last bowel movement?

  2. Are laxatives or enemas being used?

- Is there gas, belching, and/or flatulence? Frequency? (See also Flatulence, Section 2-8.)

- Bleeding

  1. Vomitus may be bright red, brown, "coffee grounds," blood tinged, or positive for occult blood.

  2. Stool may be bright red, blood tinged, dark and tarry, or positive for occult blood.

- Has there been a recent weight loss or gain?

PAST MEDICAL HISTORY

- History of gastrointestinal problems
- Therapy used and whether effective
- Allergies

PRESENT MEDICATIONS

- All medications including over-the-counter antacids, aspirin, birth-control pills, laxatives, sodium bicarbonate, etc.

HEALTH HABITS

- Smoking, alcohol, caffeine: how much and for how long?
- Nutrition: have client describe eating patterns. Is client on a special diet? Does client comply? Does it help or aggravate condition?
- Fluid intake: normal habits
- Bowel/bladder habits: compare present difficulties with normal pattern
- Menstrual cycle: last menstrual period, normal pattern, duration of periods, use of oral or other contraceptives

Physical Exam

- Prepare client by explaining the procedure, having the client empty his/her bladder, and providing privacy.
- Assist client to supine position and expose abdomen, covering breast and pubic area with a gown and bedsheet.
- Instruct client to place arms at side or across chest to lower tension on the abdomen.

INSPECTION

- Note skin color, hair distribution, jaundice, and any scars, rashes, striae, pigmentations, or surgical wounds.
- Look for asymmetry, masses, herniations, visible periostalsis, or pulsations.
- Note contour of abdomen, whether obese, flat, distended, concave, cachexic.

AUSCULTATION

- Auscultate before percussion or palpation to avoid stimulating peristalsis.
- Use the diaphragm of the stethoscope, as bowel sounds are high pitched.

- **Normal:** Bowel sounds should be heard in all four quadrants every 5 to 20 sec.

- **Abnormal:** Because bowel sounds are irregular, listening for 3–5 min is required before concluding they are hypoactive or absent.

   1. Hypoactive bowel sounds (less than one sound per minute): Listen for full 3 min. May indicate paralytic ileus, peritonitis, obstruction, hemorrhage, post abdominal surgery, mesenteric infarct, or no food in the bowel.

   2. Hyperactive bowel sounds (continuous sounds) may occur with vomiting or diarrhea, above a bowel obstruction, or just after eating.

   3. Vascular sounds may indicate aneurysm, vascular disease, heart murmur, or liver disease.

PERCUSSION

- Percuss all four quadrants, listening for areas of dullness and tympany.

- The stomach and the large and small intestines should be tympanic, except after a meal. The liver, spleen, bladder, and gravid uterus are dull.

- **Liver:**

   1. The lower border is usually at costal margin or slightly below.

   2. The upper border begins in fifth to seventh intercostal space.

   3. Normal values for length: 6–12 cm for midclavicular line; 4–8 cm for midsternal line.

PALPATION

- Light palpation: for areas of tenderness, masses, involuntary guarding, muscle tone, fluid accumulation

- Deep palpation: for normal anatomy, enlarged structures, masses and pain

   1. Liver, spleen, pancreas and urinary bladder are not normally palpable.

2. A full and distended urinary bladder is palpable as high as the umbilicus.

3. Kidneys: The lower pole of the right kidney may be palpated. The left kidney is not normally palpable except occasionally in thin individuals. Usually it is a sign of pathology if palpable.

4. Aorta: Often palpable at epigastrium slightly left of midline. It should feel like a long, thin, consistent, pulsatile mass. An enlarged area may indicate aneurysm.

5. Do not mistake normal structures for masses: feces-filled colon, distended bladder, gravid uterus, aorta, saccral promontory.

6. Techniques for assessment of abdominal fluid include bulging flank and fluid shift.

RECTAL-ANAL EXAM

- With client in lateral Sim's position, observe skin and surface characteristics of perianal area.

- Area should be smooth and clear with no tenderness, fissures, hemorrhoids, scars, ulcers, skin irritations, or rectal prolapse.

- Palpate the area for tenderness and masses.

- With gloved, lubricated index finger perform digital exam: sphincter muscle should tighten evenly around finger with minimal discomfort for client, the rectal wall should be a continuous, smooth surface with no areas of tenderness, tumors, lumps, or masses.

Laboratory Values

- CBC, electrolytes, BUN, amylase, lipase, and other studies for abnormal results or worsening trends

Diagnostic Tests

- Common tests for GI evaluation are upper GI series (barium swallow), lower GI series (barium enema), endoscopy, nuclear scans, sigmoidoscopy, ultrasonography, x-ray, cholecystogram (gall bladder series), CT scans, gastric analysis, liver biopsy, fecal analysis, duodenal drainage tests and MRI.

1-9 RECORDING CLINICAL DATA

Every hospital has its own method or standard format for recording clinical care by nurses in the medical record. The following are brief descriptions of several current documentation methods. Whatever system is used, nursing documentation must communicate the client's status, the specific care provided, and the response to that care.

The Problem-Oriented Medical Record

First suggested by Dr. L. L. Weed, this system is used in many institutions. The underlying principle is the problem-solving method (nursing process). Individual problems are identified and followed clinically in the chart in a way that is accessible to all involved in the care of the client. Medicine defines "problem" as a provable diagnosis, a potentially significant but isolated symptom, physical finding, laboratory report, or socioeconomic difficulty. In nursing, a problem is any unmet need or nursing diagnosis.

A problem list is developed from the data base and is placed prominently in the chart where it can be referred to easily, as it is the key index to the client's file (Figure 1-7). The problem list may grow or change as new data is collected. Problems are numbered for easy referral in the progress notes. As plans are implemented, client response to treatment is documented and the list is updated. Progress notes record current:

Subjective data Complaints or statements of client or family.

Objective data Information obtained through observation or measurement, i.e., vital signs, laboratory results, nonverbal behavior, etc.

Assessment Overall impression or nursing diagnosis (i.e., alteration in comfort due to presence of headache). Include etiology of problem when possible.

Plan Specific actions for further data gathering, implementing care and client/family education. Goals are stated as desired outcomes.

Implementation Record intervention, response to interventions, and progress made.

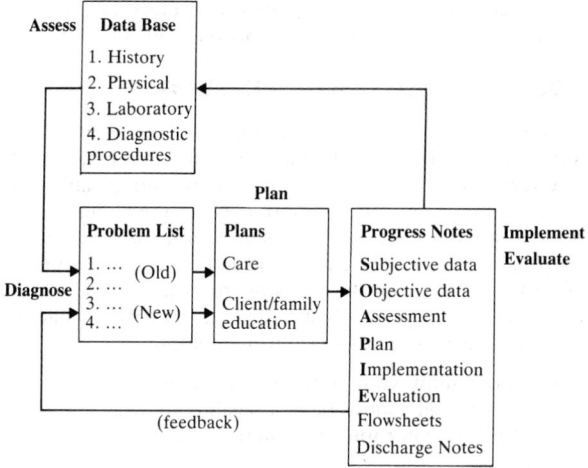

Figure 1–7. The problem-oriented medical record.

Evaluation Evaluate interventions on the basis of objective and subjective data.

Focus Charting

Introduced in the early 1980s, this method can streamline charting by reducing the format to three letters that summarize the structure: DAR. These letters represent **D**ata, **A**ction(s), and **R**esponse(s). Each entry has a symptom, a problem, nursing diagnosis or significant event placed in the left-hand column, which serves as the note's "focus." The notes, addressing the three key components, DAR, are recorded to the right of the identified problem.

Charting by Exception

In this method, only significant or abnormal findings, or exceptions to standardized, expected norms are written in the narrative notes. Key features of this method are standardized care plans, flowsheets, and at least some bedside charting. This method can reduce the amount of time spent on documentation and repetitive entries. However, the standards of care must be specific and clear in order to define the exceptions on which this method is based.

Computerized Documentation

Computerization can reduce nursing time spent on administrative tasks and make more time for client care. Bedside terminals assist in ensuring frequent entries, although terminals are more often found at the nursing station. In some systems the nurse can select actions or findings appropriate to a specific client, and generate client-specific flowsheets and care plans, thus decreasing documentation time per client per shift as much as 40–50% (Marelli, 1992). Some safeguards when using computers:

- Never allow your password to be used by someone else, as you cannot be responsible for what someone else may enter into the computer under your name.

- To protect confidentiality, never leave a computer unattended once you have logged on.

- Never delete information that has been officially entered and is part of the record. A misspelled word or inaccuracy that has not been stored yet can be deleted or corrected. However, if there is an error in information that has been stored, it must be treated much like an error in a handwritten note—mark the word "error" where the mistake begins and ends, and initial the notes.

- Printouts must be handled carefully and kept out of unauthorized hands.

Narrative Charting

Though newer forms are gaining adherents, narrative charting continues to be a predominant charting method. In fact, all the methods incorporate some use of the narrative form, such as a SOAPIE note that requires lengthy description of a client's response to nursing interventions.

Documenting

When documenting, remember the two main purposes of the medical record: 1) to communicate information to health care team members about client problems and treatment; 2) to serve as a legal record of care delivered to the client. Nurses' entries must be significant and accurate. The following are important guidelines:

FORM

- Write legibly and in ink (color per hospital policy).

- Record time and date for each entry.

- Do not skip lines between entries. Line through any blank spaces before signatures.

- Entries are to be in consecutive order chronologically. If you need to chart after the fact, write post note, the time of documenting, and the time of occurrence.

- Document events as they occur. Never chart procedures before they have been performed.

- Use correct grammar, spelling, punctuation, and syntax. Consult a dictionary if uncertain.

- The client's name must be on each record form.

- Sign each entry using your legal signature: your first initial, last name, and position (RN, LVN, etc.) Never chart for someone else nor allow anyone to chart for you.

- If you make an error, line it through with one line, initial it, and write "error" beside it.

- Never use liquid coverup or otherwise erase, destroy, or alter previously written notes.

CONTENT

- Use only those abbreviations accepted by your hospital.

- Chart observed facts. Describe client behavior in terms of what you see, hear, feel, and smell. Avoid conclusions, assumptions, labeling and judgmental wording. Avoid overuse of the word "appears."

- Chart nursing physical assessments, nursing diagnoses, goals of client care, nursing interventions, evaluation of client's progress.

- Chart exact times of client activities, treatments, procedures.

- Document changes in client condition.

- Document follow-up interventions in response to client condition.

- Record all attempts to contact physicians and the reason the physician was phoned. Document visits by the physician to the client, including details and direct quotes if pertinent.

- Record client responses to treatment. Include care given and procedures performed. Indicate that they were performed according to hospital protocol.

- Chart client care at least every 2 hr; more if the client's condition dictates.

- When charting medication errors, be as brief as possible. Do not use the word "error" or "wrong drug." Document what the client actually received, making observations, and that the physician was notified. Follow hospital policy regarding an incident report.

- If any procedure is not charted on the medical record, it is not legally considered done. Following hospital policy and thorough documentation are essential in avoiding malpractice.

Discharge Planning

Due to an increase in shortened hospital stays, discharge planning should be initiated upon admission and maintained as an ongoing process. Care plans should include thorough client teaching in order to increase self-care at home. Topics to be covered include: wound care, medications, recommended activity level and when to return to work, dietary restrictions, symptoms that should be reported, where and when to return for follow-up care, and specific concerns related to the individual's diagnosis. Assess and implement needs for home care, a social worker, hospice care, community group support, family support, or any other help that may be required.

REFERENCES

Baird S, White NE, Basinger M. Can you rely on tympanic thermometers? RN 1992; August: 48–51.

Brunner LS, Suddarth DS, eds. Textbook of medical-surgical nursing. 7th ed. Philadelphia: JB Lippincott, 1992.

Carlson JH, et al. Nursing diagnosis: a case study approach. Philadelphia: WB Saunders, 1991.

Carpenito LJ. Nursing diagnosis: application to clinical practice. 4th ed. Philadelphia: JB Lippincott, 1992.

Collins HL. Legal risks of computer charting. RN 1990; May: 81–86.

Cooper K. Measuring blood pressure the right way. Nursing '92; April: 75.

Fuller J, Schaller-Ayers J. Health assessment: a nursing approach. Philadelphia: JB Lippincott, 1990.

Ignatavicius D, Bayne M. Medical-surgical nursing. 2d ed. Philadelphia: WB Saunders, 1991.

Knapp-Spooner C, Brett J. Less is more: a med/surg flow sheet. RN 1992; March: 36–39.

Kozier B, et al. Techniques in clinical nursing. 4th ed. Menlo Park, CA: Addison-Wesley, 1993.

Lewis SM, Collier IC. Medical-surgical nursing: assessment and management of clinical problems. St. Louis: Mosby, 1992.

Lower JS. Rapid neuro assessment. American Journal of Nursing 1992; June: 38–45.

Lueckenotte AG. Pocket guide to gerontologic assessment. St. Louis: Mosby, 1990.

Marrelli TM. Nursing documentation handbook. St. Louis: Mosby, 1992.

Maslow AH. Motivation and personality. 2nd ed. New York: Harper and Row, 1970.

Matthews JP. How to use an automated vital signs monitor. Nursing '91; February: 60–64.

Raish P, Klaus B. Every nurse's guide to physical assessment: a primary care focus. New York: John Wiley and Sons, 1987.

Witherell C. Questions nurses ask about pacemakers. American Journal of Nursing 1990: December: 20–25.

CHAPTER 2

SELECTED NURSING DIAGNOSES AND NURSING INTERVENTIONS

*NANDA approved nursing diagnosis

The nursing diagnoses in this chapter have been selected because they are common problems associated with many diseases and have not been dealt with in other chapters in this volume (i.e., actual fluid volume deficits are covered in Chapter 5, Fluid and Electrolyte Balance)

Making nursing diagnoses requires assessing the data; determining the client's strengths, problems, and risks; and formulating causal relationships between the health problems and factors related to them. Nurses may write diagnoses as either two-part or three-part statements, including either just the problem and etiology, or the problem, etiology, and signs and symptoms. An example of a three-part statement is: Self-esteem disturbance related to altered body image manifested by pacing, refusing to touch body part.

An important principle to remember when making diagnoses in clinical practice is to make sure that diagnoses fall under nursing responsibility, rather than medical. For instance, terms such as hypertension, diabetes, and postpartum are medical conditions rather than human responses treatable by the professional nurse, whereas "potential for fluid volume deficit" is a nursing diagnosis category that may apply to clients with all these medical conditions. Appendix A lists the NANDA Approved Nursing Diagnostic Catagories as of 1994.

Discussion and development of nursing diagnosis categories will continue. Professionals are responsible for implementing concepts in their practice and contributing to the development of standards. New categories may be submitted for research and testing. For further instructions on this, a good reference is *Nursing Diagnosis, Process and Application* (Gordon, 1987).

More in-depth knowledge of the nursing problems in this chapter is necessary than can be contained here; included in this chapter are important reminders. And of course, nursing care plans must be individualized for each client. Making accurate nursing diagnoses based on careful assessments and determination of causes is essential to effective nursing practice. Remember the nursing process (Section 1-1) in all your daily encounters.

2-1 ACTIVITY INTOLERANCE

Activity intolerance is a person's inability to respond appropriately to activity because of difficulty with tissue perfusion. It may be caused by decreased cardiac output or inadequate nutritional status, and complicated by increased energy demands, anemia, and inability to rest and sleep due to anxiety and stress. Prolonged immobility may also cause activity intolerance as there may be accompanying decreased cardiac output and/or decreased tone and muscle loss. Any disease condition that interferes with oxygen transport can contribute to activity intolerance. The causes of activity intolerance will influence the assessments and interventions needed.

Nursing Assessment of Client with Activity Intolerance

- Assess client's awareness of fatigue, weakness, and feelings about a specific activity.

- Assess resting vital signs: BP, pulse, respirations. Assess these again in response to the activity along with skin color, mental state, and subjective feelings. After at least 3 min of rest assess these factors again. Record changes and observations.

- Compare pre-activity vital signs to the post-activity response and determine how long before client's response returns to the pre-activity level. The normal range in most people would be a return to the pre-activity rate after 10 min of rest. Report any deviations. Assess for exertional dyspnea, chest pain, diaphoresis, or dizziness.

Nursing Interventions to Reduce Intolerance

- Implement activities slowly, allowing for adequate physiological response. Gradually increase activity as tolerated.

- Have support person and assistive devices available when new activities are begun.

- Implement activities that reduce the hazards of immobility, including active and passive range of motion and exercises that minimize loss of muscle strength.

- Implement measures to promote sleep and rest:

  - Minimize environmental noise

  - Maximize bedtime rituals that promote sleepiness such as subdued lighting, soft music, backrub, reading, etc.

  - Limit sleep during the daylight hours to promote longer nighttime sleep periods

  - Schedule nursing care, activities of daily living, diagnostic tests and treatments so that adequate rest periods are allowed

  - Reduce stress anxiety by allowing expression of concerns and respond appropriately to these concerns if possible

- Implement measures to conserve energy.

  - Sit for most activities of daily living such as showering, brushing teeth, combing hair

  - Limit the number and timing of visitors if this is energy draining.

- Instruct client regarding the reason for the intolerance and how it is reduced gradually. Encourage client to increase activities and exercise daily.

- Collaborate with the client to establish realistic goals in preparation for discharge.

2-2 SLEEP PATTERN DISTURBANCE: SLEEPLESSNESS

Factors that prevent, delay or interrupt sleep may be physical, mental, emotional, environmental, or a combination of these.

Nursing Assessment for the Client with Sleeplessness

- Anxiety, fear, grief, worry, or other emotions can interfere with sleep and may be associated with hospitalization.

- Environmental stimuli, such as light, noise, offensive smells, heat or cold, or an uncomfortable bed may cause sleep disturbances.

- Physical conditions such as pain, muscle spasms, distended bladder or bowels, hunger, thirst, fever, or other irritations can contribute to sleep disturbances.

- Daytime inactivity or prolonged bed rest may contribute to sleeplessness at night. Encourage the client to be active during the day with minimal time spent in bed.

- Many medications can alter sleep patterns. Changing the medication or schedule may improve sleep. Table 7-6A on page 330 lists a few of the many medications that may affect sleep.

- Interventions by health care providers (i.e., collection of lab specimens, vital signs, medication administration), especially at night, can interfere with normal sleep patterns.

- Caffeine intake (in coffee, chocolate, tea, cola drinks) may cause sleeplessness and if so, should be avoided, particularly after 4 p.m.

- Loud snoring may be a sign of the sleep disorder sleep apnea. Snoring may be corrected by having client sleep on their side, however, an evaluation and workup for sleep apnea may be indicated. The client with sleep apnea should be assessed for the safe use of opiates, sedatives or hypnotics, as these medications may aggravate an oxygen deficit that already may be severe.

Nursing Interventions to Relieve Sleeplessness

- Intervene based on assessment of the cause of sleeplessness.

- Talk with the client about what may be causing him/her concern. Reinforce preoperative teaching or answer questions regarding the client's particular condition.

- Reduce stimuli in the environment by decreasing stimulating activities, quieting noise, and dimming the lights at sleep time.

- Encourage the client to avoid strenuous physical activities 1–2 hr prior to bedtime, as these activities can be stimulating.

- Massage the muscles, especially those of the limbs and back, as relaxed muscles relieve mental tension.

- Have the client void.

- Help the client assume the position he/she finds most restful. Assure that client's immediate environment is comfortable and restful (i.e., smooth bed linens, adequate room ventilation, comfortable air temperature).

2-3 PAIN

Pain relief is not only one of the fundamental goals of nursing, but is also the primary reason clients seek medical treatment. Nurses have the opportunity to become experts in the art and science of pain relief.

The three main aspects of pain management are pain assessment, therapeutic relief measures, and evaluation. The nurse, client and health care team work together collaboratively to develop a plan for obtaining relief. The plan is then implemented and evaluated so that another combination of measures can be enacted if the first one produces less than optimal results.

Each client must be considered individually. Perhaps the problem is medical or surgical or without specifically identified etiology. Whether the cause of pain is identified or not, the validity of the client's pain and the development of a pain management plan must be addressed. Is there underlying pathology that needs prompt attention (e.g., emergency appendectomy in the case of right-sided abdominal pain)? Or does the client simply need better positioning (e.g., leg elevation after a fractured tibia)? Pain management intervention may be pharmacologic and technologically focused, or as simple as a therapeutic conversation between client and nurse.

I. **Nursing Assessment of the Client with Pain**
   In collecting assessment data, it is important to utilize all resources. The nurse's clinical observations and the client's subjective responses provide the basis for the assessment process. Additionally the client's family and significant others can provide essential information. The medical chart and other members of the health care team should also be consulted. Collectively, the assessment data provides a foundation for the development of a pain management plan.

   A. **Objective signs that pain is present**

      1. **Behavioral signs:** Guarding, protective behavior, hands placed over painful area, pinched facial expression, clenched fists or teeth, inability to sleep or concentrate, refraining from any movement, fatigue, decreased appetite, self-focusing, shortened attention span, impaired thought process, moaning, crying, pacing, facial mask of pain (eyes lackluster, "beaten look").

      2. **Autonomic response:** Pallor, diaphoresis, ↑ or ↓ BP, ↑ respirations, ↑ or ↓ heart rate and/or stroke volume, tight muscles, dry mouth, pupillary dilatation. *Note:* Behavioral signs and autonomic responses may not be reliable indicators of whether a client is experiencing pain. These responses may diminish or completely cease as adaptation occurs. Adaptation may occur quickly; within minutes to hours, or may take longer.

   B. **Subjective assessment tool**

   • **The who, what, where, when, why and how of pain assessment.** An easy way to remember all the ways to evaluate pain is to get the "story" on the pain like an investigative reporter. Remember that pain is "whatever the experiencing person says it is" (McCaffery, 1989).

   Who (about the client) Find out about the client's occupation, lifestyle, history. Focus on previous experiences and successful management of pain.

What (character and intensity) Ask about the character of the pain. Is it burning, stabbing, throbbing, dull, aching, crampy, or crushing? Ask about the intensity. Using a rating scale is helpful (mild, moderate, or severe) or 0–10 scale: 0 = no pain to 10 = worst pain imaginable.

Where (location) Is the pain cutaneous (arising from the skin and superficial structures), somatic, deep (from the bone, nerve, muscle, or other supportive tissues), or visceral (all organs located in the body cavities)? Visceral and somatic pain may be referred to a segment of the skin (Figure 2-1). The location may vary at different times. The client may also experience pain in more than one location. It may be helpful to have the client point to the location(s) of the pain or to draw the locations on a body diagram.

When (time pattern) When and for how long does the pain occur? Is it acute or chronic? Ascertaining when the pain comes on often helps to discover the cause. Maybe it is associated with a stress-producing event or eating certain foods. Maybe it comes on in the evening when there is muscle fatigue.

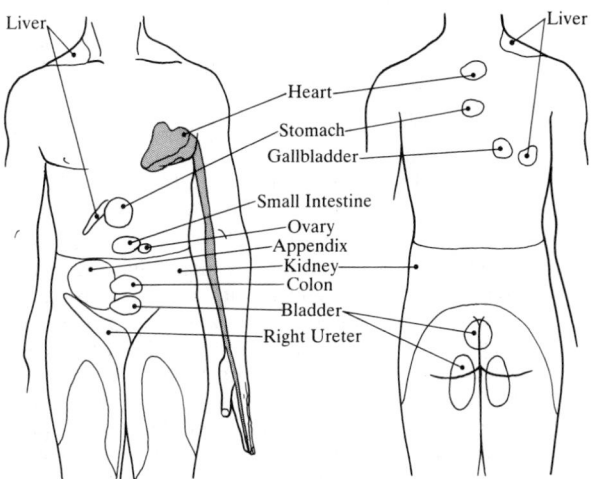

Figure 2–1. Areas of referred pain—anterior and posterior views.

Why (the cause) By assessing both the pattern and cause, it may be possible to alter certain behaviors/activities that may help in managing a client's pain. What causes the pain and/or what makes it worse?

How (the solution) How can we relieve it? Ask the client what has worked in the past. Ask what might relieve it now. Table 2-1 shows a sample of how this mnemonic can be used in pain assessment.

II. Pain Relief Measures
General:

- Notify the physician when client complains of new, unexpected or unrelieved pain, especially if other clinical signs of pathology are present, as the problem could be underlying pathology, which might require medical or surgical intervention.

- Prevent pain as much as possible by giving full dose of analgesic before pain is anticipated (e.g., postoperatively) and prepare clients thoroughly for procedures (i.e., client teaching and involvement, help clients relax, etc.)

- A combination of interventions is often more successful than one.

- Treat problems and side effects that aggravate pain, such as coughing, nausea, vomiting, anorexia, diarrhea, constipation, or anxiety.

- Pain management interventions may include one or more of the following methods: non-pharmacologic, pharmacologic, and neurosurgical. Table 2-2 lists the various therapies. These therapies are described in the remainder of this section.

- In addition, pain clinics are available in many areas that treat chronic pain clients using a holistic, interdisciplinary approach. A variety of procedures may be used based on an individualized program. Every aspect of pain and its relief is considered and clients fully participate in their own rehabilitation. Consider referral to a pain clinic when pain requires long-term management. These clients may be oncologic clients, clients with injury-related

---

TABLE 2–1. SAMPLE PAIN ASSESSMENT

OBJEC-TIVE	Client has pinched facial expression and clenched fists and BP of 140/85 mm Hg
WHO	Mr. Jones had a laminectomy 3 days ago. He states he hates to be "laid up" and wants to return to his construction job soon.
WHAT	States the pain feels like someone is stabbing him in the back. (Mild) 1 2 3 4 5 6 7 ⑧ 9 10 (Severe)
WHERE	Lower lumbar area where his incision is only (doesn't radiate).
WHEN	He states the pain is more severe when the pillows supporting his legs get out of place and also when he starts worrying about his job.

WHY	Client opinion:	"I'm not in the right position. I'm getting restless laying here in bed."
	Nursing assessment:	There are no signs of infection or bleeding in incisional area. Bladder does not appear to be distended. Client is able to move lower extremities. Right leg is rotated outward. Pillows are out of place.
	Nursing impression:	Local incisional pain postlaminectomy caused by poor body alignment, muscle spasm, anxiety, and surgical instrumentation.
HOW	Plan for relief:	1. Check for last dose of muscle-relaxing and analgesic medications.
		2. Assist client to verbalize feelings of anxiety. Assist with ambulation as this may

Table continued on following page

TABLE 2–1. SAMPLE PAIN ASSESSMENT *Continued*

    help alleviate symptoms of restlessness and anxiety.

3. Help client to a position of correct body alignment. Attend to comfort measures. Reinforce teaching about log rolling and not letting the leg rotate outward. Monitor client doing postoperative exercises three times a day.

4. Instruct client to request pain medication when pain begins, rather than waiting so that it escalates to a point that it is more difficult to control.

pain or clients experiencing pain with no identifiable cause.

Non-Pharmacologic Therapies
A. Physical therapies
1. Positioning
    a) Check this first when the client complains of pain. Injured parts may need to be elevated. Sometimes postoperative pain is due to being in the same position for too long rather than incisional pain.

    b) Use proper body alignment, positioning, and support with pillows.

TABLE 2–2. PAIN THERAPIES

NON-PHARMACOLOGIC
  A. Physical
  - Positioning
  - Application of heat, cold
  - Massage
  - Soaking
  - Transcutaneous electrical nerve stimulators (TENS)
  - Comfort measures
  - Acupressure
  B. Psychoemotional
  - Therapeutic listening
  - Distraction
  - Client teaching
  - Relaxation techniques
  - Imagery
  - Therapeutic touch
  - Psychotherapy
  - Hypnosis
  - Biofeedback

PHARMACOLOGIC
  A. Non-opiates
  - Non-steroidal antiinflammatory drugs (NSAID's)
  - Anxiolytics (anti-anxiety)
  - Steroids
  - Antidepressants
  - Membrane stabilizers (lidocaine, carbamazepine)
  - Muscle relaxants (bactofen, carisoprodol)
  B. Opiates (morphine, hydromorphone, meperidine, etc.)

NEUROSURGICAL
  - Cordotomy
  - Neurectomy
  - Rhizotomy

---

2. Application of heat and cold
  a) Do not use heat where there is a decreased sensation or movement.
  b) Do not use cold where circulation or sensation is impaired.
  c) Both heat and cold may be applied wet (i.e.,

soaks) or dry (i.e., heating pad, heat lamp, ice bag, hot water bag, or diathermy).

d) Cold is best when inflammation and swelling are just beginning; heat is better when edema is established.

e) It may be necessary to try a variety of temperatures or applications to effect pain relief.

3. **Massage**

a) Use in the early stages of inflammatory swellings and in the treatment of various forms of myalgia, fibrositis, and many other injuries. Do *not* massage if there is possibility of phlebitis. The painful area can be massaged directly or sometimes stimulation to the same area on the opposite side of the body is effective.

b) In the case of headache, the acupressure pressure point is the tissue of the hand between the large joint of the thumb and the first knuckle of the first finger.

c) Also, back rubs, foot massages, or full or partial body massages can be highly therapeutic in reducing the muscle tension and anxiety that increase pain.

d) If thromboembolism is a risk, massage should not be used. *Under no circumstance should the calf muscles of the leg be massaged.*

4. **Soaking**

a) A warm bath can relieve the pain of back strain, muscle aches, joint swelling, and inflammation. Or the painful limb can be placed in a basin of warm water.

b) Soaking not only relieves pain but speeds the healing process in local infections.

5. **Transcutaneous electrical nerve stimulators (TENS):** These have been successful in treatment of both chronic and acute pain. Electrodes that carry a small electric current are placed directly over painful areas or at trigger points along nerve pathways where pain radiates. The client is taught how to use the device and using gives the feeling of control. TENS may be contraindicated for pregnant women or clients with pacemakers or arrhythmias (consult with physician).

a) Proper placement is key in this therapy, as is skin care. Do not place electrodes over irritated areas, skin preparations, sutures, hair, or the carotid sinus.

b) Remove electrodes at least once a day and wash the area with soap and water. Before reapplying the electrodes, allow the area to air (preferably overnight), wipe it with a skin prep pad and check for redness. If an area of redness persists for more than 30 min the site must be changed and the situation reported.

6. **Comfort measures and creating a healing environment**

a) Ensure clean and comfortable bedding and bedclothes.

b) Assist with activities of daily living as appropriate

c) Assess whether the environment is contributing to anxiety/stress/pain. Intervene to decrease irritants (noise, odor, temperature).

7. **Acupressure/Acupuncture:** In these therapies, specific points on the body are stimulated with direct pressure or a needle, resulting in pain relief. The exact point may be in an entirely different location on the body from the site of pain.

B. Psychoemotional therapies

1. **Therapeutic listening**

a) Convey a caring attitude. Pay attention to the nonverbal communication as well as the verbal. Restate what client says in your own words to make sure you understand.

b) Accept nonjudgmentally what the client is experiencing but help them see ways that problems might be solved. (See also Communication and the Therapeutic Relationship, Section 12-1).

2. **Distraction:** This is more useful in mild pain than in severe pain. When undergoing a painful procedure, balance must be maintained between keeping the client informed but distracted from focusing on the pain.

a) It may be helpful if a nurse speaks quietly to client during the painful moments of a procedure.

b) Or it might help to have client say "ouch" at the painful point.

c) In chronic pain, diversionary activities that are interesting to the client need to be planned into the routine of every day, such as letter writing, reading, etc.

d) Recognize distraction at work in the case of the client who asks for a pain medication and then is seen laughing and talking on the phone.

3. Client teaching

a) Thoroughly explain procedures so that the client will be prepared and know how to have a measure of control.

b) Give client something active to do to enhance the healing process.

4. Relaxation techniques

a) Teach client to use these techniques daily (see Stress Reduction, Section 12-3), as they are powerful tools for reducing stress and promoting health and well-being. Disorders that respond particularly well to relaxation techniques are hypertension, certain arrhythmias, migraine headache, anxiety neuroses, and drug abuse.

b) Make sure the client assumes a comfortable position with shoes off, clothing loosened, bladder emptied, and all limbs supported, in a calm, quiet environment.

c) Use Quiet Breathing or Progressive Muscle Tension and Relaxation as in Section 12-3 or another technique you find helpful.

d) Meditation focuses on relaxation by having client focus inwardly and progressively relaxing themselves. This approach may use a script or tape that guides the client through the process.

5. Imagery

a) Client imagines something pleasant and holds that image before and during pain. Tapes are available that guide the client through pleasurable scenes like walking through the woods or picking flowers in an open field. Attention is paid to as many sensations as possible—the

smell of the air, the color of the flowers, the feel of the grass under the feet.
    b) A special photograph or a picture from a magazine of something that makes the client feel calm and relaxed—the ocean, a loved one, or a scene from nature can be used.
6. **Therapeutic touch:** Dolores Kreiger's method is one in which the nurse's hands interact with the client's energy field to restore imbalance in the body. An increasing number of nurses are becoming skilled in this art. Before trying it on clients nurses should receive training in this skill.
7. **Psychotherapy:** Utilizing the skills of a trained professional, the client can examine problematic areas of his/her past and present. General goals focus on decreasing stress, improved coping and increased quality of life.
8. **Hypnosis:** A treatment method in which a client focuses very intensely on a specific topic with decreased awareness of the immediate surroundings.
9. **Biofeedback:** A cognitive-behavioral therapy that assists the client in awareness and control of physiologic effects. This therapy has been used with clients with hypertension, headaches, and chronic pain.

Pharmacologic Therapies

A. Non-opiates (also see Table 2-3)
1. **Nonsteroidal anti-inflammatory drugs (NSAIDs):** This category of drugs works primarily in the periphery. They have three main effects; anti-inflammatory, analgesic, and antipyretic. NSAIDs vary as to how much action they exert. Some, like acetaminophen, are antipyretic analgesics. Others, like aspirin, are analgesic, anti-inflammatory and antipyretic. Often to achieve the desired effects, NSAIDs such as ibuprofen are ordered on a strict, regular regimen (i.e., q 6 hrs) rather than prn.

NSAIDs should be used cautiously, if at all, in clients with bleeding abnormalities, reduced kidney function, history of aspirin sensitivity, gastric

TABLE 2–3. NON-OPIOID ANALGESICS

CHEMICAL CLASS	GENERIC/TRADE NAME	USUAL DOSE	MAXIMUM DAILY DOSE	DOSING INTERVAL
paraaminophenol derivative	acetaminophen (Tylenol)	PO: 500–1000 mg	4000 mg	q 4–6h
salicylates	aspirin (ASA)	PO: 500–1000 mg	4000 mg	q 4–6h
	choline magnesium salicylate (Trilisate)	PO: 1000–1500 mg	3000 mg	q 8–12h
	difusinal (Dolobid)	PO: 1000 mg × 1, then 500 mg	1500 mg	q 8–12h
nonsteroidal anti-inflammatory (NSAID) proprionic acids	ibuprofen (Motrin, Advil)	PO: 200–800 mg	2400 mg	q 4–8h
	naproxen (Naprosyn)	PO: 500 mg × 1 then 250 mg	1500 mg	q 6–8h

			Dose	Frequency
	naproxen sodium (Anaprox)	PO: 550 mg × 1 then 275 mg	1375 mg	q 6–8h
	fenoprofen (Nalfon)	PO: 200–600 mg	3200 mg	q 6–8h
	flubiprofen (Ansaid)	PO: 100 mg	300 mg	q 6–12h
	ketoprofen (Orudis)	PO: 50–75 mg	300 mg	q 4–8h
NSAID acetic acids	ketorolac (Toradol)	IM: 60 mg × 1 then 15–30 mg PO: 10 mg	IM: 120 mg PO: 40 mg	q 6h
	sulindac (Clinoril)	PO: 150–200 mg	400 mg	q 12h
	tolmentin (Tolectin)	PO: 400 mg	2000 mg	q 6–8h
NSAID oxicams	piroxicam (Feldene)	PO: 10–20 mg	20 mg	qd

ulceration or nasal polyps. Adverse reactions include:

1) GI: nausea, vomiting, diarrhea, constipation, abdominal distress, potential for ulceration. NSAIDs should be taken with food.
2) Hematologic: decreases in hematocrit due to occult or obvious bleeding, platelet function affects, neutropenia, eosinophilia, thrombocytopenia, pancytopenia
3) Renal: decreased renal blood flow may precipitate a variety of renal disorders
4) Hypersensitivity: asthma, bronchospasm
5) Dermatologic: itching, rash, ecchymosis
6) CNS: dizziness, drowsiness, headache, tremors, confusion

2. Anxiolytics: Medications may help relieve anxiety and may help decrease pain. Includes benzodiazepines, antipsychotics and antihistamines.

3. Antidepressants: These medications can be used to provide analgesia. Dosing for analgesia is usually less than the dosing required to treat depression. They can also be used to treat the depression that often accompanies chronic pain.

4. Muscle relaxants: These may be helpful in relieving tension and spasm. Muscle relaxants can have a sedative effect that may require adjustment of the pain medication regimen.

5. Membrane Stabilizers/Anticonvulsants: Membrane stabilizers and anticonvulsants may be useful in clients with neuropathic (nerve damage) pain. This pain is usually described in terms like burning, shooting, stabbing, electrical.

6. Steroids: These medications may be helpful in relieving pain in cancer clients who experience spinal cord involvement or bone pain.

7. Antiemetics: Nausea and vomiting often accompany painful states. Medications must be given non-orally until vomiting is controlled.

B. Opiates: This group of medications includes morphine and morphine-like medications (hydromorphone, fentanyl, meperidine, etc.). The opiates work centrally and outside the central nervous system by binding to opiate receptor sites. Refer to Table 2-4

TABLE 2–4. OPIOID ANALGESICS

CLASS	DRUG	ORAL DOSE	IM DOSE (equivalent to 10 mg of IM morphine)	DURATION	COMMENTS
agonist related to morphine	morphine	20–60 mg	10 mg	3–6h	oral doses are well absorbed but metabolized on first pass through liver; can also be given SL & PR
	controlled release morphine	20–60 mg	—	8–12 h	
	hydromorphone (Dilaudid)	4 mg	1.5 mg	3–4h	
	oxymorphone (Numorphan)	no oral dose	1 mg	3–6h	
agonists related to codeine	codeine	30–60 mg	120 mg	3–6h	often formulated in combination with ASA or acetaminophen

Table continued on following page

TABLE 2–4. *Continued*

CLASS	DRUG	ORAL DOSE	IM DOSE (equivalent to 10 mg of IM morphine)	DURATION	COMMENTS
	hydrocodone (Vicodin, Lortab)	5 mg	no parenteral dose	3–4h	often formulated in combination with ASA or acetaminophen
	oxycodone (Percocet)	5 mg	no parenteral dose	3–6h	often formulated in combination with ASA or acetaminophen
synthetic opioid agonists	meperidine (Demerol)	300 mg	75–100 mg	2–4h	a toxic metabolite accumulates with repeated dosing; potential fatal drug interaction with clients taking MAO inhibitors.

synthetic opioid agonists	fentanyl	transdermal patch (72h)	0.1 mg	1–2h	
	methadone	10–20 mg	10 mg	4–6h	
	levorphanol	4 mg	2 mg	3–6h	
	propoxyphene (Darvon, Darvocet N)	65 mg as HCl 100 mg as napsylate	no parenteral dose	3–6h	often formulated in combination with acetaminophen
partial agonists	buprenorphine (Buprenex)	sublingual dose not yet available	0.4 mg	4–6h	
mixed agonist/ antagonist	pentazocin (Talwin)	50 mg	60 mg	2–4h	
	butorphanol (Stadol)	nasal spray	2 mg	3–6h	
	nalbuphine (Nubain)	none	10 mg	3–6h	
	dezocine (Dalgan)	none	10 mg	3–6h	

for a list of opioid analgesics, with prescribed doses and duration of action.

The opiates may be administered in a variety of ways in order to achieve pain management:

1. **Oral:** This route should be used when possible as it represents the simplest and most inexpensive method of delivery.
2. **IV:** This route can be used to administer continuous infusions, intermittent boluses, or client-controlled analgesia (PCA).
3. **IM:** Although this may be a common route of opiate delivery, it can be problematic. Administration with this route is painful, and drug absorption may be inconsistent.
4. **SQ:** The subcutaneous delivery of opiates may be useful for administration of small dosages if other routes are not an option. Drug absorption may be inconsistent.
5. **Intraspinal (Epidural and Intrathecal):** Although a newer form of pain management, intraspinal administration (usually epidural) can provide pain relief both in acute and chronic pain. Opiates can be administered continuously or intermittently in a bolus. Anesthetics may also be used in combination with intraspinal (epidural) opiates to provide pain relief.
6. **Sublingual/Buccal mucosa:** These represent newer yet viable alternatives for medication delivery. Further research is indicated to determine efficacy of these methods.
7. **Rectal:** This may be useful if the oral route cannot be utilized. Further research is indicated to establish dosing ranges.
8. **Topical:** Fentanyl (Duragesic) is available in a topical delivery system. It is absorbed through the skin via a "patch." It should be noted, however, that initial onset of pain relief may be delayed up to 17 hrs. when the patch is first applied. Supplemental pain medication must be given until the Duragesic starts to work.
9. **Opiate side effects**
   a) Respiratory: decreased respiratory rate due to decreased sensitivity of medullary centers to CO_2

b) CNS: dizziness, drowsiness, euphoria, dysphoria, confusion, headache, impaired physical and mental performance, decreased pupil size (miosis, pin-point pupils)

c) GI: nausea and vomiting due to stimulation of the chemotrigger zone (CTZ) in brain, abdominal distress, constipation, cough supression

d) Cardiovascular: postural hypotension, arrhythmias

e) Genitourinary: urinary hesitation, urinary retention, decreased libido

f) Hypersensitivity reactions: itching, rash, diaphoresis, laryngospasm

Neurosurgical Pain Therapies

Neurosurgical procedures may be considered when less invasive measures fail and client is suffering persistent, intractable pain of high intensity. These procedures are among the most invasive measures for the management of pain. Results obtained may be variable. Surgical interventions are to be considered only after a fully coordinated pain management plan has been implemented. These interventions are utilized infrequently in pain management.

Neurosurgical Therapies   attempt to relieve pain by interrupting nerve pathways that relay pain sensations to the brain. Surgery may be done on the peripheral nervous system, the central nervous system (the spinal cord or brain) and/or the autonomic nervous system (sympathectomy). The goal of these procedures is to relieve pain without causing the loss of other sensations. Examples of the operations performed include neurectomy, rhizotomy, and chordotomy.

III. Evaluation of Therapies

It is important to perform a complete pain assessment and history as well as a thorough reassessment. Frequency of reassessment should be appropriate for the interventions implemented and the client's condition. Assessments should be accurately documented and communicated to appropriate members of the health care team. Interventions should be tried until an optimal pain management regimen is achieved for the client. Usually a combination of therapies provide the best management strategy. Always thoroughly document the extent to which therapeutic goals have been achieved.

2-4 ANOREXIA

Loss of appetite becomes a problem when it results in nutritional and/or fluid deficits. It almost always accompanies nausea and vomiting. Disease process, treatment modalities, pain, and depression can decrease appetite. Every effort should be made by hospital staff to prevent malnutrition in clients at risk by providing nutritional support. Early intervention is important to impede the development of cachexia in clients with cancer.

Nursing Assessment of Client with Anorexia

- Compare pre-illness weight with current weight. Weight loss greater than 10% is a significant loss, 20%–30% is life-threatening. Calculate the percentage of weight loss by dividing the difference between the client's pre-illness weight and current weight by the pre-illness weight and multiply by 100.

- Ask client to describe typical breakfast, lunch, and dinner pre-illness and compare to current intake.

- Look for signs associated with malnutrition:

    - Dry, dull, thin hair; swollen face; dark areas under eyes and cheeks; dull eyes; red and swollen lips; swollen tongue that appears raw, purple, and sore; spongy gums that bleed easily; swollen thyroid glands; dry, flaky skin that appears tight and drawn; wasted muscles; swollen joints; bowed legs; heart rate above 100 beats per min; enlarged liver and spleen; burning and tingling of hands and feet; mental confusion and irritability (see also Chapter 8, Nutrition and Diets)

    - Check for decreased blood urea nitrogen, serum, albumin, protein, hematocrit, hemoglobin, cholesterol, lymphocytes, and transferrin levels

Nursing Interventions to Relieve Anorexia

- Control nausea with antiemetics, diet, and environmental measures if it is the cause of anorexia (see Section 2-5)

- Relieve other concurrent problems that might contribute to lack of appetite: sore mouth, pain, depression, constipation.

- In cancer, nausea may be caused by the cancer itself or treatments for it (radiation, chemotherapy). If client asks "Why must I eat if I don't feel like it?" emphasize the reasons for nutritional support especially during treatment:

  - To prevent or reverse weight loss

  - To maintain ability to fight infection

  - To help repair damaged tissues

  - To possibly increase positive response to treatment

  - To create an improved sense of strength and well-being

- Provide oral care before meals.

- Create a pleasant atmosphere in which the client is more likely to feel like eating:

  - Clean the unit. Remove all unappetizing sights, smells, or objects (emesis, basins, nasogastric tubes, dentures, etc.).

  - Ventilate the room to provide fresh air.

  - Provide fresh flowers, soft music, and companionship if possible.

- Serve foods with attractive color and texture.

- Serve 6–8 small meals a day with high-calorie, high-protein snacks.

- Avoid foods client has an aversion to. Red meat is frequently disliked by cancer clients. Get a dietician to consult with client as to taste changes due to illness, personal likes and dislikes, and the optimal diet. Encourage significant others to bring in favorite foods unless contraindicated.

- Measure client progress:
    - Intake and output: Give positive reinforcement for improvement in intake.
    - Measure weight daily.
    - Measure triceps skin-fold thickness to give data about fat stores; measure the thickness of the skin with calipers while pinching it at midpoint between the shoulder and elbow. Standards are men, 12.5 mm; women, 16.5 mm.

- Perform a 72-hr calorie count and consult with physician about alternative methods of providing nutrients (tube feedings, total parenteral nutrition) if nutritional status declines. (see also Chapters 6 and 8).

2-5 NAUSEA AND VOMITING

Nausea and vomiting are two of the most common symptoms of illness, along with pain and fever. Because they are associated with numerous diseases, medications, or psychogenic states, assessment of the cause is not always easy. Like pain, the mechanisms that regulate these reactions are not well understood.

Besides discomfort, which may be extreme in some cases (e.g., chemotherapy), fluid and electrolyte balance is of major concern when there is repeated vomiting or extreme nausea accompanied by no oral intake.

Nursing Assessment of Client with Nausea and Vomiting

Who: Find out about the client's history, present diagnosis, and illness pattern.

What: What is the sensation? What is the character of the vomitus? Black color may indicate bleeding, fecal odor may indicate peritonitis.

Where: Where is the client when the symptom occurs? What factors may have aggravated it (i.e., nauseating sights, smells, thoughts)?

When: When does the nausea occur—after ingesting a medication? How long has it been going on? *How long has the person been unable to take fluids?* Does it come on before, during, or after meals?

Why: Develop a hypothesis as to the cause, and work with the physician to test plans to relieve the discomfort. In many cases nonemetic medications can be substituted for emetic ones. Or antiemetic medications can be given.

Fluid status: Obtain vital signs, weight pattern, and intake and output. Assess for signs of dehydration: thready, rapid pulse, dry mucous membranes, low blood pressure (postural), decreased skin turgor, decreased urine output (see Table 5-4). Assess neurologic status as increased intracranial pressure may be present in a client who is vomiting.

Nursing Interventions to Relieve Nausea and Vomiting

- In many cases the symptoms are self-limiting. Vomiting may relieve the symptom of nausea.

- Taking medications on an empty stomach may cause nausea and vomiting. Medications including antiemetics must be given IM, IV, SQ, or via rectal suppository until nausea and vomiting have subsided.

- **Nausea and vomiting associated with cancer:** Nausea and vomiting may be complications of any cancer treatment, whether it is surgery, radiation, or chemotherapy. Prophylactic drug therapy for vomiting is much more effective than after the fact treatment. Oral therapy, suppository administration, or intermittent IV therapy can be used in selected clients.

- **Medication therapy:** Some antiemetics act directly on the vomiting center and some work through other methods. Administer antiemetics 1/2 hr to 1 hr before meals.

- Antihistamines (Benadryl, Atarax, Dramamine, Bendectine, Tigan): effective for motion sickness, Meniére's syndrome, myocardial infarction, viral hepatitis, mechanical or chemical irritation of the GI tract (not helpful in cancer chemotherapy)

- Phenothiazines (Thorazine, Compazine, Trilafon, Torecan, Stelazine): effective in nausea associated with drugs (antibiotics, cytotoxic agents, alcohol, ergots, opiates, and the inhalation anesthetics), diabetic acidosis, and radiation sickness

- Metaclopramide (Reglan) is effective for cisplatin-induced nausea and vomiting and is usually given intravenously in high doses (2–3 mg/kg every 2–3 hr). Side effects include extrapyamidal reactions, restlessness, and diarrhea.

- Corticosteroids (dexamethasone, methylprednisone): effective against nausea associated with emetic agents

- Butyrophenones (haloperidol (Haldol), droperidol): effective against nausea and vomiting associated with such potent emetic agents as cisplatin, doxorubicin, and mechlorethamine

- Selected antagonists such as Zofran (ondansetron hydrochloride) work on specific chemoreceptor sites.

- Tetrahydrocannabinol (THC) and other cannabinoids (marijuana) have been shown to be effective in relieving symptoms associated with cancer chemotherapy especially in younger clients.

- While many of the antiemetics are quite active when used as single agents, more complete control of nausea and vomiting may be achieved when drugs with different pharmacologic actions are used in combination.

- **Fluid replacement**
  - Allow oral intake according to client's ability to tolerate. Oral intake may stimulate vomiting. Therefore give very small amounts at a time until ability to tolerate is established. Try small sips of clear liquid 2 hr after the last episode of vomiting.
  - IV fluid replacement is ordered on the basis of the client's laboratory data, amount of losses, and volume of anticipated losses over 24 hr.
- **Diet**
  - Dry carbohydrates such as crackers may be tolerated as nausea subsides. Advance the diet in small increments as tolerated from clear liquids to small, frequent meals.
  - Encourage client to eat slowly.
  - Have client drink fluids an hour or so before and after meals, not with meals.
  - Have client drink cool or chilled beverages such as carbonated beverages or fruit juices slowly.
  - Choose low-fat, nongreasy foods.
  - Instruct client not to lie flat for 2 hr after meals.
- **Environmental and comfort measures**
  - Stay with client if they are vomiting.
  - Turn client's head to the side if supine to avoid aspiration of emesis.
  - Keep an emesis basin near but not within sight as it may produce more nausea.
  - Provide a clean environment, free of smells, with plenty of fresh air.
- **Psychological support**
  - Reduce anxiety that may increase nausea (see Section 12-4). Preoperative teaching has been shown to reduce postoperative nausea and vomiting.
  - Encourage rest and reduction of activity.

2-6 DIARRHEA

ACUTE

Acute diarrhea is usually self limiting, lasts from 24–48 hr, and is most frequently caused by viral infection. Other causes include bacterial infection (i.e., *Staphylococcus aureus* and other food poisonings), major alterations in diet, drug reactions, or ingestion of toxins. The sudden ingestion of large quantities of fruits and vegetables containing long-chain carbohydrates may cause acute diarrhea.

CHRONIC

Chronic diarrhea persists for several weeks or is intermittently present for weeks. Causes are irritable bowel syndrome, lactase deficiency, cancer of the colon, inflammatory bowel disease, gastrointestinal surgery, radiation, malabsorption diseases, chemotherapeutic agents, or laxative abuse.

Nursing Assessment of Client with Diarrhea

- Diarrhea is the frequent passage of loose, watery stools (generally, more than three a day).
- Frequently accompanying symptoms are abdominal pain, cramping, increased frequency of bowel sounds, urgency, and incontinence.
- Help identify the offending agent by assessing usual bowel elimination pattern, dietary habits, food intolerances, recent food and drug ingestion, travel, symptoms, and stool characteristics, including volume, color, frequency, and effect on patterns of daily living.
- Diarrhea that is tarry or burgundy colored may indicate gastrointestinal bleeding.
- Stools of high volume (more than 1 liter a day) and periumbilical, colicky pain suggest diarrhea of small intestinal origin.

- Small-volume stools, especially with bright blood, mucus, and left-sided pain suggest a diarrhea of colonic origin.

- Always assess for fluid and electrolyte status; look for signs of dehydration, rapid, thready pulse, postural hypotension, dry mucus membranes, decreased skin turgor, decreased urine output, weakness, etc. (see also Table 5-4, Fluid and Electrolyte Imbalances).

- Laxative abusers may not be willing to admit they use laxatives.

Nursing Interventions to Relieve Diarrhea

ACUTE DIARRHEA

- Antidiarrheal drugs are not recommended for routine use in acute infectious diarrhea as they would delay the natural elimination of the infection.

- Antibiotics have been implicated more frequently than any other drugs except laxatives in causing diarrhea. Other drugs include digitalis (toxicity), indomethacin, gold, guanethidine, and methyldopa. Some clients continue to have diarrhea even though the offending agent is withdrawn because of overgrowth of anaerobic organisms (see also Table 7-6C, Drugs That Can Cause Diarrhea).

- Control tube-feeding diarrhea with psyllium (Metamucil), pectin, or by adjusting the type of tube feeding (see also Tube Feedings in Section 8-5, Selected Medical Nutrition Therapies).

- Lactose-intolerant individuals must eliminate all milk and milk products from their diet, including nonfat dry milk solids in cookies, crackers, cereals, etc.

- Take stool cultures for organisms, cysts, and blood if diarrhea persists.

- Reassess for fluid and electrolyte balance. In diarrhea without undue emesis, increase fluid intake to 3000 ml/24 hr unless contraindicated.

- Diet:
    1. Clear liquid diet only during acute stage. Encourage liquids: water, apple juice, flat ginger ale.
    2. As you advance the diet, avoid milk products because a transient lactose intolerance develops when a colonic mucosa is inflamed. Avoid fat as fatty foods can cause adherence of bacteria to mucous membranes and prolong inflammatory processes.
    3. Start with cooked rice, cooked cereals, bananas, saltines, plain baked, or boiled potatoes.
    4. Add new foods slowly over a 24-to-48-hr period.
- Prevent excoriation of the anal area by keeping the area clean and dry. Petrolatum, zinc oxide, vitamin A & D ointment, sitz baths for 20 min q.i.d., heat lamp and daily inspection are measures that may help.

CHRONIC DIARRHEA

Treatment of chronic diarrhea is based on the cause or specific disease, i.e., chemotherapeutic agents, irritable bowel syndrome, ulcerative colitis. A nursing or medical textbook will have detailed information on these diseases to incorporate into your nursing care plan. These clients require a lot of emotional support.

2-7 CONSTIPATION

Normal bowel elimination can range from three bowel movements a day to three bowel movements a week, depending on the person. Constipation is considered an alteration in normal bowel function so that elimination is delayed, sluggish, and difficult and frequency is usually less than three bowel movements a week. There may be abdominal pain and bloating, pain on defecation, decreased appetite, back pain, headache, rectal bleeding, fecal impaction, and/or nausea and vomitng.

Factors that may contribute to constipation are age, diet, exercise, medication use, and ignoring the urge to defecate. Among the numerous conditions associated with constipation are dehydration, hypokalemia, hypopituitarism, hypothyroidism, multiple sclerosis, Parkinson's disease, myotonic dystrophy, paraplegia, rectal prolapse, hemorrhoids, rectal carcinoma or adenoma, fecal impaction, foreign body, volvulus, diverticulitis, Crohn's disease, ulcerative colitis, gonorrheal proctitis, anal fissure, and postoperative adhesion. Pregnancy, corrosive enemas, radiation, and chronic opiate use may also be causes.

Nursing Assessment of the Client with Constipation

- Assess normal bowel pattern. Determine chronicity. Is constipation a new problem or has it continued for a long time?

- Assess recent bowel history (last bowel movement, amount, color, consistency).

- Assess bulk in diet, fluid intake, and current fluid status.

- Review medications used for bowel care (enemas, laxatives, stool softeners), and other medications used (especially opiates).

- Determine exercise pattern. If the client has been immobilized for even a day, lack of exercise will decrease peristalsis. If client has been hospitalized for two or more days, or the client is elderly, he/she will usually require a stool softener.

- Perform a thorough physical exam, including rectal assessment. Check for abdominal pain, bloating, fecal mass.

- Observe stool sample for blood or mucus. Perform hemoccult test for blood.

- Assess knowledge deficit in client to prepare for client teaching.

Nursing Interventions to Relieve Constipation

- Formulate an individual treatment plan based on the cause (some causes listed above).

- See Table 7-6B, Drugs That Can Cause Constipation. If one may be the offending agent, see if a different medication may be substituted.

- If client is over age 45, sigmoidoscopy and barium enema may be indicated.

- If fecal impaction removal is necessary, always check with physician before removing impaction.

- Introduce or reinforce client teaching, especially prevention measures.

TEACH CLIENT ABOUT:

Diet

- ☐ The importance of balanced diet, including 6–10 g fiber/24 hr

- ☐ Six readily available foods high in fiber: whole grain breads and cereals, fresh fruits and vegetables, nuts, bran, brown rice, legumes, etc.

- ☐ Bananas, prunes, dates, figs and rhubarb are good laxatives as well as high in fiber.

- ☐ Unprocessed bran is an excellent way to increase fiber without radically altering diet. It can be added to cereals, breads, meat loaf, salads, cakes, or muffins without adding calories. Initial dose should be 1 teaspoon a day for several days, increasing by 1/2 teaspoon until 6–10 g/day is reached. (1 teaspoon bran = 1 g of fiber).

Fluids

- ☐ Importance of including 8–10 glasses of fluid in intake if not contraindicated.

Exercise

- ☐ Walking briskly 15 min every day is a good all-around exercise.

- ☐ Three conditioning exercises to strengthen muscles of abdominal and pelvic floor (particularly helpful for immobilized or bedridden clients):

  1. Sit-ups with knees bent and arms flexed behind the head to avoid undue strain on the back

2. Isometric contraction of perineal muscles

3. Pelvic tilt

☐ Long periods of sitting should be interrupted with standing periods of 5–10 min every hour.

Medication use

☐ Routine use of laxatives or enemas can cause loss of large bowel tone

☐ It is important to adhere to prescribed bowel regimen (i.e., stool softeners) when taking medications that cause constipation.

Bowel pattern

☐ Stress the importance of responding when natural urge occurs

☐ Also stress the importance of establishing regular bowel pattern, such as relaxing on toilet every day after breakfast.

2-8 FLATULENCE

Gas in the intestinal tract is made up of swallowed air, gas diffusion across the mucosa, and gas produced by bacteria. An excessive amount of air in the intestinal tract, or flatulence, can lead to intestinal distention (also called tympanites).

Any disturbance in the ability of the intestine to absorb gas or to propel it along the intestinal tract will result in distention. Causes include the ingestion of irritating foods (such as cabbage and beans), the taking of certain drugs that slow peristalsis (such as morphine), swallowing large amounts of air while eating and drinking, or abdominal surgery.

Nursing Assessment When You Suspect Flatulence

• Assess abdominal distention by observing swollen abdomen and gently percussing with fingers for a drumlike sound. Clients often complain of cramp-like pain. Particularly, assess postabdominal surgery clients for flatulence, as manipulation during surgery causes decrease in peristalsis. Distinguish between flatulence and incisional pain.

- Determine what might be the cause based on history and examination.

Nursing Interventions to Relieve Flatulence

- Eliminate the cause, when possible, to bring relief.

- Teach client to avoid activities that increase air swollowing such as chewing gum, sucking on hard candy, and smoking.

- Teach client to avoid gas-producing foods such as cabbage, beans, and fried foods.

- Encourage use of nonnarcotic analgesics once severe pain has subsided, as narcotic analgesics depress gastrointestinal motility.

- Facilitate escape of flatus by having client move about in bed and walk.

- Help client assume positions that will help flatus to move along the intestinal tract. These include lying on the abdomen, the knee-chest position, and positioning the upper body lower than the lower (gas is lighter than fluids or solids and rises). Lying on the side is also effective. Do not use a position that is contraindicated.

- A rectal tube may be indicated.

- If conservative measures fail, the physician may order a suppository.

2-9 INCONTINENCE

Clients at high risk for becoming incontinent of stool are the elderly, persons with a low level of awareness, clients with long-standing dependence on suppositories, clients with neurologic abnormalities, and clients with chronic diarrhea, hemorrhoidectomy, or rectal surgery.

Urinary incontinence is a symptom of a number of underlying conditions that affect the anatomy and innervation of the lower urinary tract. Causes include those of neurogenic origin, those of psychogenic origin, and genitourinary causes. Dehydration may be a cause.

Management of the incontinent client requires a great investment of time, energy, and resources of all the people involved. A team approach including the family is particularly important. Much understanding and emotional support is needed.

Nursing Assessment of Client with Incontinence

- Determine which category (first suggested by Adams) the client probably falls into in order to determine best approach:

  1. Mentally clear client who is willing to cooperate in efforts to regain bowel/bladder control. Change in environment or medications or bladder retaining may be all that is necessary.

  2. Client who is mentally clouded only transiently. Client who has been continent before an acute illness (such as high fever with delirium) will most likely recover quickly with implementation of a well-formulated plan.

  3. Client whose continence is beyond his/her control. The reason may be physical (i.e., inoperable neoplasm) or mental (end-stage dementia).

- Document when client is incontinent, along with fluid intake and behavior pattern.

- Assess for skin breakdown.

- Obtain current AHCPR (Agency for Health Care Policy and Research) Guidelines for Urinary Incontinence in Adults from the U.S. Department of Health and Human Services, Public Health Service, Rockville,

Maryland. The toll-free number is 1-800-358-9295. The following publications are available: Clinical Practice Guidelines (AHCPR #92-0038); A Patient's Guide (AHCPR #92-0040); Quick Reference Guide for Clinicians (AHCPR #92-0041).

Nursing Interventions to Relieve Incontinence

- Establish realistic goals for client based on assessment of ability, willingness to work toward control, and feelings about his/her condition.

- Evaluate your own response to the incontinent client and be aware of your own feelings and attitudes.

- Take a consistent approach and reinforce positive behavior.

- Establish regular bowel/bladder routine. Encourage the client to use the toilet 30 min before he or she is usually incontinent. If there is no pattern, place the client on the bedpan or commode at frequent intervals, such as every 2 hr. When the client is continent 2 hr, increase the time between voidings by 30 min each day until a 3- to 4-hr voiding pattern evolves. Try for four voidings a day and no incidents of incontinence.

- Teach pelvic floor exercises such as kegels and tensing muscles around the anus.

- Make sure client is well hydrated. Client incontinent of urine for the first time may react by restricting fluid intake. Intake should be 2000 to 2500 ml/day unless contraindicated. Limit fluid intake in the evening if night incontinence is a problem.

- Encourage use of the regular bathroom or the bedside commode rather than the bedpan, which requires an anatomical position that is almost opposite to squatting. The natural position of squatting increases intraabdominal pressure and enhances propulsion of the fecal bolus.

- Biofeedback is now being used to assist clients incontinent of urine.

2-10   URINARY RETENTION

Postoperative urinary retention occurs in approximately 13% of clients. Other predisposing factors are advanced age and decreased level of continence. Other causes may be prostate enlargement, urolithiasis, spinal cord injury, pelvic malignancy, urethral stricture, postoperative conditions, and drug use (e.g., cholinergics). Frequently, mothers immediately postpartum have difficulty voiding.

Signs and symptoms are absence of voided urine, bladder distention, overflow incontinence, and bladder pain or discomfort. Some complications are reflux of urine, elevation of intrarenal pressure, hydronephrosis, urinary tract infection, and urolithiasis.

Nursing Interventions to Induce Urination

- Check the client's chart. If the client has been NPO for a period of time, they may be dehydrated and not have the urge to void.

- Allay anxiety (see Section 12-4).

- Provide privacy.

- Relieve pain (see Section 2-3).

- Encourage the client to drink water if permitted.

- Place client in the most comfortable position; sitting for female, standing for male.

- Then try:

   1. The sound of running water to stimulate reflex action

   2. Heat applied on the abdomen (if not contraindicated)

3. Warm water poured over the genitalia into the bedpan or toilet

4. A foot bath in warm water

5. A full bath in tepid water

- If the client goes for more than 8 hr without urinating or if the bladder is distended, report this to the physician. Catheterize as a last resort.

2-11   IMPAIRED PHYSICAL MOBILITY

Preventing the complications of immobility is a very important responsibility. Almost every ill client will have his or her mobility impaired in some way. The greater the immobility, the greater the chance for complications. The goal in illness is to maintain a balance between allowing for the needed rest and getting the exercise that strengthens muscles, stimulates circulation, and promotes general functioning.

Nursing Assessment of Client with Impaired Mobility

- Identify individuals at high risk for complications: elderly or frail clients, clients immobilized for any reason (i.e., traction, arthritis, pain, surgery, paralysis, congestive heart failure, weakness), clients on cortisone, malnourished clients, clients with impaired circulation, anemia, contractures, mental deterioration, or incontinence.

- Assess client frequently. Focus assessment and reassessment on those high risk areas for the client (some clients may be at high risk for development of skin breakdown, other clients may be at greater risk for developing thrombophlebitis).

Nursing Interventions for the Client with Impaired Mobility

- Correctly position client in order to prevent complications.

- Utilize footboards, hand rolls and splints when appropriate to maintain good body alignment.

- Relieve pressure on bony prominences. Table 2-5 shows areas at high risk for skin breakdown.

- Avoid positions that compromise blood flow. For example, blood flow to the lower extremities may be compromised by crossing the legs, placing pillows under the knees or by sitting.

- Assess the need for pressure-relieving devices. Alternating pressure mattresses, or specialty beds (i.e., low air loss bed, air fluidized therapy) may be beneficial in preventing skin breakdown.

- Prevent footdrop with footboard and exercise. Prevent external rotation of the hips with trochanter rolls, pillows, exercise, and frequent position changes.

- Position client so that shearing force is minimized. Pay special attention to turning and moving client up in bed, as friction causes tissue damage. Drawsheets should be used in order to minimize friction.

- Avoid allowing the client to be positioned above 25–30° in bed for prolonged periods. A lower position decreases pressure on the sacrum and ischial tuberosities.

TABLE 2–5. AREAS AT RISK FOR SKIN BREAKDOWN

Supine Position: Occipital bone, scapula, elbow, sacrum and coccyx, heel

Prone Position: Sternum, crest of pelvis, ribs, kneecap, male genitalia

Lateral Position: Greater trochanter, shoulder, ribs, medial and lateral malleolus

Sitting: Tuberosities of pelvis

- Promote pulmonary hygiene.
  - Turn, cough, and deep-breathe (incentive spirometer) q 2 hr. while client is less active or bed-bound (see also Table 10-6).
  - Provide humidification to enhance mobilization of secretions.
  - Suction secretions if client is unable to expectorate.
  - Keep a flowchart so all shifts know when the turning and deep breathing is being done (Table 2-6).
- Institute level of activity appropriate to the client.
  - Instruct and assist client with active and passive ROM exercises three or four times a day (Tables 2-7 and 2-8).
  - Help client out of bed as soon as tolerable. Client can dangle legs, get up to the wheelchair, use the walker, and ambulate as strength improves.

2-12 IMPAIRED TISSUE INTEGRITY

Prevention and treatment of pressure ulcers is primarily a nursing responsibility. The nurse can assist in preventing ulcers by preventing the complications of immobility (see Section 2-11), incontinence and poor nutrition.

The Agency for Health Care Policy and Research (ACHCPR) has commissioned an external panel to develop guidelines for the prediction and prevention of pressure ulcers. A copy of these guidelines may be obtained through the AHCPR Clearinghouse, P.O. Box 8547, Silver Spring, MD, 20907 (or call 1-800-358-9295). Refer to AHCPR publication number 92-0047, May 1992.

Nursing Assessment of Client with Pressure Ulcers

Thoroughly assess client for skin breakdown. If breakdown is present, grade according to the following scale:

TABLE 2–6. SAMPLE 24 HR. PREVENTION CHART FOR CLIENT WITH IMPAIRED MOBILITY

MRS. JONES RM. 214

Time	Position	Cough, Deep Breathing	Exercise	Out of Bed	Bowel Movements	Intake	Output	Comments	Initials
2400	B	✓				240			MN
0200	RS	✓							MN
0400	LS	✓					150		MN
0600	A	✓				240			MN
0800	B	✓					300		KM
1000	RS	✓	passive ROM	up to commode	Ṫ			Muscle stiffness; massage given	KM
1200	LS	✓				200			KM
1400	A	✓	Passive ROM			100	250		KM
1600	B	✓							CL
1800	RS	✓	ROM active assist	Dangle		480			CL
2000	L	✓					600	Importance of ROM emphasized	CL
2200	B	✓							CL

B = back; RS = right side; LS = left side; A = abdomen.

STAGING SYSTEM
FOR BREAKDOWN*

Stage 1 Nonblanchable erythema of intact skin; the heralding lesion of skin ulceration

Stage 2 Partial-thickness skin loss involving epidermis or dermis, or both. The ulcer is superficial and presents clinically as an abrasion, blister, or shallow crater.

Stage 3 Full-thickness skin loss involving damage or necrosis of subcutaneous tissue, which may extend down to but not through underlying fascia. The ulcer presents clinically as a deep crater with or without undermining of adjacent tissue.

Stage 4 Full thickness skin loss with extensive destruction, tissue necrosis, or damage to muscle, bone or supporting structures (such as tendon, joint capsule).

Note: If the wound involves necrotic tissue, staging cannot be confirmed until the wound base is visible.

Nursing Interventions in Treating the Client with Pressure Ulcers

- There are many treatments for pressure ulcers that may yield good results. Treatment depends on the stage to which the sore has progressed.

- Once a pressure ulcer has developed, base your nursing care plan on the stage, size of the wound, and presence of infection.

- Assess causative factors such as client activity, mobility, presence or absence of sensory deficits, nutrition and hydration status, circulation and oxygenation, and skin moisture status, determining if any areas need improvement in routine.

- Assess and document the following factors: wound location, size, depth, undermining, tunneling, tissue status, (epithelialization, necrosis, infection) presence of exudate, including volume, color, consistency, and

---

*Intervention may prevent progression, or a Stage 1 lesion may be the first clinical indicator of deep tissue damage, which is irreversible.

TABLE 2–7. RANGE-OF-MOTION EXERCISES

PREPARATION

Set realistic goals before starting a ROM program for the immobilized or partially immobilized client. Goals should be based on 1) range of motion testing by the physician (a physician's order is required to do ROM if a pathologic condition is present such as arthritis, fracture, or acute cardiac condition), 2) assessment by the nurse and physical therapist, and 3) the overall condition and willingness of the client to take part in the restoration of function, or maintenance of function. The understanding and acceptance by the client of the critical need for exercise is key to effective results.

TECHNIQUE

- Place the client in a supine position with arms to the side and knees extended. Hold the extremity at the joint to support it while you are flexing, extending, rotating, adducting, and abducting. Move each joint through its free range of motion (each person has a different range) about three times, slowly, rhythmically, and smoothly.
- Start with the head and neck, go to the shoulders, elbows, wrists and fingers, then hips to toes. See Table 2-8 for the movements for each joint.
- Fear and pain may thwart the client's efforts to follow an exercise pattern. If these are not relieved, more joint stiffness and muscle contractures may follow. Work together with clients to break out of limiting patterns into rehabilitation.
- Never move a joint to the point of pain. If a painful muscle spasm occurs during ROM, move the joint to the point of resistance, and then exert gentle steady pressure until the muscle relaxes.
- Unless otherwise ordered, move the joints through their normal range three times a day.
- Advance passive exercise to active assistive, and active exercise as soon as the client is able. Then progress to resistive and isometric exercise.

---

odor. Use a plastic ruler or lesion measuring card and document changes according to agency protocol. Stage wound.

- Stage 1 ulcers will usually heal completely once the pressure on the affected area is relieved. Tissue should not be massaged, as this can increase tissue

TABLE 2–8. PASSIVE RANGE-OF-MOTION EXERCISES

JOINT	MOVEMENT
Neck	Flexion, extension, rotation
Shoulder	Flexion, extension, abduction, adduction, internal rotation, external rotation; hyperextension done in prone position
Elbow	Flexion, extension, supination, pronation
Wrist	Flexion, extension, ulnar deviation, radial deviation
Thumb and fingers	Flexion, extension, abduction, adduction, opposition
Hip	Flexion, extension, abduction, adduction, internal rotation, external rotation; hyperextension done in prone position
Knee	Flexion, extension
Ankle	Dorsiflexion, plantar flexion, eversion, inversion
Toe	Flexion, extension, abduction, adduction

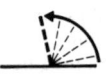 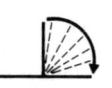 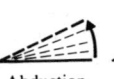 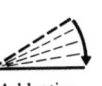 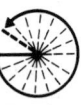

Flexion   Extension   Abduction   Adduction   Rotation

Flexion = "bending" the various joints, or decreasing the angle; extension = "straightening" out or increasing the angle of a joint; abduction = movement away from the body's center; adduction = movement of a limb toward the body's center; rotation = turning or movement of a part around its axis (e.g., the head or hips); hyperextension = extension beyond the ordinary range (e.g., the neck extending backward); dorsiflexion = backward bending of the hand or foot; plantar flexion = bending of the foot in the direction of the sole; pronation = turning downward (i.e., rotating the forearm so that the palm of the hand is down); supination = turning upward (i.e., rotating the forearm so the palm is up).

trauma. Protection from moisture is imperative. A transparent or hydrocolloid dressing may be applied until healing occurs.

- Stage 2 pressure ulcer is reversible if detected early. If irrigation is ordered, use the prescribed solution. A transparent or hydrocolloid dressing can be applied.

- Stage 3 pressure ulcer is usually irrigated daily; gauze or pouch dressings may be applied. Pressure relieving bed may be indicated. Treatment is often similar to Stage 2.

- Stage IV ulcers require debridement, intravenous fluids, and antibiotics. Consult with the physician on specific treatment orders.

- Clean wound by flushing with normal saline or using a commercially made product. Avoid using detergents since they will damage granulating tissue. Use scrupulous sterile technique.

- Special debridement measures may be required, including:

  - Use of special medications for debriding such as dextranomer (Debrisan) or collegenase (Santyl). There are many preparations on the market. Follow instructions carefully if drug is prescribed. Do not allow these substances to touch normal skin, since they do not discriminate between healthy and unhealthy tissue. Discontinue as soon as eschar is gone.

  - Whirlpool treatments are used for debridement in some institutions.

  - Surgical intervention, wound debridement, incision and drainage, grafting, or surgical removal of ulcer and affected tissues may be necessary if ulcers do not respond to conservative measures.

  - Hyperbaric oxygen therapy may be indicated to hasten metabolic and healing processes by directing a high level of oxygen to the tissues.

2-13 POTENTIAL FOR INJURY RELATED TO SEIZURES

Seizures can be classified into five basic groups, based on their causative factors:

Category	Example
Pathologic process	Vascular anomalies Space-occupying lesions (e.g., tumors, brain abscesses) Craniocerebral trauma Infection (e.g., encephalitis) Neuronal injury (e.g., anoxia from deficient oxygen supply) Epilepsy
Toxic substances	Endogenous toxins (e.g., uremia) Exogenous toxins (e.g., phenothiazines, lead ingestion, alcohol)
Metabolic disturbances	Electrolyte imbalances
Febrile state	Systemic infection
Idiopathic	Seizures occurring without any identifiable cause

Generally seizures are partial or generalized. Partial seizures arise from a localized area of the brain, usually do not spread to the entire brain, and usually do not impair consciousness.

Partial seizures include jacksonian and complex partial seizures (psychomotor or temporal lobes). A jacksonian seizure typically produces a stiffening or jerking in one extremity, accompanied by a tingling sensation in the same area. A complex partial seizure may be preceded by an aura, or sensation the client feels immediately before the seizure, such as a pungent smell, nausea and vomiting, a dreamy feeling, an unusual taste, or visual disturbance. Mental confusion may last several minutes after the seizure. Jacksonian and complex partial seizures may spread to become generalized.

Generalized seizures include absence (petit mal) seizures, which occur mainly in children and generalized tonic-clonic (grand mal) seizures. In an absence seizure there is a brief change in the level of consciousness indicated by blinking and rolling of the eyes, a blank stare, and slight mouth movements; each seizure usually lasts from 1–10 sec.

Generalized tonic-clonic (grand mal) seizures typically begin with a loud cry. The client then falls to the ground, loses consciousness, the body stiffens, and then alternates between episodes of muscular spasm (tonic phase) and relaxation (clonic phase). Tongue biting, incontinence, labored breathing, apnea, and subsequent cyanosis are not uncommon. The seizure usually stops within 2–5 min. Afterward, the client may be confused, may complain of fatigue, headache, or muscle soreness, and may fall into a deep sleep.

Nursing Interventions to Prevent Injury When Client Has History or Likelihood of Seizures

- Maintain bed in low position at all times unless side rails are up or nurse is with client.
- Make sure call light is within easy reach at all times.
- Keep side rails up at bedtime, after sedation, if client is confused, and when otherwise needed.
- Have oral airway and suction equipment at bedside.
- Pad side rails.
- Sometimes IV diazepam (Valium) is used during seizures. Ascertain if there are prn orders for Valium if seizure activity occurs.

Nursing Interventions During a Seizure

- Do not restrain the client during a seizure.
- Help the client to a side-lying position and loosen any tight clothing.
- Gently turn the head to provide an open airway.

- Place something flat and soft, such as a pillow, jacket, or hand under his head.

- Clear the area of hard or sharp objects.

- Note the time the seizure begins and ends.

- Do not force anything into the client's mouth. A tongue blade or spoon could lacerate mouth and lips or displace teeth and cause respiratory problems.

- If the client's mouth is open (teeth are not clenched) place a soft object such as cloth between teeth to protect the tongue.

- Administer IV diazepam with great caution if ordered.

- Reassure the client. After the seizure subsides, orient the client to time and place, and inform him/her that he/she has had a seizure.

- Seizure activity rarely lasts longer than 5 min. If a seizure lasts longer than 5 min it becomes status epilepticus, a critical emergency. Refer to Section 13-9, Seizures: Status Epilepticus, for nursing management.

2-14 SELF-CARE DEFICIT

A self-care deficit is defined as any limitation or inability to perform the activities of daily living such as feeding, bathing or hygiene, dressing or grooming, toileting, or an activity specific to that client. The causes of a self-care deficit may include a neurological insult (CVA, tumor, trauma), the loss or congenital absence of one or more limbs, contractures secondary to burns or prolonged immobility, or many other limitations.

Nursing Assessment of the Client with a Self-Care Deficit

- Assess and document the client's limitations in self care. See Table 2-9 for one example of a functional assessment tool.

- Develop a nursing care plan, setting realistic goals for maximum self-care. The following can be used as de-

---

TABLE 2–9. FUNCTIONAL ASSESSMENT—KATZ INDEX OF ADL*

The Index of Independence in Activities of Daily Living developed by Katz can be used to denote client functional independence or dependence in bathing, dressing, going to toilet, transferring, continence, and feeding. Independence means without supervision, direction, or active personal assistance.

A. Independent in feeding, continence, transferring, going to toilet, dressing, and bathing.
B. Independent in all but one of these functions.
C. Independent in all but bathing, and one additional function.
D. Independent in all but bathing, dressing, and one additional function.
E. Independent in all but bathing, dressing, going to toilet, and one additional function.
F. Independent in all but bathing, dressing, going to toilet, transferring, and one additional function.
G. Dependent in all six functions.

Other: Dependent in at least two functions, but not classifiable as C, D, E, or F.

---

*From Katz S et al.: Studies of illness in the aged. The index for ADL: a standardized measure of biological and psychosocial function, JAMA 185:94–99, 1963.

sirable outcomes or goals at the end of the client's hospitalization:

- Express acceptance of the need for assistance with self-care

- Be able to perform self-care to his/her optimum level

- Initiate and implement a plan to maintain personal hygiene

- Have a personal directory of community resources available for him/her

Nursing Interventions in Management of the Client with a Self-Care Deficit

- Discuss and develop ways to modify environment to optimize the client's ability to perform the activities of daily living.

- Introduce client to agencies and businesses that provide services or products that help people with client's deficit.

- Encourage independence in performance of self-care, assisting client only as necessary.

- Encourage the client to set his/her own pace during self-care.

- Offer pain medication prior to self-care activities.

- Deliver care in a safe, patient, and non-judgmental manner.

- Acknowledge and reinforce the client's accomplishments.

- Evaluate progress frequently. Reset goals if necessary.

- Discuss the home environment with the client and his/her family or significant others to help them plan for the self-care needs of the client at home.

REFERENCES

Acute Pain Management Guideline Panel. Acute pain management in adults: operative procedures or medical procedures and trauma. Clinical Practice Guidline. AHCPR Pub. No. 92-0032. Rockville, MD: Agency for Health Care Policy and Research, Public Health Service, U.S. Department of Health and Human Services, February, 1992.

Brunner LS, Suddarth DS, eds. The Lippincott manual of nursing practice. 5th ed. Philadelphia: JB Lippincott, 1992.

Bryant R. Acute and chronic wounds: nursing management. St. Louis: Mosby Year Book, 1992.

Carpenito LJ. Nursing diagnosis: an application to clinical practice. 4th ed. Philadelphia: JB Lippincott, 1992.

Goodman T, Thomas C, Rappaport N. Skin ulcers: overview and nursing implications. AORN 1990, 52:24.

Gordon M. Nursing diagnosis, process and application. New York: McGraw Hill, 1987.

Ignatavius D, Bayne M. Medical-surgical nursing: a psychophysiologic approach. Philadelphia: WB Saunders, 1991.

Kavey NB, Anderson D. Why every patient needs a good night's sleep. RN 1986; December: 16–19.

Kozier B, et al. Techniques in clinical nursing. Menlo Park, CA: Addison-Wesley, 1993.

Lewis C, Collier I. Medical-surgical nursing: assessment and management of clinical problems, St. Louis: Mosby, 1992.

McCaffery M, Beebe A. Pain: clinical manual for nursing practice, St. Louis: Mosby, 1989.

North American Nursing Diagnosis Association. Approved nursing diagnostic categories. Nursing Diagnosis Newsletter, 1994.

Osten R, et al., eds. The cancer manual. 8th ed. Boston: The American Cancer Society, 1990.

Puntillo K, ed. Pain in the critically ill. Maryland: Aspen Publishers, 1991.

Schmidling ER, et al. Treating pressure ulcers with a myocutaneous flap. Nursing, '92, 22:7, 1992.

Swearingen P. Photo atlas of nursing procedures. 2nd ed. Menlo Park, CA: Addison-Wesley, 1993.

U.S. Department of Health and Human Services, Public Health Division, AHCPR Publication No. 92-0047. Rockville, MD, May 1992.

CHAPTER 3

LABORATORY TESTING

3-1 NURSING FUNCTIONS IN LABORATORY TESTING

Laboratory data constitute one small part of the entire clinical picture upon which health care personnel base treatment decisions. Effective laboratory interpretation depends on judgments made with other data in mind, such as statements from the client, physical signs and diagnostic reports. Physicians use laboratory reports to diagnose disease, while nurses identify problems that require collaborative efforts and those that can be treated by nursing interventions. The following are general guidelines for fulfilling the nurse's role in utilizing laboratory technology:

1. Ordering

- Follow the protocols of your institution for collecting and utilizing laboratory data.

- Ordering lab tests is usually reserved for physicians. However, in some settings, ordering routine tests such as urinalysis, occult blood tests, or wound cultures may be part of basic health care given by the nurse.

- Be aware of the rationale for different tests when transcribing orders in order to ensure accuracy. Does it make sense for a client with a specific diagnosis to have this test?

2. Client preparation

- Limit factors that may affect test results, i.e., make sure specimens are drawn at the correct time of day, when the client is at rest, etc. (see Section 3-3). After checking with the physician hold drugs or foods that may cause false test results. On the lab slip, list drugs and food that the client is taking that could affect test results.

- Inform the client about the test being given and whether dietary or other instructions are to be followed. Answer any questions that may come up.

- Table 3-1 lists some tests that require special dietary preparation of the client.

Text continued on page 107

TABLE 3–1. LAB TESTS REQUIRING FOOD AND DRINK RESTRICTIONS

TESTS	# OF HOURS CLIENT SHOULD BE NPO PRIOR TO TEST (WATER IS ALLOWED)	DIETARY PREPARATION
Addis Count, 12 hr (urine)	√	No fluids to be taken during 12 hr urine collection period
Adrenocortico-tropic suppression (ACTH)	8 √	Low carbohydrate diet 48 hr prior to test
Aldosterone, urine	√	Sodium may be restricted
Alkaline phosphatase	10–12 √	
Alpha-1-antitrypsin	8	Hold oral contraceptives 24 hr prior to test
Ammonia	8–10	Refrain from smoking 8–10 hr
Amylase	1–2	
Bilirubin (total and direct), (indirect)	8	Carrots, yams, or foods high in fats should not be eaten 3–4 days before test
Blood Urea Nitrogen (BUN)	8 √	
Calcium	8 √	Hold breakfast till after test
Catecholamines (urine)		No drugs, chocolate, coffee, vanilla, walnuts, beer, chianti wines, bananas, 3–7 days before the test
Cholesterol	12 √	A low-fat meal prior to test. No alcohol for 24 hrs
Cortisol	3	Take sample before meals
C-reactive protein	8–12 √	

**TABLE 3–1. LAB TESTS REQUIRING FOOD AND
DRINK RESTRICTIONS** *Continued*

TESTS	# OF HOURS CLIENT SHOULD BE NPO PRIOR TO TEST (WATER IS ALLOWED)	DIETARY PREPARATION
Creatinine clearance (urine)	√	Meats, poultry, fish, tea, and coffee should be avoided for 6 hr prior to and during test according to physician's orders
D-xylose absorbtion (blood and urine)		No foods containing pentose, i.e. fruits, jams, jellies, pastries 24 hr prior to test
Folic Acid	8 √	No alcoholic beverages 24 hr prior to test
Fungal Organisms	12 √	
Gastrin	12	No alcoholic beverages 24 hr prior to test
Glucose—Fasting Blood Sugar	4–12 √	IV's with glucose and insulin must also be withheld
Glucose—Postprandial		Take test 2 hr after breakfast or lunch
Glucose Tolerance Test—Oral	12 (8–16) √	Normal diet 3 days prior to test. No coffee, tea, smoking or eating during test. Give 100 mg of glucose solution after obtaining FBS
17-Hydroxyindolacetic acid (urine)		No bananas, pineapple, avocados, plums, eggplant, or walnuts 3 days before the test
5-Hydroxycorticosteroids (urine)		No coffee during 24-hr collection. Encourage fluid intake during test
Immunoglobulins (Ig)	12 √	NPO sometimes not required

Table continued on following page

TABLE 3–1. LAB TESTS REQUIRING FOOD AND DRINK RESTRICTIONS *Continued*

TESTS	# OF HOURS CLIENT SHOULD BE NPO PRIOR TO TEST (WATER IS ALLOWED)		DIETARY PREPARATION
Lipase	8–12		
Lipoproteins— Lipids	12–14	√	Regular diet 3 days prior to test. No alcohol 24 hr prior
Occult Blood (stool)			Meat, poultry, and fish should be eliminated from the diet 3 days prior to test
Osmolality (urine)			A high-protein diet 3 days prior to test Restrict fluids 8–12 hr before the test
Phosphorous	8–12		Hold IV fluids with glucose 4–8 hr
Protein (Total)	8	√	
Renin	8		Note sodium content of diet on lab slip
Schilling test	8–12		No B vitamins for at least 3 days, or laxatives for at least 24 hrs. Do not perform test if client is pregnant or lactating
Theophylline levels			No coffee, tea, colas, or chocolate 8 hr prior to test
Thyroid-stimulating hormone			No shellfish several days before test
Triglycerides	12		No alcohol 3 days prior
Uric Acid	8		Restrict high-purine foods such as meats, liver, kidney, brains, heart, sweetbreads, scallops, and sardines for 24 hr pretest

TABLE 3–1. LAB TESTS REQUIRING FOOD AND DRINK RESTRICTIONS *Continued*

TESTS	# OF HOURS CLIENT SHOULD BE NPO PRIOR TO TEST (WATER IS ALLOWED)		DIETARY PREPARATION
Uric Acid (urine)			A diet high or low in purines may be ordered before and/or during time of urine collection
Vanilmandelic Acid (VMA) (urine)			Bananas, fruit juices, chocolate, tea, coffee, carbonated drinks (except ginger ale), vanilla and vanilla products, candy, mints, jelly, cheese, gelatins, and cough drops should be eliminated from the diet 72 hr prior to the test
VDRL screening test	8–12	√	No alcohol 24 hours prior to test

√ Check with your laboratory for specific protocol. This list is not all inclusive.

Data from Kee JL Handbook of laboratory and diagnostic tests with nursing implications. Norwalk, CT: Appleton-Century Crofts, 1990.

Corbett JV. Laboratory tests and diagnostic procedures with nursing diagnoses, 3rd. ed. Norwalk, CT: Appleton and Lange, 1992.

Chernecky C, Krech R, Berger B. Laboratory tests and diagnostic procedures. Philadelphia: WB Saunders, 1993.

- Allay anxiety that could affect test results, such as adrenal hormones and blood gases.

3. Obtaining and delivering specimens

- Perform peripheral tests if indicated according to protocol. Tests that require only a drop or two of blood or urine and can be carried out on the unit include: dipsticks for urine chemistry, slide tests for occult blood, specific gravity, and finger-stick blood glucose.

- In all cases specimens must be fresh, uncontaminated, and clearly labeled.

- Deliver stat tests immediately to the laboratory. Table 3-2 lists tests commonly ordered stat tests. Table 3-3 lists other tests that require immediate transport.

TABLE 3–2. LAB TESTS COMMONLY ORDERED STAT

Acetone (serum)
Alcohol
Aminophylline
Amylase
Bilirubin
Blood gases
Blood urea nitrogen (BUN)
Calcium
Cerebrospinal fluid (CSF)
Complete blood count (CBC)
Digoxin levels
Dilantin levels
Direct Coombs'
Drug screening—serum and urine
Electrolytes (sodium, potassium, chloride, bicarbonate)
Fibrin degradation products (FDPs)
Fibrinogen
Glucose
Gram stains
Innoculate media for cultures
Magnesium—serum
Partial thromboplastin time (PTT)
Prothrombin time (PT)
Platelet count
Salicylates
Transfusion reaction investigation
Type and cross match
Urinalysis (UA)

TABLE 3–3. LAB TESTS REQUIRING IMMEDIATE TRANSPORT

Acid phosphatase (ACP) (serum)
Adrenocorticotropic suppression (ACTH)—pack in ice
Ammonia (plasma)—pack in ice
Antibiotic susceptibility (sensitivity) test
Arterial blood gases—pack in ice, do not expose to air
Bilirubin (total, direct, indirect)—protect from light
Cerebrospinal fluid (CSF) (spinal tap)
Cold agglutinins (serum)—put in a warm bath 37° C
Complement C3/C4 (serum)
Cultures (blood, sputum, stool, throat, wound, urine)
Drug toxicity levels
Erythrocyte sedimentation rate (blood)
Folic acid (serum)
Partial thromboplastin time—pack in ice
Phosphorus (serum)
Potassium levels (serum)
Prothrombin time (plasma)—pack in ice
Semen examination
Urinalysis—take to lab within 30 min or refrigerate up to 2 hr

4. Reporting

- Report abnormal findings to the physician. In many cases nurses are the first to see results of lab reports. Although sometimes lab personnel call doctors with stat results, often the nurse must determine whether the physician should be notified immediately or if the report is not urgent. Normal reports may have great diagnostic importance in addition to abnormal findings, as a normal report may rule out the probability of certain disease entities.

5. Follow-up

- Keep abreast of the latest laboratory data in order to make informed assessments on your clients. Note trends that indicate the effectiveness of medical and nursing treatments.

3-2 SPECIMEN COLLECTION

I. Blood Samples
A. Venous Specimens

- Specimens should generally be collected in the morning, before breakfast.

- Wear protective gloves when performing venipuncture or other vascular access procedures as defined by hospital policy according to latest Centers for Disease Control (CDC) updates.

- Blood should not be taken from the arm of a client who has an intravenous infusion line, fistula or mastectomy. However, if no other access is available, blood may be drawn from a vein distally from the IV after the IV has been turned off for 3–5 min. Note action taken on the lab slip.

- The following guidelines will help prevent hemolysis of blood cells.

  - Make sure there is no moisture in the collection tube.

  - Dry the site after cleansing with antiseptic.

  - Use a medium- or large-gauge needle to withdraw a large volume of blood.

  - If a syringe is used the needle must have a tight fit to avoid frothing.

  - Avoid pulling back the plunger too forcefully

  - Remove the needle before slowly forcing the blood to the side of the collection tube.

  - Keep the tourniquet on no longer than 1 min

- Do not take blood from a hematoma, agitate a specimen, warm a specimen, or delay in transporting it to the lab.

B. Arterial specimens: Because potential hazards are greater in performing arterial puncture than venipuncture, arterial samples are usually only ordered for blood gas studies (ABGs).

Nursing Considerations

- Designated personnel draw ABGs in each hospital: doctors, nurses or respiratory therapists. Special kits are provided for this procedure.

- The sample may be drawn from the radial, brachial or femoral arteries. In most hospitals, only physicians are allowed to do femoral punctures, whereas nurses with special training may do radial or brachial punctures. Nurses usually obtain samples from arterial lines.

- Note three important facts on the lab slip that are important for correct interpretation of results:

  - How long the client has been receiving oxygen, and at what liter flow when specimen is taken. If not on O_2, write "room air."

  - If the client is on assisted ventilation, note as such and the settings of the respirator.

  - The temperature of the client, as a fever increases the metabolic rate.

- Notify the laboratory when the ABG's are about to be drawn.

- The specimen must be packed in ice and taken to the laboratory *immediately.* It should arrive within 5 min.

- Maintain pressure on the withdrawal site for at least 5 min if the radial site is used, 10 min or more for the femoral.

- Prolonged bleeding can occur if the client is taking anticoagulants. If there are any bleeding problems, the pressure dressing should be taped on the puncture site and left for several hours.

- See Tables 3-5 and 5-2, Arterial Blood Gas Interpretation in Acid-Base Imbalance, for normal values and interpretation.

- Pulse oximeters, which measure oxygen saturation, but not PCO_2 levels, can reduce the number of ABGs needed for monitoring the client with possible hypoxia.

- Venous blood gases may be assessed in situations where assessment of oxygenation is unnecessary.

C. **Capillary blood—finger, earlobe and heel sticks:** For some tests, such as hematocrits and blood sugars, finger sticks or earlobe sticks may be used rather than venipuncture. Heel sticks are used on infants.

- Cleanse the site with 70% alcohol, and air-dry.

- Puncture site with a sterile lancet designed for finger sticks.

- Discard the first drop, then fill the capillary tube supplied by the laboratory, or place drop of blood on special filter paper.

- Do not squeeze to get capillary blood, as tissue fluids released by squeezing dilute the sample.

- Clients needing to do finger sticks at home can buy apparatus that automatically punctures the finger to the right depth.

- Always follow guidelines from the CDC on handling blood samples safely (see Section 9-2).

II. **Urine Specimens**

The urine assay is one of the simplest assays to perform. Examination of the urine provides a great deal of information, provided the specimen has been collected properly and carefully. The nurse should be aware of the four main types of specimens as well as abnormal urine observations.

A. **The first morning specimen used for routine urinalysis and pregnancy tests**

- For routine analysis, at least 10 ml are needed.

- Specimens should be sent to the lab as soon as possible after collection to avoid the bacterial proliferation that invalidates test results.

- If delay cannot be avoided, the urine may be refrigerated for up to 2 hr.

- Test results may show up falsely positive if there is vaginal contamination, mucoid discharge, or bleeding at the time of collection.

B. Random specimen for qualitative determinations

- These can be done any time.
- Examples of assays include calcium, hemoglobin, porphobilinogen or porphyrins, hemoglobin metabolites, and some toxic substances such as salicylates.
- There are usually no food or drink restrictions.

C. Sterile specimens for microbiologic examination

- See Table 3-4, "How to Collect Culture Specimens," for the procedure for doing "clean-catch" midstream urine.
- Deliver specimens immediately to minimize overgrowth of commensal organisms and preserve the viability of the pathogens.

D. Twenty-four-hour or timed specimens: Because many substances (e.g., glucose, protein, electrolytes, and hormones) are excreted in variable concentrations during a 24-hour period, chemical quantitative determinations are more meaningful if measured over 24 hr than in a random specimen. Accuracy is essential in obtaining the collection. For best results:

- Give client both oral and written instructions
- Make sure client knows that *all* the urine is collected during the 24 hr, or the test is not valid.
- Instruct client to empty the bladder completely at a specified time and discard this first voiding.
- Begin timing the test from right after the first voiding is discarded, i.e., 8:20 a.m.
- Mark time and date of beginning test clearly on the specimen bottle.

Text continued on page 117

TABLE 3–4. HOW TO COLLECT CULTURE SPECIMENS

Collect these specimens before antibiotics are started or note drugs taken on the lab slip. Label the specimen with date, time, client's name, suspected diagnosis, and source of culture. Use strict sterile technique. Transport to the lab immediately.

TYPE OF CULTURE	AMOUNT NEEDED	PROCEDURE
Urine Clean-catch midstream	2–3 ml (15–30 if also for urinalysis)	Instruct client in how to collect specimen or supervise procedure. Males retract foreskin and cleanse glans penis; females cleanse and separate labia so urinary meatus is clearly visible, then cleanse meatus. The client then voids 25–30 ml, and collects specimen without stopping urine stream in sterile container.
Foley catheter specimen	Same as above	Cleanse specimen port of catheter with alcohol, and aspirate urine with a sterile needle, or at a point distal to the Y branch from a latex catheter. Remove needle from syringe before emptying into container.
Blood (venous or arterial)	10 ml (divided in half, aerobic and anaerobic)	2–3 specimens from both arms may be ordered within 24 hr. Cleanse aspiration site with alcohol and prep skin according to hospital policy. Using sterile syringe, collect specimen, changing needles before injecting into aerobic and anaerobic tubes. The tubes should contain a culture medium. If client is receiving penicillin, note this on the lab slip so that

TABLE 3–4. HOW TO COLLECT CULTURE SPECIMENS *Continued*

TYPE OF CULTURE	AMOUNT NEEDED	PROCEDURE
		penicillinase may be added to inactivate drug.
Wound	Small amount in syringe or one swab in test tube with culture medium	Cleanse surrounding area with a disinfectant and enough friction to void the normal flora. A pungent odor suggests the presence of anaerobes; a syringe and oxygen-free collection tubes are recommended. For a swab, firmly but gently saturate swab with exudate from infected site. Saturate with sterile saline solution if surface of wound is dry before taking culture. Wear gloves.
Sputum	2–3 ml in sterile container	Instruct client to cough deeply and expectorate into cup. Client is not to expectorate saliva. If client is not able to produce sputum, use aerosol mist spray of saline solution or water to induce sputum production. Cupping or postural drainage may be necessary.
Nasopharynx	One swab in a test tube	Gently pass swab just inside the nares.
Throat	One swab in a test tube	Depress tongue with tongue blade. With adequate lighting and without touching lips, sides of mouth or tongue, swab the area of inflammation or exudation.

Table continued on following page

TABLE 3–4. HOW TO COLLECT CULTURE SPECIMENS *Continued*

TYPE OF CULTURE	AMOUNT NEEDED	PROCEDURE
Eye	One swab in a test tube	Carefully retract lower lid and gently swab sclera. Do not touch cornea.
Vagina	One swab in a test tube	Use oxygen-free specimen container if an anaerobic specimen is needed. A cervical specimen is done if testing for gonorrhea.
Male genital tract	One swab in a test tube	Specimen should contain urethral discharge or prostatic fluid. Obtain before voiding.
Stool Ova and parasites	Walnut-sized piece or 15–20 ml of diarrhea	Collect specimen with a tongue blade into a wide mouth plastic or waxy container after client has defecated in a clean bedpan. If mucus or streaks of blood are present, include some of this material. Repeat tests are often ordered.
Rectal swab	One swab in a test tube	Rectal swabs are sometimes done for shigella or gonorrhea. Wear nonsterile gloves when touching the perineal area. Insert a sterile cotton-tipped swab 1 in. into the anal canal, move from side to side, then leave for 30 sec for the detection of organisms.
Detection of pinworms	2-in. piece of cellophane tape	Pinworm eggs are deposited on the perianal area during the night. The specimen should be taken in the morning before bathing.

**TABLE 3–4. HOW TO COLLECT CULTURE
SPECIMENS** *Continued*

TYPE OF CULTURE	AMOUNT NEEDED	PROCEDURE
CSF fluid, pleural fluid, peritoneal fluid	1 ml, aerobic and anaerobic	See Section 4-9, Procedures of Biopsy or Aspiration, for how to obtain these specimens. Notify lab that CSF, pleural, or peritoneal fluid is coming and transport immediately.

- Collect all subsequent voidings in the prepared specimen bottle, including the final one before the next designated 24 hr.

- Refrigerate or pack in ice all specimens during the collection period, unless otherwise indicated.

- Be sure to notify the next shift that the client is completing a 24-hr urine collection and post notices on the client's door, by his/her bed, and on the Kardex.

- Return the specimen bottle to the lab promptly after the collection is completed.

E. Abnormal urine observations

Color Normal urine color varies from light yellow to dark amber, depending on concentration. If the reason for abnormal urine color is not known, call it to the attention of the physician so that a test can be run. Record your observations. The following items can cause a change in the color of urine:

Drugs. Table 7-6E lists drugs that can color urine.

Foods. Beets, rhubarb and dyes used in certain foods.

Purulent matter. Urine appears cloudy.

Blood. Urine appears dark and "smoky."

Pseudomonas infections. Urine appears greenish color.

Bilirubin. Urine turns dark orange that foams on shaking.

Protein. Large amounts can cause urine to foam.

Odor Old urine smells like ammonia. Foul odor in freshly voided urine may indicate a urinary tract infection, or may be caused by food or drugs. Asparagus gives a distinct odor to the urine.

Specific gravity This test measures the concentration of urine compared to the density of water. It can be easily performed using either a urinometer or a refractometer as an indicator of fluid balance in clients. The normal adult has a wide range from dilute urine to concentrated, but the higher the reading, the more concentrated the urine. Reference values for adults are 1.001–1.040 with random samples of about 1.015–1.025. Refractometers have the added advantage of measuring protein, which may also be tested by dipstick.

III. Microbiologic Specimens (Cultures)

The success of these diagnostic tests is often dependent on the quality of the specimen. These are important rules for collecting microbiologic specimens:

- Collect specimens before antibiotics are begun if possible. If antibiotics have already been started, notify the lab, as enzymes may need to be added to test tubes to counteract the antibiotic or special tubes used.

- Use the correct specimen container. All specimens, except stool, must be collected in sterile containers, and anaerobic specimens must be collected in oxygen-free containers. Call the laboratory if there is any doubt about specimen containers or culture medium.

- Reduce the possibility of specimen contamination from indigenous or external flora as much as possible by cleaning skin before taking a blood culture, cleaning around a wound before taking a culture, making sure a throat swab touches the back of the throat only, and carefully carrying out clean-catch urine procedure. See Table 3-4 for specific specimen collection procedures.

- Collect the right amount (see Table 3-4).

- Meticulous hand washing and gloving before and after culture collection is essential to prevent exposure of others to pathogens.

- Do not contaminate outside of container with specimen. Observe universal precautions for handling body fluids.

- Send the culture to the laboratory immediately.

IV. Stool Specimens

The stool may be examined for microorganisms, parasites, or chemical determinations. Occult blood is the most common chemical determination.

- Barium sulfate in the stool may obscure examination; tests requiring barium should be scheduled after specimens are taken.

- Handle all fecal specimens with great care, as they are a potential source of infective material.

A. Cultures for bacteria, parasites: See Table 3-4.

B. Stool for occult blood (or "guaiac"): Test reagents such as "Hemoccult" are extremely sensitive:

- Have the client refrain from eating meat or fish and taking aspirin for 2–3 days before the test (check with your laboratory).

- Only a small amount of stool is needed for these tests. Many times samples of different parts of the stool will be requested.

- Newer techniques for assessing occult blood in the stool make it possible that initial screenings do not necessitate the handling of fecal material. One device is a pad thrown into the toilet after a bowel movement, and a spot on the pad changes color if there is blood in the stool. Another uses filter paper as toilet paper. Become familiar with the methods used in your facility.

- More than one specimen may be needed to detect intermittent bleeding.

- Specimens should be tested within 48 hr of collection and must be protected from sunlight.

C. **Fecal fat determinations:** The entire stool is sent to the lab for 1–5 days if the fat content of the stool is to be measured to evaluate malabsorption problems.

3-3 INTERPRETING LAB RESULTS

Factors Affecting Test Results

To achieve the most meaningful interpretations when analyzing laboratory data, hospital personnel should be aware of the factors that may affect test results:

1. **Age and sex (gender)** are two chief factors that influence laboratory norms.
2. **Pregnancy** alters the normal reference values.
3. **Proper identification** of client and specimen. If possible let the client tell you his or her own name when taking specimens, then verify with a second method, i.e., a wristband.
4. **Physical activity:** Most commonly, specimens are taken after a period of rest such as before breakfast. Some test values can be increased as much as 8–41% with strenuous exercise. Notify the lab if the client has not been at rest before the test.
5. **Posture** of the client, whether sitting or standing.
6. **Diet and hydration:**

   - Most laboratory tests do not require dietary restrictions, but those that do must be carefully adhered to. Table 3-1 lists some tests that require food and drink restrictions.

   - In addition to diet, the hydration of the client can dramatically affect test results. Tests that are particularly sensitive to and can be indicators of the hydration level are hematocrit, hemoglobin, serum aldosterone, arterial blood gases, electrolytes, BUN, osmolality, and specific gravity.

7. **Drug interference:** Drugs can alter laboratory tests in at least three ways: by changing the client's physiology, such as birth control pills (there will be an increased value in the following tests: iron, transferrin, triglycerides, ceruloplasmin, and many more); by directly interfering with chemical analysis; and drugs' toxic effects on the liver and kidneys can cause elevated organ function tests.

   • Consult a pharmacology text or laboratory handbook such as Chernecky, 1993, for details on drug interactions and effects of specific drugs on lab tests. Many drugs can cause tests to register falsely negative or positive.

   • When a client is receiving drugs known to affect laboratory values, consult with the attending physician on the advisability of discontinuing or postponing the initiation of the drug until the test is completed.

   • List drugs being taken by the client on the laboratory requisition slip.

8. **The time of day is critical in measuring hormone levels:** Note the time the specimen is collected on the lab slip.

9. **Geographical location:** Altitude may cause hematology values to be different in a city such as Denver than they would be in a population at sea level.

10. **Ethnic or racial differences:** Usually of slight importance, as a mixture of people is usually used to obtain values.

3-4 "NORMAL" REFERENCE VALUES

The values listed in Tables 3-5 to 3-11 are to be used as guidelines only for the adult client. Each hospital laboratory has their own list of reference values based on their measurements of a population sample. For the reasons listed above and other reasons, clinicians must not allow their interpretation of lab results to be restricted by the boundaries of reference values, but must take all data into consideration. Comparing a client's present values with previous values (his/her reference values) allows the observation of trends, which is key in diagnosis.

Text continued on page 144

TABLE 3–5. ARTERIAL BLOOD GASES: NORMAL LABORATORY VALUES AND INCREASED/ DECREASED INDICATIONS

TEST	REFER-ENCE VALUE	POSSIBLE ETIOLOGY	
		Increased	Decreased
ph	7.35–7.45	Alkalosis	Acidosis
pCO$_2$ arterial	35–45 mm Hg	Compensated metabolic alkalosis Respiratory acidosis Administration of high concentration of O$_2$	Compensated metabolic acidosis Respiratory alkalosis Chronic lung disease Decreased cardiac output
pO$_2$	75–100 mm Hg (dependent on age and altitude) Above 500 mg Hg while on 100% O$_2$	Polycythemia	Decreased efficiency of the lungs
O$_2$ saturation	95% or greater	O$_2$ Administration	High altitude Lung diseases
Bicarbonate (HCO$_3^-$)	24–28 mEq/l	Compensated respiratory acidosis Metabolic alkalosis	Compensated respiratory alkalosis Metabolic acidosis

TABLE 3–6. BLOOD, SERUM, PLASMA CHEMISTRY: NORMAL REFERENCE VALUES AND INCREASED/DECREASED INDICATIONS

TEST	NORMAL VALUE	POSSIBLE ETIOLOGY	
		Increased	Decreased
Acid Phosphatase, prostatic	0–0.8 U/L (0.0–13.0 nkat/L)	Prostatic cancer Paget's disease	
Alanine Aminotransferase (ALT, SGPT)	7–55 U/L (0.12–0.91 μkat/L)	Hepatocellular destruction	
Albumin	3.5–5.0 g/dl (507–725 μmol/L)	Dehydration	Chronic liver disease Malabsorption Malnutrition Nephrotic syndrome
Aldolase	0–7.5 U/L (0–117 nkat/L)	Skeletal muscle disease	Renal disease
Alkaline phosphatase	30–115 U/L (0.5–1.92 μkat/L)	Bone diseases Hyperparathyroidism Rickets	Excessive Vit. D ingestion Hypoparathyroidism
Alpha₁-antitrypsin	85–213 mg/dl (0.85–213 mg/dl)	Inflammation Arthritis Stress syndrome	Chronic lung disease (early) Malnutrition Nephrotic syndrome
Alpha₁-fetoprotein	<25 ng/ml (<25 μg/L)	Cancer of testes Cancer of ovaries Carcinoma of liver	
Ammonia (plasma)	12–55 μmol/L (12–55 μmol/L)	Severe liver disease	
Amylase	53–123 U/L (0.88–2.05 nkat/L)	Acute and chronic pancreatitis Mumps (salivary gland disease) Perforated ulcers	Acute alcoholism Cirrhosis Extensive destruction of pancreas
Bilirubin			
Total:	0.0–1.0 mg/dl (0–17 μmol/L)	Biliary obstruction Impaired liver function	
Direct:	0.0–0.4 mg/dl	Hemolytic anemia Pernicious anemia	

Table continued on following page

TABLE 3–6. BLOOD, SERUM, PLASMA CHEMISTRY: NORMAL REFERENCE VALUES AND INCREASED/DECREASED INDICATIONS *Continued*

TEST	NORMAL VALUE	POSSIBLE ETIOLOGY	
		Increased	Decreased
	(0–7 μmol/L)	Prolonged fasting Biliary obstruction	Anemia
Cholesterol			
Desirable:	<200mg/dl (<5.18 mmol/L)	Hypothyroidism Idiopathic	Diarrhea Hyperthyroidism
Border-line high:	200–239 mg/dl (5.18–6.19 mmol/L)	Hypercholesterol-emia Renal disease	Malnutrition Steroid therapy
High	≥240 mg/dl (≥6.20 mol/L)		
Copper	70–155 μg/dl (11.0–24.4 μmol/L)	Cirrhosis Female on contra-ceptives	Wilson's disease
Cortisol			
8:00 AM	5–25 μg/dl (0.14–0.69 μmol/L)	Cushing's syn-drome Pancreatitis	Adrenal insuffi-ciency Panhypopituitary states
8:00 AM	<10 μg/dl (<0.28 μmol/L)	Stress	
Creatine	0.2–1.0 mg/dl (15.3–76.3 μmol/L)	Active Rheumatoid Arthritis Biliary obstruction Hyperthyroidism Renal disorders Severe muscle disease	Diabetes
Creatine Phos-phokinase (CPK) or Crea-tine kinase (CK)	Male: 60–400 U/L (1.00–6.67 μkat/L) Female: 40–150 U/L (0.67–2.50 μkat/L)	Hypothyroidism Musculoskeletal injury or disease Myocardial infarc-tion Severe myocarditis	

TABLE 3–6. BLOOD, SERUM, PLASMA CHEMISTRY: NORMAL REFERENCE VALUES AND INCREASED/DECREASED INDICATIONS *Continued*

TEST	NORMAL VALUE	POSSIBLE ETIOLOGY	
		Increased	Decreased
Creatinine	0.6–1.5 mg/dl (53–133 μmol/L)	Severe renal disease	
Electrolytes Sodium	135–145 mEq/l (135–145 mmol/L)	Dehydration Impaired renal function Primary aldosteronism Steroid therapy	Addison's Disease Diabetic ketoacidosis Diuretic therapy Excessive loss from the GI tract Excessive perspiration Water intoxication
Potassium	3.5–5.0 mEq/l (3.5–5.5mmol/L)	Addison's disease Diabetic ketoacidosis Massive tissue destruction Renal failure	Cushing's syndrome Diarrhea (severe) Diuretic therapy Gastrointestinal fistula Pyloric obstruction Starvation Vomiting
Chloride	95–105 mEq/l (95–105mmol/L)	Cardiac decompensation Metabolic acidosis Respiratory alkalosis Steroid therapy Uremia	Addison's disease Diarrhea Metabolic alkalosis Respiratory acidosis Vomiting
Bicarbonate	20–30 mEq/l (20–30 mmol/L)	Compensated respiratory acidosis Metabolic alkalosis	Compensated respiratory alkalosis Metabolic acidosis
Calcium	8.5–11.0 mg/dl (4.5–5.5 mEq/l) (2.1–2.6 mmol/L)	Acute osteoporosis Hyperparathyroidism Vitamin D intoxication	Acute pancreatitis Hypoparathyroidism Liver disease Malabsorption syndrome Renal failure Vitamin D deficiency

BUN 7-18

Table continued on following page

**TABLE 3–6. BLOOD, SERUM, PLASMA
CHEMISTRY: NORMAL REFERENCE VALUES
AND INCREASED/DECREASED INDICATIONS**
Continued

TEST	NORMAL VALUE	POSSIBLE ETIOLOGY	
		Increased	Decreased
Magnesium	1.5–2.5 mEq/l (0.75–1.25 mmol/L)	Addison's disease Hypothyroidism Renal failure	Chronic alcoholism Hyperparathyroidism Hyperthyroidism Severe malabsorption
Ferritin (serum)	20–300 ng/ml (20–300 μg/L)	Sideroblastic anemia Infection Inflammation	Iron deficiency anemia
Folic acid	3–25 ng/ml (7–57 nmol/L)		Alcoholism Hemolytic anemia Inadequate diet Malabsorption syndrome Megaloblastic anemia
Glucose, fasting	70–120 mg/dl (3.89–6.66 mmol/L)	Acute stress Cerebral lesions Cushing's disease Diabetes mellitus Hyperthyroidism Pancreatic insufficiency	Addison's disease Hepatic disease Hypothyroidism Insulin overdosage Pancreatic tumor Pituitary hypofunction Postgastrectomy dumping syndrome
Glucose Tolerance Test (GTT)			
Fasting	70–120 mg/100 ml (3.89–6.66 mmol/L)	Diabetes mellitus	Hyperinsulinism
30 min	30–60 mg/dl above fasting (1.67–3.33 mmol/L)		

**TABLE 3–6. BLOOD, SERUM, PLASMA
CHEMISTRY: NORMAL REFERENCE VALUES
AND INCREASED/DECREASED INDICATIONS**
Continued

TEST	NORMAL VALUE	POSSIBLE ETIOLOGY Increased	Decreased
60 min	20–50 mg/dl above fasting (1.11–2.78 mmol/L)		
120 min	5–15 mg/dl above fasting (0.28–0.83 mmol/L)		
180 min	Fasting level or lower		
Human Growth Hormone	2.0–6.0 ng/ml (2.0–6.0 µg/L)	Acromegaly Pregnancy	
Insulin	4–24 µU/ml (29–172 pmol/L)	Acromegaly Adenoma of islet cells Untreated mild cases of Type II diabetes	Diabetes mellitus Obesity
Iron	50–150 µg/dl (9.0–26.9 µmol/L)	Excessive RBC destruction	Iron-deficiency anemia
Iron-binding capacity (IBC)	250–410 µg/dl (45–73 µmol/L)	Iron-deficient state Oral contraceptives Polycythemia	Cancer Chronic infections Pernicious anemia Uremia
Lactic acid	5–20 mg/dl (0.56–2.2 mmol/L)	Acidosis Congestive heart failure Shock	

Table continued on following page

TABLE 3–6. BLOOD, SERUM, PLASMA CHEMISTRY: NORMAL REFERENCE VALUES AND INCREASED/DECREASED INDICATIONS *Continued*

TEST	NORMAL VALUE	POSSIBLE ETIOLOGY Increased	Decreased
Lactic dehydrogenase (LDH)	95–200 U/L 80–120 U (Wacker) (95–200 U/L)	Congestive heart failure Hemolytic disorders Hepatitis Metastatic cancer of the liver Myocardial infarction Pernicious anemia Pulmonary embolus Skeletal muscle damage	
Lactic dehydrogenase isoenzymes			
LDH-1	20%–35% (0.20–0.35)	Myocardial infarction Pernicious anemia	
LDH-2	30%–40% (0.30–0.40)	Pulmonary embolus Sickle cell crisis	
LDH-3	15%–25% (0.15–0.25)	Malignant lymphoma Pulmonary embolus	
LDH-4	0%–10% (0–0.10)	Lupus erythematosus Pulmonary infarction	
LDH-5	4%–12% (0.04–0.12)	Congestive heart failure Hepatitis Pulmonary embolus and infarction Skeletal muscle damage	

TABLE 3–6. BLOOD, SERUM, PLASMA CHEMISTRY: NORMAL REFERENCE VALUES AND INCREASED/DECREASED INDICATIONS
Continued

TEST	NORMAL VALUE	POSSIBLE ETIOLOGY	
		Increased	Decreased
Lipase	0.2–1.5 U/ml (0.2–1.5 U/ml)	Acute pancreatitis Hepatic disorders Perforated peptic ulcer	
Osmolality	280–296 mOsm/kg (280–296 mmol/kg)	Chronic renal disease Diabetes mellitus	Addison's disease Diuretic therapy
Phosphorous, inorganic	2.8–4.5 mg/dl (0.90–1.45 mmol/L)	Healing fractures Hypoparathyroidism Renal disease Vitamin D intoxication	Diabetes mellitus Hyperparathyroidism Vitamin D deficiency
Proteins			
Total	6.0–8.0 g/dl (60–80 g/L)	Burns	Agammaglobulinemia
Albumin	3.5–5.5 g/dl (35–50 g/L)	Cirrhosis	Liver disease
Globulin	2–3.5 g/dl (20–35 g/L)	Dehydration	Malabsorption
Renin			
Supine position	1.4–2.9 ng/ml/hr (0.39–0.81 ng/L sec)	Renal hypertension Volume decrease, i.e. hemorrhage	Increased salt intake Primary aldosteronism
Upright position	0.4–4.5 ng/ml/hr (0.11–1.25 ng/L sec)		
Testosterone	Male: 400–1200ng/dl (13.9–41.6 nmol/L) Female: 25–90 ng/dl (0.87–3.1 nmol/L)	Polycystic ovary Virilizing tumors	Hypofunction of testes

Table continued on following page

**TABLE 3–6. BLOOD, SERUM, PLASMA
CHEMISTRY: NORMAL REFERENCE VALUES
AND INCREASED/DECREASED INDICATIONS**
Continued

TEST	NORMAL VALUE	POSSIBLE ETIOLOGY	
		Increased	Decreased
T3 Uptake	25–35% (0.25–0.35)	Hyperthyroidism Metastatic neoplasms	Hypothyroidism Pregnancy
T3	110–230 ng/dl (1.7–3.5 nmol/L)	Hyperthyroidism	
T4 thyroxine	5–12 μg/dl (64–154 nmol/L)	Hyperthyroidism Thyroiditis	Cretinism Hypothyroidism
Thyroid stimulating hormone	0.3–5.4 μU/ml (0.3–5.4 mU/L)	Myxedema Primary hypothyroidism	Secondary hypothyroidism
Transaminases			
SGOT	7–40 U/L (0.12–0.67 μkat/L)	Liver disease Myocardial infarction Pulmonary infarction Acute hepatitis	
SGPT	5–36 U/L (0.08–0.6 μkat/L	Liver disease Shock	
Triglycerides	40–150mg/dl (0.45–1.69 mmol/L)	Diabetes mellitus Hyperlipidemia Hypothyroidism Liver disease	Malnutrition
Urea Nitrogen (BUN)	10–30 mg/dl (1.8–7.1 mmol/L)	Increased protein catabolism (fever, stress) Renal disease Urinary tract infection	Malnutrition Severe liver damage

TABLE 3–6. BLOOD, SERUM, PLASMA CHEMISTRY: NORMAL REFERENCE VALUES AND INCREASED/DECREASED INDICATIONS
Continued

TEST	NORMAL VALUE	POSSIBLE ETIOLOGY	
		Increased	Decreased
Uric acid	Female: 2.5–5.5 mg/dl (268–387 μmol/L) Male: 4.5–6.5 mg/dl (149–327 μmol/L	Eclampsia Renal failure Gout Gross tissue destruction High protein weight reduction diet Leukemia	Administration of uricosuric drugs
Vitamin A	15–60 μg/dl (0.52–2.09 μmol/L)	Excess ingestion of vitamin A	Vitamin A deficiency
Vitamin B12	200–1000 pg/ml (148–738pmol/L)	Myeloid leukemia	Extreme vegetarianism Malabsorption syndrome Pernicious anemia Total or partial gastrectomy
Zinc	50–150 μg/dl (7.6–22.9 μmol/L)		Alcoholic cirrhosis

TABLE 3–7. HEMATOLOGY: NORMAL LABORATORY VALUES AND INCREASED/DECREASED INDICATIONS

TEST	NORMAL VALUE (SI units in parentheses)	POSSIBLE ETIOLOGY	
		Increased	Decreased
Bleeding Time (Simplate)	3.0–9.5 min (180–570 sec)	Defective platelet function	
(Ivy)	1–6 min (60–360 sec.)	Thrombocytopenia Aspirin ingestion	
Erythrocyte count			
Male:	$4.4–6.0 \times 10^6/\mu l$ ($4.5–6.0 \times 10^{12}/L$)	Dehydration High altitudes	Anemia Leukemia
Female:	$4.0–5.0 \times 10^6/\mu l$ ($4.5–5.0 \times 10^{12}/L$)	Polycythemia vera	Posthemorrhage Severe diarrhea
Erythrocyte Indices			
Mean corpuscular volume (MCV)	82–98 fl (82–98fl)	Macrocytic anemia	Microcytic anemia
Mean corpuscular hemoglobin (MCH)	27–33 pg (27–33 pg)	Macrocytic anemia	Microcytic anemia
MCHC (mean corpuscular hemoglobin concentration)	32%–36% (0.32–0.36)	Spherocytosis	Hypochromic anemia
Erythrocyte sedimentation rate	Male: <15 mm/hr (<15 mm/hr) Female: 0–20 mm/hr (0–20 mm/hr)	*Moderate increase:* Acute hepatitis Myocardial infarction Rheumatoid arthritis *Marked increase:* Severe bacterial infections	Malaria Severe liver disease Sickle-cell anemia

**TABLE 3–7. HEMATOLOGY: NORMAL
LABORATORY VALUES AND
INCREASED/DECREASED INDICATIONS**
Continued

TEST	NORMAL VALUE (SI units in parentheses)	POSSIBLE ETIOLOGY	
		Increased	Decreased
Fibrinogen	200–400 mg/dl (2.0–4.0 g/L)	Malignancies Pelvic inflammatory disease Burns (after first 36 hr) Inflammatory disease	Burns (during first 36 hr) DIC Severe liver disease
Fibrin degradation products	<10 µg/ml (<100mg/ liter)	Acute DIC Massive hemorrhage Primary fibrinolysis	
Hematocrit	Male: 40%–54% (0.40–0.54)	Dehydration High altitudes	Anemia Hemorrhage
	Female: 38%–47% (0.38–0.47)	Polycythemia	Overhydration
Hemoglobin	Male: 13.5–18.0 g/dl (135–180 g/L)	COPD High altitudes	Anemia Hemorrhage
	Female: 12.0–16.0 g/100ml (120–160 g/L)	Polycythemia	
Lupus erythematosus (LE preparation)	No LE cells seen (No LE cells seen)	Lupus erythematosus Rheumatoid arthritis	
Partial thromboplastin time, activated (PTT)	30–45 sec* (30–45 sec)*	Heparin therapy Hemophilia Liver disease	
Prothrombin time	12–15 sec*	Anticoagulant therapy	

Table continued on following page

TABLE 3–7. HEMATOLOGY: NORMAL LABORATORY VALUES AND INCREASED/DECREASED INDICATIONS
Continued

TEST	NORMAL VALUE (SI units in parentheses)	POSSIBLE ETIOLOGY	
		Increased	Decreased
(Protime, PT)	(12–15 sec)*	Deficiency of clotting factors Inadequate vitamin K in diet Liver disease	
Platelet count	150,000–400,000/μl (150–400 × 10⁹/L)	Acute infections Chronic granulocytic leukemia Chronic pancreatitis Cirrhosis Collagen disorders Polycythemia Post-splenectomy	Acute leukemia DIC Thrombocytopenic purpura
Reticulocyte count	0.5%–1.5% of RBC 0.005–0.015 of RBC	Hemolytic anemia Polycythemia vera	Hypoproliferative anemia Macrocytic anemia Microcytic anemia
Sickle cell preparation	Negative (Negative)	Sickle-cell anemia	
White Blood Cell (Leukocyte) count	4,500–11,000/μl (4.0–11.0 × 10⁹/L	Inflammation Infections	Aplastic anemia Side effects of chemotherapy

TABLE 3–8. IMMUNOLOGY-SEROLOGY: NORMAL REFERENCE VALUES AND INCREASED/DECREASED INDICATIONS

TEST	REFERENCE VALUES	POSSIBLE ETIOLOGY	
		Increased	Decreased
Autoantibodies			
Anti-DNA antibody	Negative at 1:10 dilution	Systemic lupus erythematosus	
Antinuclear antibody	Negative at 1:8 dilution	Chronic hepatitis Rheumatoid arthritis Systemic lupus erythematosus	
Anti-RNP	Negative	Mixed connective tissue disease Rheumatoid arthritis Systemic lupus erythematosus Sjögren's syndrome Scleroderma	
Anti-Sm	Negative	Systemic lupus erythematosus	
Antistreptolysin-O	≤166 Todd units	Acute glomerulonephritis Rheumatoid fever Streptococcal infection	
C-reactive protein (CRP)	Negative or ≤ 1.2 mg/dl	Acute infections Inflammation Widespread malignancy	
Complement components			
C1q	11–21 mg/dl (0.11–0.21 g/L)		Acute glomerulonephritis Systemic lupus erythematosus
C3	80–180 mg/dl (0.8–1.8 g/L)		Rheumatoid arthritis
C4	15–50 mg/dl (0.15–0.5 g/L)		Endocarditis Serum sickness

Table continued on following page

**TABLE 3–8. IMMUNOLOGY-SEROLOGY:
NORMAL REFERENCE VALUES AND
INCREASED/DECREASED INDICATIONS**
Continued

TEST	REFER-ENCE VALUES	POSSIBLE ETIOLOGY	
		Increased	Decreased
Coombs' or Anti-human globulin (AHG)			
Direct	Negative	Acquired hemo-lytic anemia	
Indirect	Negative	Anti-RH antibodies in pregnant women Blood incompata-bilities Presence of irregu-lar antibody serum Transfusion reac-tion	
Immuno-globulin			
IgA	90–400 mg/dl (0.9–4.0 g/L)	Cirrhosis Rheumatoid arthri-tis IgA myeloma Autoimmune disor-ders	Hereditary telan-giectasia Malabsorption syn-dromes Burns
IgD	0.5–12 mg/dl (5–120 mg/L)	Chronic infection Connective tissue disease	
IgE	<1 mg/dl (<10 mg/L)	Anaphylactic shock Atopic disease (allergies)	
IgG	650–1800 mg/dl (6.5–18.0 g/L)	Hepatitis Rheumatoid arthri-tis Scleroderma IgG monoclonal gammopathy Lupus erythemato-sus	Congenital defi-ciencies Acquired deficien-cies Nephrotic syn-dromes Burns Immunosuppres-sion

**TABLE 3–8. IMMUNOLOGY-SEROLOGY:
NORMAL REFERENCE VALUES AND
INCREASED/DECREASED INDICATIONS**
Continued

TEST	REFER-ENCE VALUES	POSSIBLE ETIOLOGY Increased	POSSIBLE ETIOLOGY Decreased
IgM	55–300 mg/dl (0.5–3.0 g/L)	Biliary cirrhosis Hepatitis Rheumatoid arthritis Acute infections	Congenital and acquired antibody deficiencies Lymphocytic leukemia Protein-losing enteropathies
Rheumatoid factor	Negative or titer < 1:20	Rheumatoid arthritis Sjögren's syndrome Lupus erythematosus	
Thyroid antibodies	≤ 1:10 titer	Hashimoto's thyroiditis Thyroid carcinoma Early hypothyroidism Pernicious anemia Lupus erythematosus Graves' disease	

**TABLE 3–9. URINE CHEMISTRY:
NORMAL REFERENCE VALUES AND
INCREASED/DECREASED INDICATIONS**

TEST	REFERENCE VALUES (SI units in parentheses)		POSSIBLE ETIOLOGY Increased	POSSIBLE ETIOLOGY Decreased
Acetone	Random	Negative	Diabetes mellitus High-fat, low-carbohydrate diets Starvation states	

Table continued on following page

**TABLE 3–9. URINE CHEMISTRY:
NORMAL REFERENCE VALUES AND
INCREASED/DECREASED INDICATIONS**
Continued

TEST	REFERENCE VALUES (SI units in parentheses)	POSSIBLE ETIOLOGY Increased	Decreased
Aldosterone	24 hr	2–26 µg/day (5.5–72.1 nmol/day)	*Primary aldosteronism:* Adrenocortical tumors *Secondary aldosteronism:* Cardiac failure Cirrhosis Large dose of ACTH Salt depletion	ACTH deficiency Addison's disease Corticosteroid therapy
Amylase	24 hr	1–17 U/day (1–17 U/day	Acute pancreatitis	
Bence Jones protein	Random	Negative	Multiple myeloma Biliary duct obstruction	
Bilirubin	Random	Negative	Hepatitis	
Calcium	24 hr	100–250 mg/day (2.5–6.3 mmol/day)	Bone tumor Hyperparathyroidism Milk-alkali syndrome	Hypoparathyroidism Malabsorption of calcium and vitamin D
Catecholamines	24 hr			
Epinephrine		<20 µg/day (118 nmol/day)	Pheochromocytoma Progressive muscular dystrophy	
Norepinephrine		<100 µg/day (<591 nmol/day)		
Chloride	24 hr	110–250 mEq/24 hr (110–250 mmol/day)	Addison's disease	Burns Excess perspiration Vomiting Diarrhea Menstruation

**TABLE 3–9. URINE CHEMISTRY:
NORMAL REFERENCE VALUES AND
INCREASED/DECREASED INDICATIONS**
Continued

TEST	REFERENCE VALUES (SI units in parentheses)		POSSIBLE ETIOLOGY Increased	Decreased
Copper	24 hr	<30 µg/ day (0.5 µmol/ day)	Cirrhosis Wilson's disease	
Creatine	24 hr	<100 mg/ day (<763 µmol/day)	Carcinoma of the liver Endocrine diseases Infections, burns Muscular dystrophy Skeletal atrophy	Hypothyroidism
Creatinine	24 hr	0.8–2.0 g/day (7.7–17.7 mmol/day)	Anemia Leukemia Muscular atrophy *Salmonella*	Renal disease
Creatinine clearance	24 hr	85–135 ml/min (1.42–2.25 ml/sec)		Renal disease
Estrogens Female:	24 hr			
Ovulation peak		28–100 µg/day (104–370 nmol/day)	Gonadal or adrenal tumor	Agenesis of ovaries Endocrine disturbances
Luteal peak		22–80 µg/ day (81–296 nmol/day)		Ovarian dysfunction
Pregnancy		Up to 45,000 µg/ day (Up to 166,455 nmol/day)		

Table continued on following page

**TABLE 3–9. URINE CHEMISTRY:
NORMAL REFERENCE VALUES AND
INCREASED/DECREASED INDICATIONS**
Continued

TEST	REFERENCE VALUES (SI units in parentheses)		POSSIBLE ETIOLOGY Increased	Decreased
Meno-pause		1.4–19.6 μg/day (5.2–72.5 nmol/day)		
Male:		5–18 μg/day (18–67 nmol/day)		
Glucose	Random	Negative	Diabetes mellitus Low renal threshold for glucose resorption Physiological stress Pituitary disorders	
Hemoglobin	Random	Negative	Extensive burns Glomerulonephritis Hemolytic anemias Hemolytic transfusion reaction	
17-Hydroxy-corticoste-roids	24 hr	3–12 mg/day (8.3–33 μmol/day)	Adrenal cancer Cushing's syndrome	Addison's disease Hypofunction of anterior pituitary
5-Hydroxyin-doleacetic acid	24 hr	2–9 mg/day (10.5–47.1 μmol/day)	Malignant carcinoid syndrome	

**TABLE 3–9. URINE CHEMISTRY:
NORMAL REFERENCE VALUES AND
INCREASED/DECREASED INDICATIONS**
Continued

TEST	REFERENCE VALUES (SI units in parentheses)	POSSIBLE ETIOLOGY	
		Increased	Decreased
17-Ketoste-roids			
Male:	10–22 mg/day (35–76 μmol/day)	Autonomous tumor of adrenals Cushing's syndrome	Adrenal cortical insufficiency Diabetes mellitus Hypogonadism
Female:	6–16 mg/day (20.8–55 μmol/day)	Adrenal hyperplasia Interstitial cell tumor of testes Hyperpituitarism Severe stress	Hypopituitarism
Ketone bodies	24 hr	20–50 mg/day (0.34–0.86 mmol/day)	Marked ketonuria	
Lead	24 hr	< 100 μg/day (<0.48 μmol/day)	Lead poisoning	
pH	Random	4.0–8.0 (4.0–8.0)	Chronic renal failure Compensatory phase of alkalosis Salicylate intoxication Vegetable diet	Compensatory phase of acidosis Dehydration Emphysema
Phosphorous, inorganic	24 hr	0.9–1.3g/day (29–42 mmol/day)	Fever Hypoparathyroidism Nervous exhaustion Rickets TB	Acute infections Nephritis

Table continued on following page

TABLE 3–9. URINE CHEMISTRY: NORMAL REFERENCE VALUES AND INCREASED/DECREASED INDICATIONS
Continued

TEST	REFERENCE VALUES (SI units in parentheses)		POSSIBLE ETIOLOGY	
			Increased	Decreased
Protein (dipstick)	Random	Negative	Congestive heart failure Nephritis Nephrosis Physiologic stress	
Protein (quantitative)	24 hr	<150 mg/day (<0.15 g/day)	Cardiac failure Inflammatory processes of urinary tract Nephritis Nephrosis Toxemia of pregnancy	
Sodium	24 hr	40–250 mEq/day (40–250 mmol/day)	Acute tubular necrosis	Hyponatremia
Specific gravity	Random	1.003–1.030 (1.003–1.030)	Albuminuria Glycosuria	Diabetes insipidus Dehydration
Uric Acid	24 hr	250–750 mg/day (1.5–4.5 mmol/day)	Gout Leukemia	Nephritis
Urobilinogen	24 hr	0.5–4.0 mg/day (0.8–6.8 μmol/day)	Hemolytic disease Hepatic parenchymal cell damage Liver disease	Complete obstruction of bile duct
Uroporphyrins	Random	Negative	Porphyria	
Vanilmandelic acid	Random	1.8 mg/day 1.5–7 μg/mg creatine (5–40 μmol/day)	Pheochromocytoma	

TABLE 3–10. CEREBROSPINAL FLUID: NORMAL LABORATORY VALUES AND INCREASED/DECREASED INDICATIONS

TEST	REFERENCE VALUE (SI units in parentheses)	POSSIBLE ETIOLOGY	
		Higher	Lower
Pressure	60–150 mm (60–150mm)	Hemorrhage Intracranial tumor Meningitis	Head injury Spinal tumor Subdural hematoma
Blood	Negative (Negative)	Intracranial hemorrhage	
Cell count (age dependent)	WBS: 0–8 cells/µl (0–8 × 10^6/L) RBS: 0 (0 × 10^6/L)	Inflammation or infections of the CNS	
Chloride	100–130 mEq/l (100–130 mmol/L)	Uremia	Bacterial infections of CNS (meningitis, encephalitis)
Glucose	45–75 mg/dl (2.5–4.2 mmol/L)	Diabetes mellitus Viral infections of CNS	Bacterial infections and TB of the CNS
Protein			
Lumbar	15–45 mg/dl (0.15–0.45 g/L)	Guillain-Barré syndrome Poliomyelitis Traumatic tap Syphilis of CNS	
Cisternal	15–25 mg/dl (0.15–0.25 g/L)		
Ventricular	5–15 mg/dl (0.05–0.15 g/L)	Acute meningitis Brain tumor Chronic infections Multiple sclerosis	

TABLE 3–11. DRUG TOXICITY LEVELS

	TOXIC LEVELS		
DRUG	**Conv. Units**	**SI Units**	**COMMENTS**
Alcohol (ethanol)	>0.30% Marked intoxication >0.40% Severe toxic effects with alcoholic stupor		0.10% is legal limit for driving in most states. 0.08% for California
Chlordi-azepoxide (Librium)	>10µg/ml	>33µmol/L	
Diazepam (Valium)	>1.0 mg/L	>3.5µmol/L	≥2.0 mg/L lethal
Digoxin (Lanoxin)	>2.5ng/ml	>2.6 nmol/L	
Digitoxin	>30ng/L	>39 nmol/L	
Dilantin	>30mg/L	>120µmol/L	
Gentamycin (Garamycin)			
Peak	>10mg/L	>22 µmol/L	
Trough	>2 mg/L	>4 µmol/L	
Lithium	>2.0 mEq/L		Therapeutic range, 0.5–1.5 mEq/L (or 0.5–1.5 mmol/L) is close to toxic range, hence rational for monitoring
Meperidine (Demerol)	>200 g/dl	>8.09 µmol/L	
Phenytoin (Dilantin)	>30mg/L	>120 µmol/L	
Phenobarbital	>60µg/ml		Long-acting and cumulative
Propanolol (Inderal)	>200 ng/ml	>771 nmol/L	
Quinidine	>10 µg/ml		
Theophyllin (Amino-phylline)	>25 µg/ml		
Salicylate	>20 mg/dl	>1.45 mmol/L	>60 mg/dl lethal

REFERENCES

Anderson S. ABG's: six easy steps to interpreting blood gases. Am J Nurs 90(8):42–45, 1990.

Barnett R, et al. Medical usefulness of STAT tests. Am J Clin Path 1978; 69:520–523.

Chernecky C, Krech R, Berger B. Laboratory tests and diagnostic procedures. Philadelphia: WB Saunders, 1993.

Corbett JV. Laboratory tests and diagnostic procedures with nursing diagnoses. 3rd ed. Norwalk, CT: Appleton and Lange, 1992.

Jordan CD, et al. Case records of the Massachusetts General Hospital: normal reference laboratory values. N Engl J Med 1992; 327 (10): 718–724.

Kee JL. Handbook of laboratory tests with nursing implications. Norwalk, CT: Appleton and Lange, 1990.

Lewis SM, Collier IC. Medical-surgical nursing: assessment and management of clinical problems. 3rd ed. St. Louis: Mosby, 1992.

Pagana KD, Pagana TJ. Diagnostic testing and nursing implications: a case study approach. 3rd ed. St. Louis: Mosby, 1990.

Wallach J. Interpretation of diagnostic tests. 5th ed. Boston: Little, Brown, 1992.

DIAGNOSTIC PROCEDURES

Proper preparation for diagnostic procedures is essential in preventing the inconvenience or even trauma of having to repeat tests. Emotional support and client teaching before, during, and after diagnostic procedures is crucial, as some tests can be more traumatic than surgery. Clients particularly want to know what sensations to expect. Nursing assessment and care after tests help prevent complications.

Preparations vary in different institutions. *The policy in one's own facility must always be followed.*

Complete Table 4-1, Checklist for Diagnostic Procedures, whenever your client has tests ordered (some endoscopic procedures require surgical checklist [see Section 4-8]).

Nursing diagnoses likely to be related to most or all laboratory tests include:

1. Knowledge deficit related to test procedure and health problems

2. Anxiety related to possible positive test result

3. Potential for non-compliance related to inadequate understanding of necessity of procedure

4. Potential for ineffective coping related to test results and disease process

5. Potential for altered family processes related to health problems

6. Potential for alteration in comfort related to non-invasive or invasive test procedures

TABLE 4–1. CHECKLIST FOR DIAGNOSTIC PROCEDURES

Client Teaching
- ☐ The date, time, and expected duration of the scheduled procedure
- ☐ What will happen during the test and what is expected of him or her
- ☐ The importance of cooperation

Allergy and Other Contraindications
- ☐ Obtain and document all allergies on the front of the chart. Ask particularly about seafood, iodine, and contrast dyes, anesthetics.
- ☐ Notify radiology and physician of any allergies
- ☐ Check for contraindications, e.g., for pregnancy. If there is any question of pregnancy, these tests are contraindicated, with the exception of ultrasound. Other tests are contraindicated in specific situations, e.g., liver biopsy in the case of abnormal blood coagulation studies. A history of repeated x-ray studies or other exposure to radiation should be reported to the physician before more x-rays are done.

Written Consent
- ☐ The consent form is on the front of the chart per hospital policy, signed by the client or a designated family member (not always required for noninvasive procedures)

Physical Preparation of the Client
- ☐ Remove all jewelry within the area to be examined; put valuables in the safe or dipose of per hospital policy
- ☐ Client has complied with dietary restrictions and bowel and bladder preps have been completed
- ☐ Record baseline vital signs
- ☐ Client has voided and is wearing a hospital gown with no metal snaps
- ☐ Administer ordered premedications
- ☐ Client rests in bed with side rails up after the medications are given

4-1 RADIOGRAPHY (SIMPLE X-RAYS) AND FLUOROSCOPY

Simple X-Rays

X-ray studies are generally for screening purposes, and are followed by more extensive diagnostic tests if warranted.

CHEST X-RAY

The most commonly ordered diagnostic procedure. Portable chest X-rays generally are not as good quality as those in the radiology department. Transport is preferable if possible.

Common views:

1. AP anterior posterior "flat plate": The x-ray beam passes through the body's anterior to posterior surface; position done during portable chest radiography.

2. PA: Client is preferably upright. X-ray beam passes through the body's posterior to anterior surface (PA preferred over AP whenever possible).

3. Lateral: X-rays are taken through the left or right side of the chest.

4. Oblique: Various views are slanted or inclined at specific angles.

5. Recumbent lateral ("decubitus"): Helps to localize fluid in the pleural space.

HEART X-RAY

Can detect cardiomegaly, aneurysms, anomalies of the vessels. The PA, left lateral, and left anterior oblique (LAO) with 60-degree rotation views are most commonly ordered. Client usually stands and is asked to take a deep breath and hold it while films are taken.

ABDOMEN AND KUB (KIDNEY, URETER, AND BLADDER)

A paper gown is worn and client lies in a supine position on a tilted x-ray table. Check with radiology as to NPO restriction.

SKULL X-RAY

Hairpins, glasses, and dentures are removed. Skull fractures, head trauma, tumors, bone defects, etc. can be detected.

For All X-Rays

- If there is any question of pregnancy, x-ray studies should be avoided, especially during the first trimester. If a chest x-ray is deemed necessary for a pregnant client, a lead apron covering the abdomen and pelvic areas must be worn. Ideally, women in their child-bearing years should follow the 14-day rule: X-rays should be taken only during menses or 14 days after.

- X-rays usually take 10–15 min, but there may be a waiting period of half an hour or so before and 10–15 min afterward. Explain that the waiting period after is to make sure the films are readable; if more pictures need to be taken it is not an indication of abnormality.

- Food and drink are not restricted with simple x-ray, except for the abdominal, where fasting for 8 hr is sometimes requested.

- Metal and jewelry must be removed because they show up on film and obscure body structures in the area they cover.

Fluoroscopy

This allows physicians to view organs in motion. The client stands in front of a fluorescent screen, the x-rays penetrate the client and strike the screen. Unfortunately, the client usually receives more radiation with fluoroscopy than with standard radiation so it should not be used if a simple x-ray would suffice. The thorax, abdomen, and heart are usually the areas evaluated.

- Obtain a history of radiation. All radiation is cumulative. Notify the physician of prolonged exposure to x-rays. All radiation exposure should be held to the lowest practicable level.

- Abdominal fluoroscopy requires the client be NPO after midnight the night before the test and a laxative is ordered that evening. Barium sulfate is swallowed.

- Fluoroscopy of the heart requires the same procedure as cardiac catheterization (see Section 4-2).

- Videotapes of the procedure allow movements to be studied at later times (cineradiography).

4-2 RADIOGRAPHIC PROCEDURES USING RADIOPAQUE IODINE, CONTRAST DYE OR AIR (RADIOGRAMS)

Structures in the body of lower density (soft tissue, blood vessels, etc.) require a radiopaque substance in order to be outlined on x-ray film. The danger of allergic reaction to the contrast medium is always present, especially when the dye is injected intravenously. Therefore, when preparing client for these tests:

- Consider kidney function prior to contrast injection. Many institutions require BUN and creatinine results prior to radiograms. If client is on dialysis, the study can be scheduled just prior to the regular dialysis appointment.

- Carefully complete Table 4-1, taking careful histories of allergy to seafood, iodine, or contrast dye taken in the past.

- Always keep emergency drugs and equipment immediately available.

- Premedication is very effective for clients with prior reaction or possibility of reaction.

Angiography (Arteriography) and Digital Subtraction Angiography (DSA)
CEREBRAL, PULMONARY, RENAL

A catheter is inserted into either the femoral, brachial, carotid, or antecubital arteries and a contrast dye is injected to allow visualization of the blood vessels by fluoroscopy. Tumors, hematomas, cysts, aneurysms, thrombosis, congenital defects, or general vascular status is evaluated. (Cardiac angiography is called cardiac catheterization).

Digital subtraction angiography (DSA) uses a computer to display certain parts of images at one time. Sometimes angioplasty is performed immediately following the test. Contraindications include pregnancy, renal disease, and hypersensitivity to local anesthetics, iodine, radioactive dye, or shellfish.

PREPARATION

Consent form	Yes
Food or fluid restriction	NPO 8 hr before test. Some hospitals allow liquids
Medications to be withheld	Anticoagulants, 8–12 hr before test
Premedications	Sedative or analgesic 1 hr before test. Steroids or antihistamine if history of allergy
Bowel or bladder prep	Have client void before premedications; laxative or enema noc of test for renal angiography, if ordered
Length of test	1–2 hr
Other	Double check for allergies to shellfish, iodine, or radiographic dye. Check recent coagulation times. Obtain baseline vitals, including peripheral pulse (dorsalis pedis, femoral, radial). Explain that the client will feel a warm, flushed sensation and salty taste in mouth when the dye is injected. Remove dentures and metallic objects. Shave injection site. IV may be standard before test in case emergency drugs are needed.

POST-TEST

Vital signs	BP, P, R, q 15 min × 4, q 30 min × 4, q 1 hr × 4. Check peripheral pulses, report weakness or absence immediately. Do not use extremity with injection site for BP.
Assess for, and report if present	Swelling, hematoma at injection site. Note temperature and color of extremity, changes could mean arterial occlusion. Dysphagia, respiratory distress, confusion, or slurred speech could be transient ischemic attack. Watch for delayed reaction to contrast dye.
Activity	Bed rest 12–24 hr
Food and fluids	Encourage oral intake of fluids unless contraindicated. Monitor intake and output.
Other	Apply pressure at injection site until bleeding stops. Check site when taking vital signs. Cold compresses as ordered if edema or pain is present. Monitor ECG tracings, urine output, IV fluids. Coughing is not abnormal after respiratory angiography.

Bronchography

Dye is injected into the tracheobronchial space via a catheter. The trachea, bronchi, and entire bronchial tree can then be visualized. Foreign bodies, obstructions, tumors, cysts, or bronchiectasis can be detected. Performed often with bronchoscopy. May be performed under general or local anesthesia.

PREPARATION

Consent form	Yes
Food or fluid restrictions	NPO 8–12 hr pre-test
Premedications	Sedative and atropine 1 hr before test
Bowel or bladder prep	Void before premedications
Length of test	1 hr
Other	Check for allergies. Meticulous oral hygiene the night before test and in the morning is very important. Postural drainage is performed 3 days before the test, and expectorants (e.g., potassium iodide) given. Encourage client to cough out secretions 2–3 days before and after test. Reassure client, as some tend to be fearful that airway will be blocked. Inform them they may have a sore throat as a result of irritation by the catheter (order lozenges).

POST-TEST

Vital signs	Monitor frequently. Temperature may be elevated for 2–3 days post-test.
Assess for, and report if present	Laryngeal edema, dyspnea, hoarseness, apprehension, delayed allergic reaction to the dye, rhonchi, fever
Activity	Resume normal activity after 24 hr.
Food and fluids	May resume when gag reflex is present (test with tongue blade at back of throat) usually 2 hr post-test. Start with ice chips, sips of water.

POST-TEST *Continued*

Medications	Offer throat lozenges.
Other	Have client perform postural drainage post-test. Monitor respiratory status.

Cardiac Catheterization (Cardiac Angiography)

In left cardiac catheterization, the catheter is inserted into the brachial or femoral artery and is advanced retrogradely through the aorta to the coronary arteries and/or left ventricle with the guidance of fluoroscopy. The patency of the coronary arteries and/or functions of the aortic and mitral valves and the left ventricle can be observed after the dye is injected.

In right cardiac catheterization, the catheter is inserted into the femoral or antecubital vein and threaded through the inferior vena cava into the right atrium to the pulmonary artery. Right atrium, right ventricle, and pulmonary artery pressures can be measured and blood samples from the right side of the heart can be obtained. The functions of the tricuspid and pulmonary valves can be observed.

Though rare (less than 2% incidence rate), complications that can occur are myocardial infarction, arrhythmias, cardiac tamponade, pulmonary embolism, and cerebral embolism.

PREPARATION

Consent form	Yes
Food or fluid restrictions	NPO 6–8 hr before test or per hospital policy
Medications to be withheld	Check with physician to see if routine medication may be given with a small sip of water. Oral anticoagulants are discontinued or dosage is reduced.

PREPARATION *Continued*

Premedications	Heparin may be ordered to prevent thrombi. A sedative or tranquilizer (i.e., diazepam [Valium]) and/or an analgesic is usually given ½ to 1 hr pre-test, but client remains awake.
Bowel or bladder prep	Void before premedications
Length of test	1½–3 hr
Other	Double-check for allergy as test is contraindicated if allergies are present. Obtain baseline vitals, including dorsalis pedis, femoral and radial pulses, marking location on skin. Record height and weight (used to calculate amount of dye needed). Injection site should be shaved and cleansed. Remove dentures. Explain that the client will feel hot, flushing sensation and metallic taste when dye is injected. If coronary angiography is done, explain that the client may feel momentary chest pain while dye is injected, but no damage will result. A KO IV will be started in the cardiac room.

POST-TEST

Vital signs	BP, P, R q 15 min × 4, q 30 min × 4, 1 hr × 4. Check peripheral pulses below insertion site. Temp. q 4 hr while awake for several days.
Assess for, and report if present	Bleeding or hematoma at catheter site. Maintain pressure dressings and sandbags and immobilize the extremity for 3–8 hr or per hospital policy. Check skin color. Assess cardiac status; dysrhythmias, chest pain.

POST-TEST *Continued*

Activity	Bed rest for 8 hr. Client should remain flat for 6 hr if femoral artery was used. The HOB can be slightly elevated if the brachial artery was used.
Food and fluids	Encourage fluid intake unless contraindicated (e.g., in congestive heart failure)
Medications	Narcotics or analgesics, antibiotics as ordered

Cholangiography (IV)

A contrast agent is injected intravenously while the client is lying on a tilting x-ray table. The biliary ducts (hepatic ducts within the liver, the common hepatic duct, the cystic duct, and the common bile duct) can then be examined for detection of calculi, strictures, or leaking anastomosis(es). Used as alternative to oral cholecystography when client cannot tolerate oral iodopaque tablets or has active intestinal inflammation.

PREPARATION

Consent form	Yes
Food or fluid restrictions	NPO 8 hr pre-test. Some encourage fat-free liquids pre-test.
Medications to be withheld	Morning insulin may be withheld.
Premedications	If ordered
Bowel or bladder prep	Laxative noc before, enema that morning (check exact orders).
Length of test	X-rays are taken at 30 min–3 hr intervals up to 8 hr after injection of dye.
Other	Double-check for allergy to iodine, seafood, or dye. Explain

PREPARATION *Continued*

purpose and procedure thoroughly and prepare client for possible lengthy procedure. Client may want to bring reading material. Explain that a burning or flushing sensation may be experienced when dye is injected.

POST-TEST

Vital signs	As ordered (e.g., q 15 min × 4, q 30 min × 4). Notify MD if temp. > 100°F (37.9°C).
Assess for, and report if present	Signs of allergic reaction. Check infusion site for signs of phlebitis—pain, redness, swelling, apply warm compresses as ordered. Dysuria is not uncommon as contrast medium is excreted.

Cholangiography (Percutaneous Transhepatic)

See IV cholangiography. The contrast medium is directly instilled into the biliary tree so that a suspicion of biliary obstruction can be confirmed or denied.

PREPARATION

Consent form	Yes
Food and fluids	Fat-free diet 1 day pre-test. Liquid breakfast day of procedure, with NPO after 8 a.m.
Premedications	Sedative or tranquilizer as ordered. Prophylactic antibiotic 24 to 72 hr pre-test if ordered.
Bowel or bladder prep	Laxative noc before, cleansing enema that a.m. if ordered
Length of test	1–2 hr

PREPARATION *Continued*

Other	Check for iodine allergy. Inform client to stay in bed 6 to 8 hr after the test. Transient pain may be experienced during injection of dye. Obtain baseline prothrombin time, clotting time, and platelet counts.

POST-TEST

Vital signs	q 15 min × 4, q 30 min × 4, q 1 hr × 4. Notify MD if temp. is 100°F (37.9°C) or over.
Assess for, and report if present	Signs of allergic reaction to contrast dye—e.g., nausea, vomiting, hives, rash, flushing. Check injection site for clean dry dressing, bleeding, swelling, tenderness. q 1 hr × 4, then q 4 hr × 24 hr. Observe for signs of septicemia, peritonitis, hemorrhage, tension, pneumothorax.
Activity	Bedrest 6–8 hr post test, with right side-lying position.

Cholangiography (T-Tube)

T-tube cholangiography is also known as post-operative cholangiography. It is usually performed 7–10 days after exploratory gallbladder or duct surgery, cholecystectomy, or liver transplant for the evaluation of the biliary ducts. Contrast medium is injected into the T-tube that was inserted in the common bile duct for drainage during surgery. Gallstones missed during surgery that could cause occlusion of the duct can in this way be visualized.

PREPARATION

Consent form	Yes
Food and fluids	NPO 4–6 hr

PREPARATION *Continued*

Premedications	If ordered
Bowel or bladder prep	Cleansing enema may be ordered
Length of test	½ hr or less
Other	Assess for allergy to dye, seafood, or iodine. The T-tube is usually removed after the procedure if findings are normal.

POST-TEST

See IV cholangiography	Assess site of T-tube removal for redness, edema, pain, or drainage q 1 hr. × 4, then q 4 hr × 24 hr. A T-tube left in place should be reconnected to drainage.

Cholecystography (Oral) (Gallbladder Radiography, Gallbladder Series)

Contrast dye is taken orally 12–14 hr before test so that absorption by the gallbladder can take place. A series of radiographic films are taken of the right upper quadrant of the client's abdomen with the client in several positions. Gallstones can the be visualized upon x-ray. Though this test is still sometimes used, ultrasound is currently the modality of choice in evaluating the gallbladder.

PREPARATION

Consent form	Yes
Food and fluids	Fat-free meal the evening before test per hospital policy. NPO after premedications, except sips of water.
Premedications	6 radiopaque tablets, 5 min apart, with full glass of water (240 ml) 12 hr before test, then NPO.

PREPARATION *Continued*

Bowel or bladder prep	No laxatives till after test. Sometimes saline enema is ordered the morning of test.
Length of test	45 min–1 hr or another 1–2 hr if post fatty films are taken.
Other	Check for allergies to iodine, seafood, radiopaque dye. Inform client tests may be repeated. Report any vomiting and diarrhea to the MD, as test may be cancelled due to hypermobility of bowel. Liver disease with bilirubin > 1.8 mg/dl, or inadequate client preparation may require that the test be cancelled or other methods used.

POST-TEST

Vital signs	Routine
Assess for, and report if present	Allergic reaction to iopanoic acid (Telepaque) tabs. Mild dysuria is common.
Food and fluids	If second part of series is ordered, client will receive meal in radiology department.

Hysterosalpingography (Hysterosalpingogram)

In this radiologic examination of the uterus and fallopian tubes, the contrast substance is injected into the cervical canal. From there it flows into the abdominal area and into the uterus and fallopian tubes. It should be done on the seventh to ninth day after the menstrual cycle begins. The client must not be pregnant, have active bleeding, or an acute infection. Adhesions, malformations, foreign bodies, trauma, infection, and tubal patency may be examined.

PREPARATION

Consent form	Yes
Food and fluids	Not restricted
Premedication	Mild sedative such as diazepam (Valium) may be ordered.
Length of test	15–30 min
Other	Make sure client is not pregnant, menstruating, or actively infected (if so, test must be canceled). Check for allergies to radiographic dye or shellfish. Explain that mild cramping and dizziness is normal during test, but to tell examiners if it is continuous or severe.

POST-TEST

Vital signs	Routine vs q 15 min × 2, then q 30 min × 2
Assess for, and report if present	Signs and symptoms of infection e.g., fever, increased pulse, pain. Assess for signs of gross bleeding, vaginal discharge, report immediately.
Other	Explain that there may be some bloody discharge for 3–4 days after the test. Report excessive or prolonged bleeding immediately. Complications of this test include uterine perforation, vascular injection of the dye, hypersensitivity, and infection.

Intravenous Pyelography (IVP, Excretory Urography)

In this test the entire urinary tract is visualized. A radiopaque substance is injected intravenously and a series of x-rays are taken at specific times. It is useful for locating stones and tumors and for diagnosing kidney diseases (e.g., polycystic kidney, renovascular hypertension). Emergency drugs (epinephrine, vasopressors, etc.) and equipment (tracheostomy set, suction machine, oxygen) should be readily available to treat anaphylaxis, as hypersensitivity to the dye can occur. An intradermal skin test to determine client tolerance may be indicated.

PREPARATION

Consent form	Yes
Food and fluids	NPO 8–12 hr pre-test if general anesthesia will be used (NPO after dinner); mild dehydration OK. Sips of water may be indicated for those with poor renal output or for the aged or debilitated.
Premedications	Antihistamine or steroid if history of allergy to iodine, seafood, or dye. A sedative may be ordered just prior to procedure. Skin test may be ordered to determine hypersensitivity.
Bowel or bladder prep	Laxative noc before, cleansing enema a.m. of test
Length of test	30–45 min
Other	Record baseline vitals. Check for allergy to radiopaque dye, iodine, or shellfish. Inform clients of possible flushing sensation during or following injection of dye. Monitor BUN levels; notify doctor if greater than 40 mg/dl, as test may be canceled.

POST-TEST

Vital signs	Monitor at the end of the procedure, then every 4 hr × 24 hr.
Assess for, and report if present	Delayed reaction to contrast dye (dyspnea, rash, flushing, hives),

POST-TEST *Continued*

	oliguria. Check for bladder distention, anuria oliguria, gross hematuria, or persistent hematuria after third voiding is abnormal. Report any signs of infection: fever, chills, dysuria, flank pain.
Food and fluids	Encourage fluids and monitor urine output. Ureteral and/or Foley catheter may be in place after the exam.
Medications	Administer analgesic as ordered.

Lymphangiography (Lymphangiogram, Lymphography)

In this examination of the lymphatic system—the lymphatic vessels and lymph nodes—contrast oil substance is injected into the lymphatic vessels of each foot. The hands may also be used to visualize axillary nodes and supraclavicular nodes. Malignant lymphoma (Hodgkin's disease) metastasis to the lymph nodes or lymphadenopathy may be identified in this manner. It is contraindicated if the client has allergy to iodine, severe chronic lung disease, cardiac disease, or advanced liver or kidney disease. Lipid pneumonia may occur if the dye flows into the thoracic duct and sets up microemboli in the lungs. The 24 hour post-injection film series are the most important part of the exam. The contrast can stay in the lymph nodes 6–9 mos.

PREPARATION

Consent form	Yes
Food and fluids	Not restricted
Premedications	A sedative may be ordered.
Bowel or bladder prep	Void before test
Length of test	2½–3 hr. with second set of films taken 24 hr later

PREPARATION *Continued*

Other	Check for allergies to iodized oil, dye, or shellfish. Record baseline vitals. Contrast dye is injected intradermally between the toes, with local anesthetic. Inform client that the dye discolors the urine and stool for several days; the skin may have bluish tinge for 24–48 hr

POST-TEST

Vital signs	BP, pulse, respirations q 15 min × 4, q 30 min × 2, q 1 hr × 4 or until stable
Assess for, and report if present	Dyspnea, pain, or hypotension, which could be due to microemboli from spillage of the contrast dye. Assess incisional site for infection. Check for leg edema.
Activity	Bed rest for 24 hr or as ordered with legs elevated.
Other	Dressing is not usually changed for 48 hr.

Myelography (Myelogram)

This procedure involves the examination of the spinal subarachnoid space (spinal canal). In clients who are hypersensitive to radiopaque contrast dye, air is injected into the lumbar area so that spinal lesions (intervertebral disks, tumors, cysts, etc.) can be visualized. This test is contraindicated if increased intracranial pressure is suspected or if client has multiple sclerosis.

PREPARATION

Consent form	Yes
Food and fluids	NPO 4–8 hr pre-test. May have light breakfast if test is in p.m.

PREPARATION *Continued*

Medications withheld	If metrizamide is to be used as contrast dye, discontinue use of phenothiazines 48 hr before test.
Premedications	A sedative and/or narcotic analgesic and atropine as ordered
Bowel or bladder prep	Cleansing enema night before or a.m. of test
Length of test	1 hr
Other	Check for allergy to iodine, seafood, or dye. If increased intracranial pressure is suspected, CT scan of the brain should be performed to rule it out. Client may have slight burning sensation when dye is injected into lumbar area. Inform client of need to either lie flat for 8 hr or for at least 6 hr after test at 30–45° degrees.

POST-TEST

Vital signs	BP, pulse, respirations q 30 min × 4, q 1 hr × 4 or until stable
Assess for, and report if present	Meningitis: headache, fever, stiff neck, irritability, photophobia, convulsions
Activity	Prone or supine position, flat, for 6–8 hr or head of bed at no more than 45 degrees if oil based contrast is used (used rarely). Sitting may be allowed if metrizamide (water soluble) is used.
Food and fluids	Encourage fluids to help replace lost spinal fluid and decrease chance of postlumbar puncture headache. Monitor urinary output. Should void within 8 hr.

POST-TEST *Continued*

Medications to be withheld	Do not administer phenothiazines for nausea and vomiting if water soluble contrast was used.
Other	Explain rationale for postoperative procedure and emphasize importance. Instruct client in preventing back injury, i.e., principles of good body mechanics, proper lifting techniques.

Pneumoencephalography (Pneumoencephalogram)

Visualization of the cerebral ventricles and cisterns is accomplished by repeatedly replacing small amounts of spinal fluid with air, oxygen, or carbon dioxide in the lumbar area. This test is only done when tumors of the posterior fossa are suspected. In most other cases, CT scan or cerebral angiography is preferred. Hypotension and headaches occur frequently. Strict bed rest with the head kept flat, increased fluid intake, and analgesics are required for 12–24 hr after the test. This procedure is contraindicated if increased intracranial pressure is present.

PREPARATION

Consent form	Yes
Food and fluids	NPO 8 hr pre-test
Premedications	A sedative for those who will receive general anesthesia. Demerol should not be used.
Bowel or bladder prep	Void before test
Length of test	1–2 hr
Other	Remove dentures and jewelry. Explain purpose and procedure thoroughly. Inform client of need to lie flat in bed for 12–24 hr afterward to help prevent head-

PREPARATION *Continued*

	ache. IV TKO is usual in case emergency drugs are needed. Record baseline vitals.

POST-TEST

Vital signs	BP, pulse, respirations and neuro checks q 15 min × 4, q 30 min × 4, q 1 hr × 4.
Assess for, and report if present	Nausea, vomiting, headache, increased intracranial pressure, fluid leak at lumbar puncture site
Activity	Flat in bed or if necessary elevate the head no more than 30 degrees for 24 hr or as ordered. Instruct the client to move slowly from side to side every 2 hr and to avoid quick movements, as they could cause nausea or increase the headache.
Food and fluids	Encourage high fluid intake to restore lost spinal fluid.
Medications	Administer analgesics for headache as needed.
Other	Be supportive of the client and family. Allow visitors, but visits should be short, as the client needs quiet time.

Pyelography, Antegrade (Antegrade Pyelogram)

A radiographic contrast examination of the bladder and ureters accomplished by injecting radiographic dye percutaneously into the renal pelvis or calyx. It is most commonly performed when retrograde pyelography is contraindicated or when dye injected via retrograde pyelography is prevented from traveling completely through the ureters to the upper collecting system of the urinary tract.

PREPARATION

Consent form	Yes
Food and fluids	NPO 4 hr pre-test
Premedications	Sedative as ordered
Bowel or bladder prep	Cleansing enema 4 hr before test. Void before test.
Length of test	30 min
Other	Assess for allergies to iodine, shellfish, or radiographic dye. Instruct the client to remain as motionless as possible during the procedure. Assess baseline vitals. This test is contraindicated in persons with clotting orders. Be aware of baseline PT/PTT.

POST-TEST

Vital signs	BP, pulse, and respirations q 15 min × 4, q 30 min × 4, q 1 hr × 4, then q 4 hr × 24 hr
Assess for, and report if present	Signs of hematoma formation or frank bleeding at surgical incision area, infection (fever, tachycardia, tachypnea, chills, or pain) Assess hourly for patency of nephrostomy tube, if placed × 24 hr
Activity	Rest as tolerated.

Pyelography, Retrograde (Retrograde Pyelogram)

Retrograde pyelography is an invasive radiographic (fluoroscopic) examination of the kidneys from a distal direction via the ureters. During cystoscopy, radiopaque contrast material is injected into catheters passed into the ureters. Mucous membranes absorb only minimal amounts of the iodine radiopaque contrast material, minimizing the

complications of hypersensitivity reactions or delayed excretion of the dye in renal impairment that are associated
with intravenous dye injection. Renal calculi, neoplasm, renal stricture, or renal malfunction can be detected through
this method.

PREPARATION

Consent form	Yes
Food and fluids	NPO 8 hr pre-test. Sometimes fluids are not restricted unless general anesthesia is used. Client should not be dehydrated before test (report signs if present to MD).
Premedications	Sedative 1 hr pre-test
Bowel or bladder prep	Laxatives and cleansing enemas as ordered.
Length of test	1 hr
Other	Check for allergy to iodine, sea-food, or radiopaque dye. Explain purpose of test and procedure, including that the client will be in stirrups. Though there may be pressure at the insertion of the cytoscope and client may feel the urge to urinate, there is usu-ally little to no pain or discom-fort. Obtain baseline vital signs.

POST-TEST

Vital signs	BP, pulse, respirations q 15 min × 4, q 30 min × 2, vs. q 4 hr while awake, 1–3 days.
Assess for, and report if present	Allergic reactions to contrast dye—skin rash, urticaria, flush-ing. Signs of infection—fever, chills, abdominal pain. Blood-tinged urine is normal; report gross hematuria and/or severe pain.

POST-TEST *Continued*

Food and fluids	Monitor urinary output. Report if <200 ml/8 hr. A ureteral and/or Foley catheter may be left in place after the examination.
Medications	Give analgesic as ordered for pain; report if severe.

Venography (Lower Limb) (Phlebography)

This is examination of the deep leg veins after injection of contrast dye or a radionuclide to identify venous obstruction due to deep-vein thrombosis. If a thrombus formation is not treated, it can lead to femoral and iliac venous occlusion, or the thrombus can lead to embolus and cause pulmonary embolism. Venography is frequently done after Doppler ultrasonography to confirm a positive or questionable deep-vein thrombosis.

PREPARATION

Consent form	Yes
Food and fluids	NPO 4 hr pre-test. Some departments allow clear liquids.
Medications to be withheld	Anticoagulants may be temporarily discontinued.
Premedications	Skin test and/or steroids 2–3 days before test if history of allergy. A sedative may be given if there is extreme apprehension, or low pain threshold.
Bowel or bladder prep	None
Length of test	½ hr–1 hr
Other	Check for allergy. Inform client there may be a slight burning when the dye is injected into the foot.

POST-TEST

Vital signs	q 15 min × 4, q 30 min × 6, then q 1 hr. Check pulse in the dorsalis pedis, popliteal and femoral arteries for volume, intensity, and rate.
Assess for, and report if present	Observe for signs of latent allergic reaction. Check injection site for bleeding, hematoma, infection, embolism, thrombophlebitis
Other	Elevate leg as ordered. If venogram is positive for deep-vein thrombosis, the MD will most likely order bed rest, heparin infusion, leg elevation, and warm, moist compresses.

4-3 RADIOGRAPHIC TESTS USING BARIUM SULFATE

Barium Enema (X-Ray Examination of the Colon)

The large intestine is examined in this procedure for the presence of polyps, an intestinal mass, diverticuli, an intestinal structure/obstruction, or ulcerations. Barium sulfate (single contrast) or barium sulfate and air (double contrast) is given slowly through a rectal tube into the large colon. The filling process is monitored by fluoroscopy, then x-rays are taken. The colon must be free of fecal material so that the barium will outline the large intestine. This test is contraindicated if client has severe ulcerative colitis, suspected perforation, or tachycardia.

PREPARATION

Consent form	Not usually required
Food and fluids	Check with your x-ray department. Usually, clear liquid diet

PREPARATION *Continued*

	18–24 hr pre-test. NPO after dinner. Encourage fluid intake for 24 hr pre-test.
Premedications	Castor oil (2 oz) or magnesium citrate (10–12 oz) between 4 and 8 p.m. evening before
Bowel or bladder prep	Cleansing enema or laxative suppository such as bisacodyl (Dulcolax) may be ordered noc before test; saline enemas till clear (maximum of three) 6 a.m. of test.
Length of test	½–1 hr
Other	Thoroughly explain procedure to client; give written instructions. Notify doctor if client has severe abdominal cramps or pain before test. Abdominal x-rays, ultrasound studies, radionuclide scans, and proctosigmoidoscopy should be done before the barium enema.

POST-TEST

Vital signs	Per hospital routine
Assess for, and report if present	Abdominal cramps, lack of stools
Medications	A laxative, such as milk of magnesia or magnesium citrate or an oil retention enema should be given to help expel barium. May need to be repeated.
Food and fluids	Breakfast or lunch is given. Encourage fluid intake.
Bowels	Client should expel barium in the bathroom immediately after the test.
Other	Inform client that stools will be light in color for several days.

POST-TEST *Continued*

> Tell client to notify you or the physician if there is no stool within 2 or 3 days, as barium may cause fecal impaction.

Barium Swallow (Upper GI, Gastrointestinal Series, Small-Bowel Series)

An examination of the esophagus, stomach, and small intestine for inflammation, ulcerations, hernias, and tumors. The client is given a barium meal orally (or a water-soluble contrast agent such as diatrizoate meglumine [Gastrografin]) and the barium is observed as it passes through the digestive tract by means of fluoroscopy.

PREPARATION

Consent form	Usually not required
Food and fluids	NPO and no smoking 8–12 hr pre-test. A low-residue diet is ordered for 2–3 days pre-test.
Medications to be withheld	Held noc before or notify radiologist. Narcotic and anticholinergic drugs are withheld for 24 hr to avoid intestinal immobility.
Premedications	No
Bowel or bladder prep	Laxatives may be ordered the night before the test.
Length of test	1–2 hr; 4–6 hr if bowel series is included. Follow-up film (24 hr post-test) may be ordered.
Other	Explain that the client swallows a chalk-flavored (chocolate, strawberry) barium meal or

PREPARATION *Continued*

	meglumine diatrizoate (Gastrofin) in calculated amounts (16–20 oz). Record vitals. Note any epigastric pain.

POST-TEST

Vital signs	Per hospital routine
Assess for, and report if present	Epigastric pain or discomfort
Food and fluids	Give late breakfast or lunch after checking with x-ray department to make sure films are complete. Increase fluid intake 24–48 hr after the test unless contraindicated.
Bowels	Administer ordered laxative (e.g., milk of magnesia).
Other	Inform client that stools will be light in color for several days. Tell client to notify you or the physician if there is no stool within 2 or 3 days, as barium may cause fecal impaction.

4-4 SCANS

Nuclear Scanning

Radioactive isotopes, sometimes called radionuclides, are substances that emit small amounts of energy. In the nuclear medicine department, rectilinear scanners, or scintillation (gamma) camera detectors can record the images they make in the body on x-ray film. The substances concentrate heavily in areas of hyperfunction (forming a "hot" spot) and less so in areas of hypofunction (showing a "cold" spot) on film. Tumors, masses, obstructions, emboli, scar tissue, and other abnormalities can be detected safely and painlessly with nuclear scanning. Because the dosages for diagnostic work are low, the precautionary measures required for radium therapy are not necessary.

- Adhere to instructions from the nuclear medicine laboratory concerning the client and the procedure. The client should arrive on time.

- Obtain written consent if required in your institution. Usually a consent form is not needed unless the radionuclide is > 30 mCi.

- Inform the client that the injected radionuclide will not affect family, visitors, other clients, or hospital staff members. The dose of radiation is usually less than the amount of radiation received from diagnostic x-ray. The radionuclide is excreted from the body in about 6–24 hr.

- Adhere to instructions from the nuclear medicine lab as to specified times to return to the lab. Refer to Table 4-2 for preparations for specific nuclear scans and imaging times.

- Obtain a brief health history in regard to recent exposure to radioisotopes, allergies that could cause an adverse reaction, pregnancy, breastfeeding, and drugs.

- Instruct client to remove jewelry or any metal object.

- List restricted drugs containing iodine that the client is taking on the request slip. This is important if the radionuclide is iodine.

Computerized Axial Tomography (CT or CAT Scan)

The CT scanner produces a narrow x-ray beam that examines body sections from many different angles. A computer then solves multiple simultaneous equations to determine x-ray absorption at different points. In this way a three-dimensional picture of the structure being studied is obtained.

CT is used for scanning the head, abdomen (stomach, small and large intestines, liver, spleen, pancreas, bile duct, kidney, and adrenals), pelvic (bladder, reproductive organs, and small and large bowel within pelvis), and chest (lung,

TABLE 4–2. PREPARATIONS FOR RADIONUCLIDE SCANNING TESTS (NUCLEAR MEDICINE)

SCAN	PURPOSE	CLIENT PREPARATION	LENGTH OF SCAN
Bone	To diagnose metastatic bone disease, osteomyelitis, and fractures	Encourage fluids (6–8 glasses of water) and frequent voiding during the 3 hr after injection	About 1 hr. Views are taken 2–3 hr after injection
Brain	To detect an intracranial mass or disorder: tumors, abscesses, cancer metastasis to the brain, head trauma (subdural hematoma)	No food/fluid restrictions. 10 gtts. of Lugol's solution are given the night before or 1 hr before the scan, or potassium perchlorate 200 mg to 1 g given 1–3 hr before the scan	45 min–1 hr
Heart	To identify cardiac hypertrophy (cardiomegaly)	NPO may be required from midnight to study	15–30 min imaging for a myocardial infarction and 1 hr during the imaging for ischemic heart disease
Kidney	To detect renal dysfunction, transplant rejection, renovascular hypertension, or hydronephrosis	Check MD's orders to see if antihypertensives such as captopril (Capoten) enalapril (Vasotec), or other medications should be held. Client should be well-hydrated	About 1 hr
Liver and Spleen	To diagnose tumors or traumatic injuries of the liver or spleen	NPO after midnight may be ordered. Scan cannot usually be done within 48–72 hr of barium studies.	About 1 hr
Lung	To diagnose pulmonary embolism; to assess pulmonary status before surgery	A chest x-ray will be needed for comparison with the scanning result and can be done before or after the scan. Pain or dyspnea could make lying on the scanning table difficult; client may sit for parts of test.	1–1½ hr depending on the client's ability to cooperate

TABLE 4–2. PREPARATIONS FOR RADIONUCLIDE SCANNING TESTS (NUCLEAR MEDICINE) *Continued*

SCAN	PURPOSE	CLIENT PREPARATION	LENGTH OF SCAN
Thyroid	To diagnose thyroid nodules, abnormal thyroid function, and thyroid cancer	Instruct the client not to take any iodine compounds or eat any foods containing iodine 3 days before test. NPO 8 hrs prior to test if radioactive tracer is given po. Thyroid and antithyroid drugs and x-ray contrast mediums will also interfere with the test. Iodine preparations, thyroid hormones, phenothiazines, corticosteroid, aspirin, sodium nitroprusside, cough syrups containing iodides, and multivitamins are usually discontinued. Check with MD.	If an iodine scan or uptake has been requested, the client will have to return 24 hr after the initial scan.

Data from Kee JL. Laboratory and diagnostic tests with nursing implications. 2nd ed. Norwalk, CT: Century-Crofts, 1990.

heart, mediastinal structure). Iodized contrast dye is used in some cases and not in others.

PREPARATION FOR ALL CT SCANS

- Obtain signed consent if required in your facility.

- Client may be required to be NPO for 4–8 hr pre-test if contrast dye is used. Check with physician. Full liquid breakfast may be allowed if test is scheduled for p.m.

- Check for allergies to iodine, radiopaque contrast dye and shellfish. If allergies exist, test is contraindicated. Alternatively, the client may be given steroids or antihistamines several days before the test or IV during the scan.

- IV infusion or heparin lock may be required before test.

- If contrast dye is injected IV, inform clients that they may experience a warm, flushed sensation in the face or body, and/or a salty or metallic taste in the mouth. Nausea is not uncommon. Sensations may last for perhaps 1–2 min.

- Inform client that test is not painful, however lying motionless is required.

- Test usually takes 30 min to 1½ hr.

BODY SCAN

- Remove jewelry, snaps, and other radiopaque objects.

- Inform the client of the necessity of lying motionless during the scan, fully explaining the procedure including IV and contrast dye if used.

- CT scan is contraindicated in client who is unable to lie motionless, or is allergic to iodine.

BRAIN SCAN (CEREBRAL SCAN)

- Remove hairpins, clips, jewelry and earrings before test.

- A mild sedative or analgesic may be ordered for restless clients or for those who have aches and pains of the neck and back. Client must lie motionless.

- Explain to client that the head is positioned in a cradle, and immobilized with a rubberized strap during the test.

- CT of the head takes 30 min without contrast media and 1–1½ hr with the use of contrast.

CHEST CT

- A chest x-ray may be required before test.

- IV contrast media is given frequently in the left arm.

ABDOMINAL AND PELVIC CT

- Oral contrast dye is needed to outline stomach and bowel.
- Client may drink fluids prior to test.

SPINE CT

- Contrast media is not usually required.
- CT of spine may be done post-myelography.
- NPO status is not usually required.
- Spinal x-rays taken prior to CT scan should be available.

POST-TEST CARE FOR ALL CT SCANS

- Observe for signs and symptoms of a severe allergic reaction to the dye (i.e. dyspnea, tachycardia, hypotension, palpitations, itching, urticaria). Keep emergency drugs and equipment readily available.
- Observe for delayed allergic reaction to the contrast dye (i.e., skin rash, urticaria, headache, and vomiting). An oral antihistamine may be ordered for mild reactions.
- Client may resume pre-test level of activity and diet unless contraindicated.

MRI Scan (Magnetic Resonance Imaging)

A noninvasive procedure that uses magnetism and radio waves to make images of cross sections of the body. Physicians can distinguish normal, cancerous, atherosclerotic, and damaged tissue masses in these images. Since MRI was first introduced in 1983 for tissue visualization, the imaging quality has greatly improved. There is no risk of radiation, the procedure is painless and there are no known side effects. The Food and Drug Administration has classified MRI into class II, which includes low risk devices.

PREPARATION

- No metal must enter the chamber. Have clients remove jewelry, clothing with metal fasteners, glasses, hair clips, etc. Client with metal prostheses such as heart valves, surgical clips, orthopedic screws, cardiac pacemakers, neurologic aneurysm clips, or intraocular metal foreign bodies (i.e. shrapnel), cannot undergo MRI.

- Inform the MRI technician if the client is pregnant, as the test should not be done in this case unless absolutely necessary.

- Prepare client psychologically, as the equipment for this test is overwhelming. Explain that the machine looks like a narrow tunnel with a pallet that slides in and out of the core. The client will lie flat on the pallet with a clear plastic cylinder around his/her head if a head scan is being done. The client enters the tunnel head first.

- Instruct client to lie completely still throughout the test. Suggest closing the eyes and pretending to be lying in a meadow or on the beach.

- There will be muffled drumbeat noises during the test.

- If excessive anxiety is present, a sedative may be ordered without compromising test results.

- Have client void

- Length of test: 15–90 min

POST-TEST

- Routine vitals

- Pre-test activities may be resumed unless contraindicated

Positron-Emission Tomography (PET Scan)

The PET scanner makes images showing the metabolic activity (glucose metabolism) in cross sections of the brain.

Before the test, the client is infused with radioactive oxyglucose, a substance the body uses as if it were glucose. The oxyglucose emits radioactivity in the form of positrons, which are picked up and transformed into visual images by a computer. Researchers are using PET scans to study stroke, epilepsy, migraine headaches, metabolic brain disorders such as Parkinson's disease, the chemistry of nerve transmission of the brain, schizophrenia, Alzheimer's disease, depression, and cranial tumors.

PREPARATION

- Consent form is often required.

- The client must not drink large quantities of fluid or caffeine-containing beverages within 2 hr of test.

- Inform the client of the necessity to lie motionless in an enclosed space for 1–3 hr. A cassette tape to listen to during the study may be helpful.

- Have client eat a meal 3–4 hr before test. Diabetic clients should take their final dose of long-lasting insulin before this meal.

- Thoroughly prepare client for this test as excessive anxiety can ruin the results. Sedatives may not be used, as they interfere with test results.

- Explain:

  - The client will relax in a supine position on the scanning table. Two IVs are usually started. A radioisotope will be infused in one IV and the other will be used to draw blood samples. The client will be asked to follow directions very carefully from this point. The physicians will use blood samples to compare the radioisotopes and blood gas levels in the client's blood to the pictures of activity in the brain.

  - Client must remain motionless throughout the study, and may be blindfolded so that sensory stimuli will be limited.

- Warn client not to stand up too suddenly after the test, as postural hypotension can result.

- Encourage client to increase fluids soon after the test in order to clear the radioactive isotope from the bladder.

4-5 BREAST EXAMS

Thermography

Thermography (mammothermography) is an infrared photographic test usually used for detection of cancerous lesions in the breast, abscesses, and fibrocystic disease. An advantage of it is that it does not expose the client to radiation. Because it is accurate only 80% of the time, however, it is used mainly for screening purposes in diagnosing lesions of the breast. It must always be used in conjunction with other clinical examinations. It should not be performed if the client is pregnant or menstruating.

PREPARATION

- Obtain menstrual history. If the client is pregnant, menstruating, or close to her period, she should not have the test, as vascularity of the breasts increases at these times.

- Instruct the client

  - Avoid smoking 4–6 hr pre-test, avoid very hot or very cold drinks immediately pre-test

  - Remove jewelry and metal

  - Remove ointments or powders on the breasts

  - Wear gown with opening in the front

  - Client will be asked to sit in a cool room (68°F) for 10–15 min before the test to equalize body temperature.

  - Client's hands will be place over her head or on her hips while photos are being taken.

  - Length of test: usually 10–15 min

Mammography (Mammogram)

A soft tissue radiographic examination of the breast used to detect breast masses, tumors, calcifications, fibrocysts, or cancer. Women age 40 and over should have a screening mammogram annually, according to American Cancer Society Guidelines.

PREPARATION

Consent form	Yes
Length of test	20 min
Other	Instruct client not to use talcum powder prior to the test, and that the procedure may cause minor discomfort.

POST-TEST

	Inform the client that results must be interpreted by a radiologist.

4-6 ULTRASONOGRAPHY (ECHOGRAPHY)

With ultrasound, body structures can be visualized on film without the use of x-rays. Sound waves introduced via a transducer are reflected or "echoed" off tissues and recorded on oscilloscope. Polaroid film, and/or videotape.

Ultrasound examinations are fast, relatively inexpensive and not known to cause any physical harm to the client. Sometimes a more invasive procedure (CT scan, radionuclide scanning, or radiographic procedure with contrast dye) may be ordered to confirm abnormal sonographic results. Sonography is safe even in pregnancy.

1. Ultrasound of the *brain* is also called *echoencephalography*. It is used for quickly checking the brain midline and ventricles.

2. Ultrasound of the *heart,* also called *echocardiography,* is a safe way to evaluate the size, shape, and position of the heart and also movement in the valves and the chambers.

3. *Abdominal aneurysms* can be detected with 98% accuracy with *sonography of the abdominal aorta.*

The umbilicus is used as a midpoint, so U + 7 cm would mean 7 cm above the umbilicus.

4. *Doppler ultrasonography* evaluates the *major arteries* of the *arms* and *legs* for blood flow. Deep-vein thrombosis or partial arterial occlusion can be detected.

5. *Abdominal ultrasonography* can include examination of the gallbladder, kidneys, liver, pancreas, spleen, and pelvic structures.

PREPARATION

- Length of test: up to 1 hr

- Food and drink restrictions will vary for abdominal aorta, Doppler, heart, kidney, obstetric (pelvic) and thyroid ultrasound studies.

- Abdominal ultrasonography (gallbladder, liver, pancreas, spleen): the client must be NPO for 8–12 hr before the test. Clients having a gallbladder sonogram should eat a fat-free meal the evening before the test.

- Obstetric and pelvic ultrasonography: instruct the client to drink 3–4 glasses of water and postpone voiding until after the test. Bladder must be full.

- Remove dressings at the site of the ultrasound; if dressing cannot be removed, note it on the request slip.

POST-TEST

- After ultrasound, cleanse remaining lubricant from the skin.

4-7 ELECTROGRAPHIC PROCEDURES

Electrographic procedures use electrodes to measure electrical activity of the brain (EEG), the heart (ECG), or skeletal muscles (EMG), in order to evaluate function.

Electroencephalogram (EEG)

Electrodes are applied to the scalp at predetermined measured positions and the brain-wave activity is measured on moving paper. In this way, neoplasms, seizure disorders, cerebrovascular accidents, head trauma, nervous system infections, Alzheimer's disease, dementia, and brain death can be detected. This test may be performed while the client is awake, drowsy, asleep, undergoing stimuli such as flashing bright lights or in more than one of these different ways.

PREPARATION

- Length of test: approximately 1½–2 hr

- Thoroughly explain procedure to client and give reassurance if needed that there is no electrical danger.

- Wash the client's hair the evening before the test and avoid any hair additives, as oil or cosmetics can affect results.

- If a sleep EEG is ordered, limit the client's sleep to 4–5 hr the night before the test.

- Withhold medications as ordered. Medications that could affect results are usually withheld for 5 hr pretest (e.g., anticonvulsants, barbituates, tranquilizers, sedatives).

- A meal should be eaten before the test, as hypoglycemia could affect results, but have client avoid coffee, teas, colas, and alcohol 5 hr before the test.

- The client will have up to 25 electrodes attached to a cap placed on the scalp while in a comfortable position. Client may then be asked to follow several commands, which may include opening and closing the eyes, blinking, swallowing, hyperventilating, or responding to bright lights.

POST-TEST

- After the test, check with the neurologist about resuming medications that were withheld.

- Remove the paste from the client's head with acetone or by washing the client's hair.

- Unless sedated, the client can resume former activities.

Electrocardiogram (ECG, EKG, Cardiogram)

The electrocardiogram records electrical activity of the myocardium. Electrodes are placed on both legs, both arms, and the chest (see Fig. 4-1 for placement). The standard ECG consists of 12 leads: 6 limb leads (I, II, III, aVF, aVL, and aVR) and 6 chest (precordial) leads (V_1, V_2, V_3, V_4, V_5, and V_6). The conduction system is usually as follows: the SA node (sinoatrial or sinus node) sends an electrical impulse through the atrium, causes atrial contraction (atrial depolarization), the impulse travels to the AV (atrioventricular) node and the bundle of His and travels down the ventricles, causing ventricular contraction (ventricular depolarization). Repolarization and recovery occur when the atria and the ventricles relax.

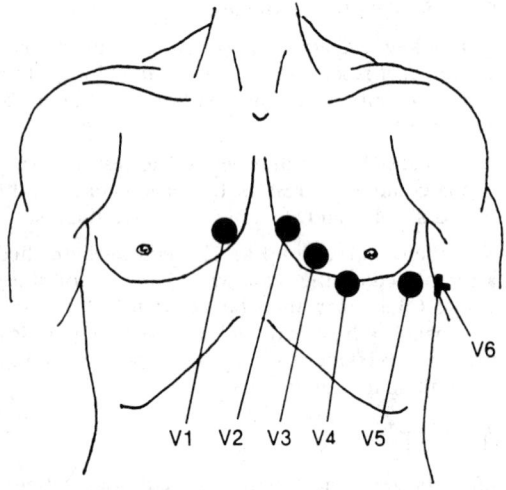

Figure 4–1. Anatomical placement for precordial chest leads for an electrocardiogram. (From Johnson R. Swartz MH. A simplified approach to electrocardiography. Philadelphia: Saunders, 1986;15. Reprinted wtih permission.)

The P wave records atrial depolarization. The QRS complex reflects ventricular depolarization and the ST segment, T wave, and U wave record ventricular repolarization. A normal ECG means that cardiac electrical conduction is normal, but the client could still have heart disease, which involves other problems.

PREPARATION

- Explain purpose and procedure. Food and drink are not restricted. The procedure is painless.

- Length of test: 15 min

- Record all medications the client is taking. Knowing the drugs the client is on may help the physician determine improvement and changes from previous ECG readings.

- Instruct the client to relax and breathe normally and lie still during the test. As body movement and electromagnetic interference can distort the tracing, tell client not to tighten muscles, grasp bed rails, or talk during the tracing.

- As electrodes must be placed directly on the skin, ask client to remove nylon stockings and clothing from the waist up. Give female clients a gown.

- Assist client to supine position.

- Strap electropads with electropaste to the four extremities. Insert color-coded lead wires into the correct electrodes (e.g., white, right arm, etc). Attach chest leads (see Fig. 4-1).

- Tell the client to inform you of any chest pain during the procedure. Mark the ECG tracing at the time the client has chest pain if it occurs and report to MD.

- After the tracing, remove the electropaste or jelly, and cleanse the electrode disks with alcohol.

Electromyogram (EMG)

In this procedure, needle electrodes are inserted into the skeletal muscles so that electrical activity can be heard over a loudspeaker, viewed on an oscilloscope, and recorded on paper all at the same time. Normally, there is no electrical activity when the muscle is at rest, but in neuro-muscular disorders, abnormal patterns can be observed. The EMG can be in two parts, with both nerves and muscles studied. In this way, neuropathy and myopathy can be differentiated.

The procedure is not painful except there may be temporary discomfort when the needles are inserted. The client should tell the technician if the discomfort persists.

PREPARATION AND POST-TEST

- Make sure consent form is signed.

- Food and drinks are not restricted, with the exception of coffee, tea, colas, other caffeine drinks, alcohol, and tobacco 3 hr pre-test.

- Check with MD about withholding medications that could affect results—muscle relaxants, cholinergics, anticholinergics. Record these on requisition slip.

- Draw blood for serum enzymes prior to the test if ordered.

- Instruct client to follow technician's instructions carefully—relax muscles at the directed times.

- An analgesic is sometimes ordered.

- Length of test: usually 1 hr or longer

4-8 ENDOSCOPIC PROCEDURES

Endoscopy uses a lighted tube to visualize the inside of body cavities. Some of these procedures are performed under a general anesthetic. More often local anesthetic is used (proctoscopy is frequently done on an outpatient basis). Most clients find the intrusion of a lighted tube into the body a traumatic experience. Emotional support and thorough examination of purpose and procedure are essential.

When a client goes for an endoscopic procedure, the preparation is similar to preparation for surgery. Indeed, some minor surgical procedures are frequently performed during endoscopy such as the removal of polyps or the removal of tissue for biopsy. If your client is undergoing general anesthesia, complete a pre-operative checklist such as Table 10-3 prior to the test, in addition to specific preparations listed in the following pages. Complete Table 4-1, Checklist for Diagnostic Procedures, emphasizing thorough client teaching if local anesthetic will be used.

The major complications of endoscopy are perforation and hemorrhaging. The signs may develop immediately post-test or after a period of hours. Pain, abdominal distention, hypotension, or bleeding should be reported to the physician immediately.

Bronchoscopy

The direct inspection of the larynx, trachea, and bronchi through a metal bronchoscope or a flexible fiberoptic bronchoscope called a bronchofibroscope. A catheter can be inserted through the bronchoscope so that specimens can be collected from the tracheobronchial tree.

PREPARATION

Consent form	Yes, also pre-op checklist
Food and fluids	NPO 6 hr pre-test or 8–12 hr if having general anesthesia
Premedications	As ordered. Atropine is frequently ordered to dry secretions.
Bowel or bladder prep	Void and relax before premedications.
Length of test	1 hr
Other	Oral hygiene before the test is important. Remove dentures, jewelry, contact lenses. Instruct client to practice breathing in and out through the nose with the mouth open. Take baseline vitals, prepare vital-signs flow chart. There may be hoarseness and/or a sore throat after the test.

POST-TEST

Vital signs	BP, pulse, respirations q 15 min × 4, q 30 min × 4, q 1 hr × 4, temp. q 4 hr × 24 hr
Activity	Elevate head of bed to semi-Fowler's position. If the client is unconscious, turn head to the side.
Assess for, and report if present	Laryngeal edema, dyspnea, hoarseness, bronchospasms, pneumothorax, cardiac arrhythmias, bleeding from biopsy site, shortness of breath, excessive hemoptysis (client may have some blood-tinged sputum, which is normal, but report it if excessive).
Food and fluids	Start with ice chips, when gag reflex is present (usually takes 2–8 hr). Test gag reflex by touching posterior pharynx with a tongue blade or sterile swab.
Medications	Offer throat lozenges.
Other	No smoking for at least 6–8 hr, as it may cause coughing and bleeding. Have emergency suction equipment for oral and nasal airways and tracheostomy tray at bedside.

Colonoscopy

A long flexible fiberscope (colonoscope) is inserted anally and advanced with extreme caution through the rectum, the sigmoid colon, and the large intestine to the cecum. The origin of lower intestinal bleeding, diverticular disease, ulcerative colitis, polyps, or tumors can be diagnosed. Polyps are often removed with the use of an electrocautery snare, thus avoiding surgery. This test is contraindicated in near-term pregnancy, after recent abdominal surgery, after acute myocardial infarction, in severe active ulcerative colitis, or in a confused/uncooperative client. It is not recommended within 2 wk of a barium study. Procedure may vary in different institutions.

PREPARATION

Consent form	Yes
Food and fluids	Clear liquid diet 2–3 days pretest; NPO 8 hr pretest
Premedications	A sedative/tranquilizer and/or narcotic may be ordered to promote relaxation.
Bowel or bladder prep	Laxative given (castor oil or magnesium citrate) the noc before the test. Warm water or saline enemas until returning fluid is clear (maximum of 3) in the morning. If Golytely is used, follow those instructions.
Length of test	½–1½ hr
Other	Lab work (hemoglobin, hematocrit, prothrombin time, partial thromboplastin time, platelet count) should be done 2 days before, and results should be on the chart. Explain procedure thoroughly. Client will be in Sim's position on left side. Encourage relaxation and deep breathing when colonoscope is inserted.

POST-TEST

Vital signs	q ½ hr × 4, q 1 hr × 4, or until stable
Assess for, and report if present	Excessive anal bleeding, abdominal hemorrhage, severe cramps, purulent rectal drainage, or fever must be reported immediately. Perforation is a rare but serious complication. Check for abdominal distention.

POST-TEST *Continued*

Activity	Bed rest 2–8 hr post-test
Food and fluids	Resume normal diet
Other	Inform the client that flatus may be a result of air insertion and that minor amounts of blood in the stool are expected after polyp removal.

Colposcopy

Examination of the vagina and cervix using a binocular instrument (colposcope), which has a magnifying lens and a light. This procedure is done when the result of a client's Pap smear has been positive or there is other reason to suspect a cervical lesion. Typical epithelium, leukoplakia vulvae, and irregular blood vessels can be identified and a biopsy specimen can be taken.

PREPARATION

Consent form	Yes
Food and fluids	No restrictions
Premedications	None
Length of test	15–20 min
Other	Inform client that she should not experience any pain. Test is performed in lithotomy position (legs in stirrups).

POST-TEST

Vital signs	Routine
Assess for, and report if present	Excessive bleeding from biopsy site
Other	Inform client that she may have some bleeding for a few hours because of the biopsy. She may use tampons. But if bleeding be-

POST-TEST *Continued*

comes heavy and it is not her
menstrual cycle, it should be reported immediately. No sexual
intercourse for a week or so until biopsy is healed.

Cystoscopy

The direct visualization of the bladder wall and urethra
is accomplished with the use of a cystoscope (a tubular
lighted telescopic lens). Tissue samples can be obtained
and small renal calculi can be removed from the ureter,
bladder, or urethra. This test is also indicated to determine
the cause of hematuria or the cause of urinary infection.
Usually performed by a urologist, a retrograde pyelography
may also be performed during the cystoscopy. Local or general anesthesia may be used.

PREPARATION

Consent form	Yes. Pre-op checklist if general anesthesia
Food and fluids	Full liquid breakfast the morning of test if local anesthetic is used; for general anesthetic, NPO 8 hr pre-test
Premedications	A narcotic analgesic 1 hr before test; sometimes 3-4 glasses of water are given before test.
Length of test	½–1 hr
Other	Record baseline vitals. Inform client whether anesthesia is local or general. There should be little or no discomfort. Test is per- formed in lithotomy position (legs in stirrups). Obtain history concerning presence of cystitis or prostatitis which could result in sepsis following the proce- dure.

POST-TEST

Vital signs	BP, pulse, respirations q 15 min × 4, q 30 × 2, q 1 hr × 4; temp. q 4 hr while awake, for several days
Assess for, and report if present	Complications: hemorrhaging, perforation of the bladder, urinary retention. Anuria may indicate blood clots. Report gross hematuria immediately (blood-tinged urine is not uncommon post-test). Report signs of infection (fever, chills, increased pulse rate, pain).
Food and fluids	Monitor intake and output for 48 hr post-test. Encourage fluid intake if output is <200 ml/hr.
Medications	Analgesic may be ordered. Antibiotics may be given prophylactically.
Other	Inform client that a slight burning sensation when voiding is considered normal, but increased fluid intake will help to decrease dysuria. Apply heat to lower abdomen to relieve pain and spasm as ordered. A warm sitz bath may be therapeutic.

Gastroscopy (Esophagoscopy, Duodenoscopy, Endoscopy)

This test allows the MD to visualize the lumen of the upper GI tract. Esophagitis, hiatal hernia, esophageal varices, esophageal stenoses, achalasia, gastritis, ulcers, neoplasms, diverticula, duodenal ulcer, and other problems can be visualized directly. This test is performed under local anesthesia in a gastroscopic room of the hospital or clinic. If the esophagus, the stomach, and the duodenum are included in the endoscopic examination, the procedure is called esophagogastroduodenoscopy. A camera can be attached to the fiberoptic endoscope, and suction may be applied for the removal of secretions and foreign bodies. Main complications are perforation and hemorrhage.

PREPARATION

Consent form	Yes. Also complete Table 4-1.
Food and fluids	NPO 8–12 hr pre-test; Gastric lavage performed in an emergency
Premedications	Sedative/tranquilizer, narcotic analgesic 1 hr before test; can be titrated IV
Length of test	1 hr or less
Other	Remove dentures, jewelry, and clothing from neck to waist. Explain procedure, ie. that throat will be sprayed with anesthetic. Take baseline vitals. Keep emergency drugs and equipment available for severe laryngospasm or reaction to drugs or anesthetic.

POST-TEST

Vital signs	BP, pulse, respirations q 15 min × 4, q 30 min × 4, q 1 hr × 4; temp. q 4 hr while awake for 48 hr
Assess for, and report if present	Complications: hemorrhaging, perforation of the GI tract—pain, dyspnea, fever, tachycardia, subcutaneous emphysema in the neck
Food and fluids	NPO 2–4 hr post-test. Check gag reflex before offering food and fluids by touching posterior pharynx with a tongue blade.

POST-TEST *Continued*

Medications	Offer throat lozenges.
Other	Inform client of possible flatus or "burp-up gas," which is normal (air is instilled during the procedure). Client should not drive for 12 hr post test due to anesthetic.

Laparoscopy

The direct inspection of the surfaces of the internal organs such as the liver, uterus, gallbladder, pancreas, and lymph nodes by use of a lighted scope-type instrument inserted into the abdominal cavity. Used to diagnose ascites, biopsy, cholangiography, cirrhosis, dysmenorrhea, ectopic pregnancy, endometritis, fever of undetermined origin, gallbladder disease, infertility, jaundice, lymphoma staging, malignancy staging, pancreatic disease, and pelvic inflammatory disease (PID).

PREPARATION

Consent form	Yes
Food and fluids	NPO for 12 hr pre-test
Premedications	Anesthesia may be given.
Bowel or bladder prep	Cleansing enema 4 hr before test. Void before test.
Length of test	30 min
Other	Assess for allergies before tests. Prepare surgical site with a shave. Bandage inguinal and umbilical hernias.

POST-TEST

Vital signs	BP, pulse and respirations q 15 min × 4, q 30 min × 4, q 1 hr × 4
Activity	Rest as tolerated.

POST-TEST *Continued*

Assess for, and report if present	Signs of infection in surgical incision area for 24 hr. Hemorrhage, nausea, puncture of the intestinal loop, and subcutaneous emphysema

Proctoscopy (Proctosigmoidoscopy, Sigmoidoscopy)

This is examination of the anus, rectum, and sigmoid colon with a proctoscope, or a sigmoidoscope. It is indicated when there are changes in bowel habits, chronic constipation, bright blood or mucus in the stool or as part of the annual physical examination in clients over 40 yr old.

PREPARATION

Consent form	Yes
Food and fluids	Light dinner, light breakfast or NPO 8 hr pre-test. Heavy meals, vegetables and fruits should be avoided within 24 hr of the test.
Premedications	Client may take prescribed medications by 6 a.m. the morning of the test with MD's permission.
Bowel or bladder prep	A saline, warm tap water, or Fleet enema the a.m. of test; bisacodyl (Dulcolax) given if enemas are contraindicated. If Golytely Prep is used, follow instructions carefully.
Length of test	15–30 min
Other	If client has had barium study within 3 days, notify MD. Client will be in Sim's position or knee-chest position. Instruct client to breathe deeply when scope is inserted. Take baseline vitals. Have equipment for specimen collection ready: culture tubes, slides

PREPARATION *Continued*

	with jar containing 95% ethyl alcohol, and a jar with 10% formalin.

POST-TEST

Vital signs	As ordered or q 30 min × 4, at least
Assess for, and report if present	Signs of bowel perforation: pain, abdominal distention, shock-like symptoms; report immediately
Activity	Encourage client to rest for several hours post-test.
Other	Be particularly supportive.

4-9 PROCEDURES OF BIOPSY OR ASPIRATION

These procedures are similar in that in all cases specimens are obtained using sterile technique and local anesthetics. Nurses assist the physician in preparing the client, organizing the necessary equipment, supporting the client during the procedure, and assessing for complications afterward. These procedures are usually completed at the bedside.

Nursing interventions are similar for all these tests. Important variations are in the equipment to be assembled, positioning of the client and potential problems to assess for during and after the procedure. Be particularly supportive when clients must undergo these tests as they can be frightening. Complete the checklist found in Table 4-3 when assisting with any of these procedures.

Thoracentesis

The aspiration of fluid or air from the pleural space for diagnostic or therapeutic purposes. Therapeutically, it may be used to relieve lung compression and prevent or treat infection. Fluid is aspirated (≤1200 ml) slowly with a 50-

ml syringe. Lab tests performed on the fluid may include specific gravity, white-cell count, red-cell count, protein concentration, glucose concentration, amylase content, and culture and sensitivity.

PROCEDURE

- Complete the checklist found in Table 4-3.

- Assess for any bleeding disorder, as this must be corrected before thoracentesis is performed.

- Equipment needed:

  > Sterile thoracentesis tray
  > Sterile gloves
  > Local anesthetics (procaine hydrochloride or Novocaine 1%)
  > Skin prep tray with antiseptic
  > Pail or drainage tube and bag
  > Hospital drape, towels
  > Collection bottles with heparin
  > Sterile dressing for puncture site—4 × 4 gauze pads, tape, povidone, iodine

- Positioning: The client should be in an upright position, sitting comfortably, leaning slightly forward, with arms elevated on a pillow or a bedside stand.

- Physically support the client when the physician inserts the needle.

- Afterward, take vitals q 15 min × 4, q 1 hr × 4, then q 4 hr × 24 hr.

- Assess chest sounds with vital signs.

- Observe for:

  - Pneumothorax: a chest x-ray is usually ordered after this procedure. Watch for syncope, vertigo, dyspnea, tightness in the chest, uncontrollable cough, blood-tinged frothy mucus, or rapid pulse.

  - Infection: fever, pleuritic pain, purulent drainage, redness, and tenderness at puncture site

  - Fluid and electrolyte imbalances, hemorrhage, shock, cardiac distress

---

**TABLE 4–3. CHECKLIST FOR PROCEDURES
OF BIOPSY OR ASPIRATION**

☐ Make sure the consent form is signed.

☐ Reinforce physician's explanation of what the procedure entails, the purpose, and what is expected of the client. Explain importance of remaining immobile during aspiration.

☐ Take a history of allergy to local anesthetics and other drugs, document it on the chart, and notify the physician.

☐ Order equipment and assemble it at bedside (see specific procedures for variations in equipment).

☐ Have client void before the procedure.

☐ Take baseline vital signs.

☐ Help the client get into the appropriate position for the test (see specific procedures).

☐ Maintain sterile technique.

☐ Observe client carefully during procedure for signs of distress.

☐ Support emotionally. Perhaps distraction or deep breathing would be helpful if there is discomfort.

☐ Apply sterile pressure dressing to puncture site post test and assess for bleeding and crepitus q 5 minutes × 6.

☐ Assist with specimen collection and labeling. Send specimens to lab immediately.

☐ Position client correctly afterward and maintain bed rest if required.

☐ Assess frequently afterward for fluid and electrolyte status, emotional state, and signs of specific complications (see specific procedures).

Abdominal Paracentesis

Abdominal paracentesis is a procedure that removes excess acidic fluid from the abdomen via a puncture with a sterile needle through the abdominal wall. Therapeutically, it is done to release tense ascites causing respiratory embarrassment. Diagnostic procedures performed on the fluid include culture for bacteria, cytologic testing, cell counts, and determination of protein concentration.

PROCEDURE

- Complete the checklist found in Table 4-3.
- Equipment needed:

    Sterile paracentesis tray
    Sterile gloves
    1–2% lidocaine (xylocaine)
    Skin prep
    Pail or drainage bag
    Sterile towels and drapes
    Specimen bottles for lab
    Sterile dressing for puncture site
    Scultetus binder

- Positioning: either Fowler's position or sitting on edge of bed with feet and arms supported on overbed table
- Afterward, assist client to position of comfort and maintain bed rest
- Monitor vital signs for evidence of hemodynamic changes q 15 min × 4, q 1 hr × 4, then q 4 hr × 24 hr.
- Observe for:
    - Leakage from insertion site, subcutaneous emphysema, and scrotal edema
    - Fluid and electrolyte imbalances (hypovolemia): tachycardia, cool moist skin, postural hypotension, shock due to fluid shift. Albumin may be ordered to replace lost proteins.
    - Measure abdominal girth and weight
    - Infection (peritonitis): fever, abdominal pain, redness, purulent drainage at puncture site

Liver Biopsy

Percutaneous needle biopsy of the liver provides information about the cause, nature, activity, severity, and prognosis of liver disease. It should not be performed on clients with a prothrombin time elevated more than 3 sec above

control or in those with a platelet count of less than
50,000/μ. Hemorrhage is a major risk of this procedure as
the liver is a highly vascular organ.

PROCEDURE

- Complete the checklist found in Table 4-3.

- Check the chart to see that coagulation studies are
  complete and current within 24 hr—prothrombin
  time, partial thromboplastin time, platelet count,
  blood type, and cross match. Notify physician if there
  are abnormal results, as biopsy may be contraindicated in persons with coagulation defects, rigid
  pleural space infection, or ascites.

- Keep the client NPO in case surgery is indicated after
  the procedure.

- Equipment needed:

    Menghini needle, other needles per physician
    Stylex syringes 3 ml, 5 ml, 20 ml
    Scalpel with No. 11 stainless steel blade
    1% lidocaine
    Sterile gloves
    Skin prep
    Sterile towels and drapes
    Dressings—4 3 × 3's and bandage for puncture
        site
    Specimen tubes for culture, jar with formalin
    Extra pillow, sandbags

- Teach client breathing technique used in procedure:
  inhale, exhale, hold breath for 15 sec.

- Administer sedatives 30–60 min before procedure if
  ordered.

- Positioning: either supine or left lateral position with
  right arm abducted

- Support the client during the 10–15 sec the needle is
  inserted and the client holds breath.

- Apply pressure dressing over the puncture site after
  removal of the needle.

- Position client in a right lateral position with sandbags under the side to control bleeding.

- Instruct the client to maintain the position for 2 hr and bed rest for 12 hr or as physician instructs.

- Take vital signs frequently: q 15 min × 4, q 30 min × 2, then q 1 hr × 4, q 4 hr × 24.

- Observe for:

  - Pneumothorax: shortness of breath, chest pain, decreased breath sounds

  - Hemorrhage: blood-soaked dressings, tachycardia, diaphoresis, restlessness, pain, decreased BP

  - Infection (peritonitis): fever, abdominal pain, nausea, shortness of breath, tenderness, firm abdomen

  - Bradycardia and hypotension: transient effects due to vagal stimulation during biopsy which may be treated with atropine.

Bone-Marrow Aspiration

Because red and white blood cells and platelets are manufactured in the bone marrow, the aspiration of this tissue is diagnostic for most blood dyscrasias. The sites most commonly used are the sternum and the iliac crest. Marrow may also be aspirated from the tip of the lower thoracic or lumbar spinal process. Bone marrow aspiration is contraindicated in hemophilia, hemostasis, and coagulation defects.

PROCEDURE

- Complete the checklist found in Table 4-3.

- Equipment needed:

  Bone marrow aspiration tray, including aspiration needle with stylet
  Syringes
  Sterile gloves
  Local anesthetic (1% procaine or lidocaine)
  Skin prep
  Sterile towels, drapes

Dressings for puncture site
Specimen containers

- Check the chart to see if coagulation studies have been completed: prothrombin time, partial thromboplastin time, platelet count, and blood typing and cross match. Notify physician if there are abnormal results.

- Administer sedatives if ordered. Support emotionally. Notify physician if client seems particularly anxious.

- Positioning: Supine if sternum is used, on opposite side if iliac crest is used

- Instruct client to remain immobile. Inform him or her there may be momentary but sharp pain or deep pressure when marrow is aspirated.

- Apply pressure over puncture site until bleeding stops, then a sterile dressing.

- Position client comfortably. Keep on bed rest for 24 hr, or as instructed.

- Take vital signs frequently (q 15 min × 4, q 30 min × 2, q 1 hr × 4).

- Assess often for bleeding, infection, or other complications.

Synovial-Fluid Aspiration

The synovial fluid will appear yellow, cloudy, milky, greenish, bloody, or grayish if pathology is present. Normally, it appears straw-colored, clear, or slightly cloudy. Trauma, osteoarthritis, rheumatic fever, systemic lupus, gout, rheumatoid arthritis, tuberculosis, and sepsis are some conditions in which synovial-fluid examination is helpful in diagnosis.

PROCEDURE

- Complete the checklist found in Table 4-3.
- Administer ordered sedatives and/or analgesics.

- Equipment needed:

    Spinal needle
    Syringes
    Alcohol swabs
    Iodophore prep
    Sterile saline
    Sterile specimen containers—tubes for culture, cytology, clot, and glucose
    Required additives (check with laboratory—usually heparin or EDTA for cytology, potassium oxalate for glucose)

- After the procedure, support affected limb on a pillow. Maintain joint rest for 12 hr, or as directed.

- Apply ice to affected joint for 24–48 hr unless contraindicated.

- Observe for infection: redness, swelling, crepitation, fever, drainage, pain.

- Maintain appropriate isolation if infection is suspected.

Lumbar Puncture (Spinal Tap)

The aspiration of cerebrospinal fluid from the subarachnoid space is useful in the diagnosis of central nervous system infections (e.g., meningitis, syphilis), hemorrhage, increased intracranial pressure, and meningeal carcinomatosis. It is also used to administer anesthesia, reduce intracranial pressure in pseudotumor cerebri, and give medications in the treatment of intracranial infections or neoplasms.

PROCEDURE

- Complete the checklist found in Table 4-3.

- Assess neurologic status.

- Equipment needed:

    Lumbar puncture set
    Sterile gloves

1% Lidocaine hydrochloride, 2 ml
Skin prep
Sterile fenestrated drape, towels
4 culture tubes for specimen collection
Bandage for puncture site

- Positioning: Explain importance of client cooperation in positioning. The client is placed on the side with a pillow under the head. The knees are then brought up to the chest and the head is flexed as much as possible.

- Explain to client that the injection of the anesthetic may sting a little. During the procedure there may be some brief pain down the legs or a feeling of pressure, but it is normal. Emphasize the importance of maintaining the correct position.

- Communicate frequently during the procedure to lessen anxiety. Perhaps the client can focus on a pleasant image or on breathing.

- After applying sterile dressing to puncture site, return client to supine position with head flat.

- Instruct the client to lie no higher than at 30 degrees (head of bed elevation) for up to 8 hr to prevent headache.

- Transport proper labeled specimens to lab immediately, discarding first specimen as it is likely to be contaminated with blood.

- Take vital signs frequently—q 15 min × 4, q 30 min × 4, q 1 hr × 4.

- Assess for and report changes in neurologic status, respiratory difficulty, or changes in motor function. Assess puncture site for redness, swelling, or drainage every 4 hr × 24 hr.

REFERENCES

Chernecky CC, Krech RL, Berger B. Laboratory tests and diagnostic procedures. Philadelphia: W.B. Saunders, 1993.

Collier I, and Lewis S. Medical-surgical nursing: assessment and management of clinical problems. St. Louis: Mosby, 1992.

Corbett JV. Laboratory tests and diagnostic procedures with nursing diagnoses. Norwalk, CT: Appleton and Lange, 1992.

Kee JL. Handbook of laboratory and diagnostic tests with nursing implications. Norwalk, CT: Appleton and Lange, 1990.

Johnson R, Swartz MH. A simplifed approach to electrocardiography. Philadelphia: W.B. Saunders, 1986.

McDonagh A. Getting your patient ready for a nuclear medicine scan. Nursing '91; February: 53–57.

Pagana KD, and Pagana T. Diagnostic testing and nursing implications: a case study approach. St. Louis: Mosby, 1990.

CHAPTER 5

FLUID AND ELECTROLYTE BALANCE

5-1   **Normal Functions**

5-2   **Imbalances**

Because even mild or moderate illness can upset the mechanisms that regulate fluid balance, every client in the clinical setting is a potential candidate for imbalance. Every system in the body is involved in maintaining homeostasis. Whenever any system is impaired, the danger of imbalance exists. Help avoid life-threatening situations by being extra vigilant whenever a client is receiving IV therapy, is severely debilitated, has GI disturbances or kidney disease. Elderly clients are particularly at risk, as they have diminished fluid reserves. Help clients maintain stability by:

- Constant assessment of fluid and electrolyte status
- Providing or restricting appropriate fluids and electrolytes
- Careful observation and measurement of fluids ingested and excreted (intake and output)
- Accurately recording and reporting this information
- Teaching clients basic principles for maintaining balance

5-1   NORMAL FUNCTIONS

Body Fluids and Daily Requirements

Sixty percent of total body weight is water. Water is essential as a solvent and is required in virtually every chemical reaction in the body. Daily balance depends on an equal ratio between ingested and excreted fluids. An intake of approximately 2.6 liters is considered adequate for a 24 hr period, with 1500–2000 ml ingested orally if possible (Table 5-1). Individual requirements change in illness. For example, acute renal failure and inappropriate antidiuretic hormonal secretion are two cases where requirements may decrease. However, more commonly, requirements increase, such as in febrile states, poorly controlled diabetes, upper respiratory tract, and other infections.

INTRACELLULAR FLUID (ICF)

Two-thirds of body water is inside the cells. The intracellular fluid contains needed nutrients and is the environment for chemical reactions in the cells. The predominant electrolytes are potassium (K^+), magnesium (Mg^{++}), and phosphate ($HPO_4^=$).

EXTRACELLULAR FLUID (ECF)

One-third of body water is outside the cells in either the interstitium or plasma. The extracellular fluid functions as transporter of water (H_2O); oxygen (O_2); electrolytes; and nutrients to the cells. It also removes wastes such as carbon

TABLE 5–1. NORMAL FLUID BALANCE FOR AN ADULT IN A 24-HR PERIOD

INTAKE		OUTPUT	
Beverages	1200 ml	Urine	1500 ml
In food	1100 ml	Skin and lungs	1000 ml
Produced in	300 ml	(insensible)	
metabolism		In feces	100 ml
	2600 ml		2600 ml

dioxide (CO_2) and protein breakdown products. Enzymes, hormones, RBCs, and WBCs are also transported via the ECF. The predominant electrolytes are sodium (Na^+) and chloride (Cl^-).

Figure 5-1 shows fluid and solid proportions in total body weight.

TRANSCELLULAR FLUIDS

Joint fluid, aqueous humor, cartilage, and connective tissue fluids, intraocular fluid, bone, and cerebral spinal fluids are sometimes referred to as transcellular fluids. Their volumes are relatively small.

FLUID SPACING

Fluid spacing refers to how fluid is distributed in the body. *First* spacing means that there is a normal distribution of fluid in both the extracellular and intracellular compartments. *Second* spacing is an excess accumulation of interstitial fluid (edema). *Third* spacing is fluid accumulation in the interstitium in areas that normally have no fluid or a minimum amount of fluid. It occurs due to imbalance between osmotic and hydrostatic pressures of the vasculature

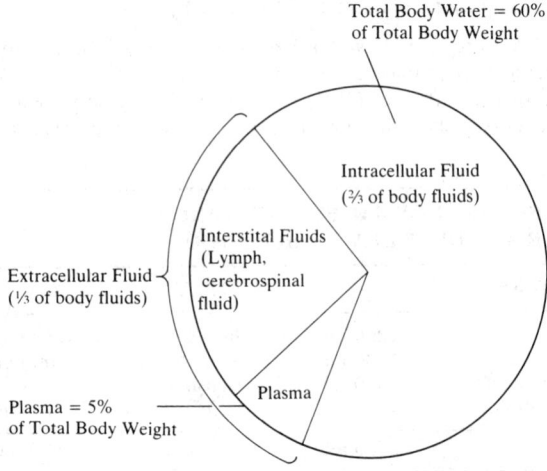

Figure 5–1. Approximate proportions of fluids in the body.

and interstitium. Some examples of third spacing are ascites, sequestration of fluid in the bowel with peritonitis, and edema associated with burns. Third spacing is problematic because fluid is shunted away from the normal fluid compartments, especially the vasculature, which may produce hypovolemia. Albumin or another colloid may be administered to try to pull fluids into the vessels through oncotic pressure, but this treatment is controversial.

Electrolytes

Electrolytes are substances that develop electrical charges when dissolved in water, as opposed to those such as proteins and glucose that do not. Positively charged ions are the cations: sodium (Na^+), potassium (K^+), calcium (Ca^{++}), and magnesium (Mg^{++}). Negatively charged ions are anions: chloride (Cl^-), bicarbonate (HCO_3^-) and phosphate ($HPO_4^=$). Cations and anions are balanced in each compartment, although the ICF and ECF have different compositions of water and electrolytes. The ECF contains a greater proportion of Na^+, Ca^{++}, and HCO_3^-, while the ICF has more K^+, Mg^{++}, and $HPO_4^=$.

Electrolytes hold fluid within compartments, help maintain the acid-base relationship essential for enzyme activities, aid in transmission of neuromuscular impulses, and facilitate protein and carbohydrate metabolism.

Normal values for serum electrolytes are expressed in milliequivalents per liter, which is a measure for comparing relative concentrations of ions in solution.

Sodium (Na^+)	135–145 mEq/liter
Chloride (Cl^+)	95–105 mEq/liter
Potassium (K^+)	3.5–5.0 m Eq/liter
Bicarbonate ($HCO3^-$)	20–30 m Eq/liter
Phosphate (PO_4^-)	0.8–1.4 mEq/liter
Calcium (Ca^{++})	4.5–5.5 mEq/liter
Magnesium (Mg^{++})	1.5–2.5 mEq/liter

Osmolality

The ICF and ECF fluid compartments have equal osmolality, or number of dissolved particles per unit of water (expressed as milliosmoles). Normal body fluid osmolality is 275–295 mOsm/kg. Water always moves from an area of lower concentration of particles to an area of higher concentration, or "water follows salt." Diffusion, active transport, filtration, and osmosis are mechanisms by which fluids and electrolytes shift through the cell membrane in order to maintain balance in the compartments.

Diffusion occurs when molecules move from an area of higher concentration to one of lower concentration, with no external energy required. Net movement of molecules stops when the concentrations are equal in both areas. For example, if a drop of red food coloring were dropped into a glass of water, the water would soon be pink.

Active transport is the movement of molecules from areas of low concentration to areas of high concentration across a concentration gradient with external energy required. The energy source for the pump is adenosine triphosphate (ATP), produced in the mitochondria of cells.

Filtration forces a fluid through a filter because of a difference in pressure between the two sides of the filter. Hemodialysis utilizes this process when blood is pumped next to a filter, and the pressure is lower on the dialysis side of the filter. Excess water in the blood is driven across the membrane and discarded.

Osmosis is the flow of water between a membrane permeable to water but not solute particles. The water moves from the area that is more dilute to the area that is less dilute. No external energy is required.

These four processes control the movement of fluids and electrolytes between the intracellular and extracellular spaces, and are very important in maintaining the chemical stability of cells. The all-important concept of osmolality is particularly important to remember when IV fluids are administered. The three types of IV fluids are:

Isotonic solutions: i.e., normal saline (0.9% NaCl). The same electrolyte concentration as plasma. The ICF and ECF remain balanced.

Hypotonic solutions: i.e., 0.45% NaCl. A lesser electrolyte concentration than plasma. Water will not necessarily remain in the vasculature.

Hypertonic solutions: i.e., 50% DW. A greater concentration than plasma, this solution will pull water into the vasculature.

See also Table 6-4 for osmolality, tonicity and electrolyte composition of commonly used IV solutions.

Acid-Base Balance

Crucial to the health of cells is the maintenance of normal concentration of hydrogen and bicarbonate ions. The ph scale (Figure 5-2) measures the concentration of H^+ ions in a solution. The more acidic a solution, the lower the pH reading. The more alkaline, the higher the reading.

The pH of water, or a neutral pH, is 7.0. The ECF is normally slightly alkaline with a pH value of 7.35–7.45. The ICF is slightly acid, but its exact pH is not known.

Highly efficient control mechanisms protect the body from harmful changes in acidity. The buffer systems (bicarbonate-carbonic acid, protein and phosphate systems) act chemically to bind or release H^+ as the situation requires. The lungs and kidneys remove H^+ permanently from the body.

The lungs act quickly (within minutes) to get rid of excess H^+ by increasing the excretion of CO_2 (an acid) through hyperventilation. In the event of alkalosis, the lungs will decrease the breathing rate in order to conserve CO_2. If for some reason the breathing rate was decreased, the mechanisms would work like this: $\downarrow$ breathing rate$\rightarrow \uparrow CO_2 \rightarrow \uparrow$ carbonic acid$\rightarrow$acidosis$\rightarrow \uparrow$ breathing rate$\rightarrow \downarrow CO_2 \rightarrow \downarrow$ carbonic acid$\rightarrow$ normal pH

Although the kidneys are slower, requiring hours or days to neutralize excess acid or base, the renocardiovascular system is extremely effective in health in bringing pH back to normal. Not only do the kidneys excrete excess H^+ ions, strong acids, drugs, and toxins, but they also regulate the concentration of specific electrolytes and water in the ECF and produce HCO_3^- as it is needed as a buffer.

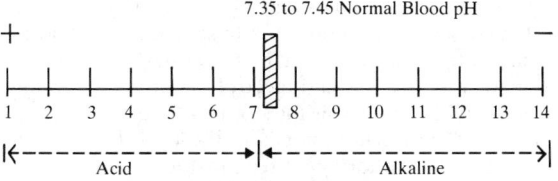

Figure 5–2. The pH scale.

**TABLE 5–2. ARTERIAL BLOOD GAS
INTERPRETATION IN ACID-BASE IMBALANCE**

CONDITION	pH	pCO$_2$	HCO$_3$
Acidosis			
Respiratory	↓	↑	Normal or ↑
Metabolic	↓	Normal or ↓	↓
Alkalosis			
Respiratory	↑	↓	Normal or ↓
Metabolic	↑	Normal or ↑	↑

The pH of urine can vary widely because of this function. Although usually slightly acid, urine pH can range from 4.7–8.

Arterial blood gas measurement is crucial in assessment of acid-base imbalance. Table 5-2 gives a brief sketch of what happens to normal reference values in acidosis and alkalosis. Refer to Table 3-5 for normal values for arterial blood gases.

Body Systems Important in Maintaining Homeostasis

All systems help with homeostasis. But along with the respiratory and urinary systems, the endocrine, GI, and nervous systems play particularly important roles in maintaining stability.

Endocrine Adrenals secrete aldosterone, which conserves Na$^+$, Cl$^-$, and water, and facilitates excretion of K$^+$. ADH (antidiuretic hormone) from the pituitary is all-important in water conservation. The parathyroids aid in Ca^{++} and HPO$_4^=$ metabolism.

GI Absorbs dietary fluids and 7–9 liters of glandular and GI tract secretions a day. The liver is important in protein, carbohydrate and fat metabolism; it also secretes bile, of which water and electrolytes are major components, and is a reservoir for storing blood.

Nervous The thirst center is in the hypothalamus. The volumetric monitoring system in the midbrain affects ADH release, thirst, and aldosterone release.

5-2 IMBALANCES

If any of the factors listed in Table 5-3 are present, extra vigilance is required. Imbalances are usually multiple.

Nursing Assessment for Prevention and Treatment of Fluid and Electrolyte Imbalance

- Assess vital signs frequently and note trends (see Section 2-4)

- Record daily weights—One liter of water weighs 1 kg (2.2 pounds). If a client drank 240 ml of fluid, weight gain would be 0.24 kg (0.5 pound). A client on diuretic therapy who loses 2 kg in 24 hr has experienced a fluid loss of about 2 liters. A sudden weight change is the best indicator of fluid volume deficit or excess. Measure weight at the same time daily and in similar clothes.

TABLE 5–3. CAUSES OF FLUID AND ELECTROLYTE IMBALANCE

CLIENT INABILITY	RISK FACTORS	DISEASE STATES	IATROGENIC FACTORS
Lack of access to adequate fluids, diet Lack of knowledge of proper fluids, diet Debilitation prevents adequate intake	Vomiting Diarrhea Burns Draining wounds Ulcers Fever Excessive perspiration Heat exposure Edema	Endocrine disorders Cardiac disease GI disorders Impaired renal functioning Impaired respiratory functioning Neurologic damage	IV therapy Low-sodium diet GI suctioning Paracentesis Thoracentesis Medications (diuretics, laxatives, sodium bicarbonate) Diagnostic dye studies NPO status

- Measure and record fluid intake and output, overall, and for 24 hr (normal urine output is 1 ml (kg/hour)

- Observe client's neurologic status as changes may be related to fluid/electrolyte shifts (see Section 1-5)

- Check respiratory status for altered breathing patterns (see Section 1-6)

- Decreased-skin turgor may indicate dehydration, though this is less predictive in the elderly

- Be alert for noticeable swelling or tightening of rings, shoes, clothes

- Assess relevant laboratory data:

  - Blood chemistries: electrolytes, pH, pCO_2, CO_2, serum osmolality, BUN, plasma proteins, HCt, serum creatinine

  - Arterial blood gases

  - Urinalysis: electrolytes, specific gravity, pH, sodium

  - EKG

  - Chest x-ray

- Remember that medications such as diuretics, antacids, antihypertensives, digitalis, and morphine may significantly alter fluid regulation.

- Review client's dietary history to determine approximate levels of sodium, protein, and sugar intake (dietary analysis is best referred to a registered dietician).

- Check for history of any psychiatric or eating disorder involving compulsive behavior affecting fluid intake.

Nursing Interventions for the Prevention and Treatment of Fluid and Electrolyte Imbalance

- Use Tables 5-3, 5-4, and 5-5 to help determine causes, signs, and symptoms, and treatment of fluid, electrolyte and/or acid-base imbalances to make an accurate

Text continued on page 222

TABLE 5–4. FLUID AND ELECTROLYTE IMBALANCES

IMBALANCE	CAUSES	WARNINGS	INTERVENTIONS TO RESTORE BALANCE
H_2O			
↓ Extracellular fluid volume (deficit)	Blood loss ↑ Diuresis Fluid sequestration in body cavity Inadequate fluid intake	Weight loss ↓ BP (postural)/CVP Thready, rapid pulse ↓ Skin turgor Dry mucous membranes Collapsed neck veins ↓ Urine output ↑ Hematocrit ↑ Albumin	↑ Isotonic fluids ↑ H_2O intake
↑ Extracellular fluid volume (excess)	↑ Isotonic IV solutions Renal disease Heart failure Liver damage Long-term steroid therapy	Rapid weight gain ↑ BP, ↑ CVP Full pulse Edema Cough, moist rales Distended neck veins Dyspnea ↓ Hematocrit	↓ Isotonic fluids ↓ Dietary Na^+ ↓ H_2O intake Diuretics Amicon diafilter*
Na^+			
↓ Serum osmolality ($Na^+ < 135$ mEq/liter)	↑ Hypotonic solutions (e.g., 5% D/W) Tap-water enemas	Absence of thirst ↓ Temperature Thready, rapid pulse Polyuria (ex-	↓ Plain water ↑ Sodium chloride

Table continued on following page

TABLE 5–4. FLUID AND ELECTROLYTE IMBALANCES *Continued*

IMBALANCE	CAUSES	WARNINGS	INTERVENTIONS TO RESTORE BALANCE
	Vomiting GI suction- ing Renal disease Hyperaldo- steronism	cept in renal disease) Malaise Confusion Seizures	
↑ Serum os- molality (Na^+ > 145 mEq/ liter)	↑ Hyper- tonic solu- tions ↓ H_2O in- take Renal disease ↑ Sweating Watery diar- rhea Prolonged fever	↑ Thirst ↑ Tempera- ture Pulse Oliguria Dry mucous membranes Confusion Seizures	↑ Water intake ↓ Sodium chloride intake
K^+ Hypokalemia (K^+ < 3.5 mEq/liter)	K^+-wasting diuretics IV replace- ment fluids without K^+ Vomiting Diarrhea Gastric suctioning Excessive dieting	Weak pulse Muscle weakness Anorexia, nausea, vom- iting Loss of re- flexes Lethargy Confusion ↓ BP (pos- tural) Cardiac ar- rhythmias	Administra- tion of K^+, IV or orally Client teach- ing: replace- ment K^+ and foods high in K^+
Hyperkalemia (K^+ > 5 mEq/ liter)	Renal failure ↑ IV intake of K^+ Massive tis- sue injury (e.g., burns)	Oliguria Muscle weakness Nausea, vomiting, diarrhea	Administra- tion of IV calcium, glu- cose, and in- sulin or bi- carbonates

TABLE 5–4. FLUID AND ELECTROLYTE IMBALANCES *Continued*

IMBALANCE	CAUSES	WARNINGS	INTERVENTIONS TO RESTORE BALANCE
	Rapid transfusion of stored blood K^+ supplements given with K^+ sparing diuretics	Intestinal colic $\downarrow$ BP (postural) Bradycardia Cardiac arrhythmias	Cation exchange resin (Kayexelate) Renal dialysis
Ca^{++}			
Hypocalcemia ($Ca^{++} <$ 4.5 mEq/liter)	Parathyroid removal or deficiency Intestinal malabsorption Burns $\downarrow$ Dietary intake	Numbness Tingling Muscle cramps Abdominal cramps Muscle twitches Tetany	$\uparrow$ Calcium intake, IV or orally
Hypercalcemia ($Ca^{++} >$ 5.5 mEq/liter)	Immobility Hyperparathyroidism Bone metastasis Multiple myeloma $\uparrow$ Dietary intake	Muscle weakness Bone pain Pathologic fractures Intractable nausea and vomiting Kidney stones Tissue calcifications Cardiac arrhythmias	Administer isotonic fluids, diuretics, calcitonin, corticosteroids, or phosphate
M^{++}			
Hypomagnesemia ($M^{++} <$ 1.5 mEq/ liter)	Alcoholism Malabsorption Diuretic therapy	$\uparrow$ BP Muscle twitches Hyperactive reflexes	$\uparrow$ Magnesium intake, IV or orally

Table continued on following page

TABLE 5–4. FLUID AND ELECTROLYTE IMBALANCES *Continued*

IMBALANCE	CAUSES	WARNINGS	INTERVEN-TIONS TO RESTORE BALANCE
	Vomiting, diarrhea GI suctioning	$\downarrow$ Serum Ca^{++} and K^+ values Convulsions Cardiac arrhythmias	
Hypermagnesemia (M^{++} > 2.5 mEq/liter)	Epsom salt overdose Renal failure Overcorrection of hypomagnesemia	$\downarrow$ BP Lethargy Flushing Loss or weakness of deep tendon reflexes Coma	$\downarrow$ Dietary M^{++} IV calcium dialysis administration
$HPO_4^=$ Hypophosphatemia ($HPO_4^=$ < 1.8 mEq/liter)	Malnutrition Malabsorption Antacids Alcoholism	Mental irritability Muscle weakness Seizures Coma	$\uparrow$ Phosphate intake, IV or orally
Hyperphosphatemia ($HPO_4^=$ > 2.6 mEq/liter)	Renal failure Hypoparathyroidism Acromegaly	Manifestations similar to hypocalcemia Kidney stones	$\downarrow$ Dietary phosphate Phosphate-binding antacids Dialysis

$\uparrow$ = excessive or increased; $\downarrow$ = deficient or decreased.
*Has been available in the United States since 1983. See Am J Nurs, November 1983.

nursing diagnosis. The collaborative efforts of the health team may be required.

- Provide ordered fluids according to client condition. Set goals for oral intake, for instance, 1000 ml/day

TABLE 5–5. ACID-BASE IMBALANCES

IMBALANCE	CAUSES	WARNINGS	INTERVENTIONS TO RESTORE BALANCE
H^+, HCO_3^-			
Respiratory alkalosis ($pCO_2 < 30$) $pH > 7.45$	Anxiety Pain Damage to respiratory center in brain Hypoxemia Excessive mechanical ventilation Hyperventilation from any cause	Numbness Tingling Lightheadedness Altered consciousness Tetany ↓ Serum K^+ ↑ RR	Oxygen administration (if there is hypoxemia) Assistance to slow breathing (if not hypoxemic) Adjustment of mechanical respirator
Respiratory acidosis ($pCO_2 > 50$) $pH < 7.35$	Depression of respiratory center by disease, drugs Lung diseases High-spinal-cord injury Congenital thoracic cage abnormalities Shallow breathing from any cause	↑ BP, pulse (early) Headache Blurred vision Muscle contractions Lethargy → coma Cardiac arrhythmias High serum K^+	Improve depth of ventilation Mechanical ventilation
Metabolic alkalosis ($HCO_3 > 30$ mEq/liter) $pH > 7.45$	Loss of acid by vomiting, GI suctioning, draining, or draining fistula Ingestion of bicarbonate of soda or other antacids Hypokalemia	Irritability Disorientation Lethargy Muscle twitching Cramps Slow, shallow breathing Tetany Cardiac arrhythmias	Isotonic-fluid administration Acetazolamide
Metabolic acidosis ($HCO_3 < 20$ mEq/liter) $pH < 7.35$	Diabetic ketoacidosis Chronic kidney failure Starvation Severe diarrhea Salicylate poisoning	Apathy Disorientation ↑ BP, pulse (early) Rapid, deep breathing Hyperkalemia Cardiac arrhythmias	IV bicarbonate administration

shift, 800 ml/evening, 300 ml/noc shift, and maintain a urine specific gravity within normal range.

- Teach client about proper fluid intake and diet.
    - See Table 8-9 for foods high in potassium, and Section 8-5 for sodium restricted nutrition therapy.
    - Teach client how to monitor intake and output, and correct use of medications.
- Continue assessment, planning, implementation, and evaluation of client and treatment plan.

Fluid Volume Deficit

Fluid volume deficit is a loss of both water and solutes. It may be due to:

Isotonic dehydration General fluid and electrolyte losses or inadequate intake of fluids and electrolytes. Causes: hemorrhage, vomiting, diarrhea, profuse salivation, fistulas, abscesses, ileostomy, cecostomy, frequent enemas, profuse diaphoresis, burns, severe wounds, long-term NPO status, diuretic therapy, GI suction.

Hypertonic dehydration Water loss exceeds solute ·loss. Causes: hyperventilation, watery diarrhea, renal failure, ketoacidosis, diabetes insipidus, excessive fluid replacement (hypertonic), excessive sodium bicarbonate administration, tube feedings, dysphagia, impaired thirst, unconsciousness, fever, impaired motor function, systemic infection with fever.

Hypotonic Loss is relatively rare and usually associated with chronic illness which involves loss of solutes from the ECF in excess of water loss. Causes: excessive fluid replacement, renal failure, chronic or severe malnutrition.

NURSING ASSESSMENT OF CLIENT WITH FLUID VOLUME DEFICIT

Look for output greater than intake, dry skin/mucous membranes, increased serum sodium and other abnormal lab values, increased urine specific gravity, decreased or increased urine output, decreased skin turgor, thirst, nausea, anorexia, increased pulse rate.

NURSING INTERVENTIONS FOR CLIENT WITH FLUID VOLUME DEFICIT

- Monitor intake; assure at least 1500–2000ml/24 hr unless contraindicated. Assess likes and dislikes, provide favorite fluids within dietary restrictions, giving small amounts frequently.

- Monitor output; assure at least 1000–1500 ml/24 hr.

- Rate of fluid replacement and type of fluids used is dependent on degree and type of dehydration present, and existing cardiac, pulmonary, or renal problems. Commonly used intravenous fluids are:

  1. Isotonic fluids such as 0.9% saline (NS) or Ringer's lactate

  2. Hypotonic fluids such as .25% saline or .45% saline

  3. Hypertonic fluids such as 3% saline

- Protein replacement (Albumin) may be needed in client who has lost proteins (colloids) from the vascular space.

- Administer drug therapy as ordered to help or correct underlying causes of dehydration, such as antidiarrheals, antiemetics, or antipyretics.

- Weigh daily at same time of day with same type of clothing.

- Assess client's understanding of reason for maintaining fluid balance and teach accordingly. Teach that coffee, tea, and grapefruit juice are diuretics and can contribute to fluid loss.

- Involve client in maintaining intake and output log if possible.

- Assess lab values and specific gravity to monitor status.

Fluid Volume Excess

The two kinds of overhydration are:

Isotonic or hypervolemia   Fluid volume is increased in the ECF. If mild to moderate, it rarely has serious consequences, and the kidneys are usually able to handle the temporary overload. Circulatory overload, pulmonary and interstitial edema may occur if severe.

Hypotonic, or water intoxication All body fluid compartments become overly saturated with fluid and solutes become diluted. Usually associated with heart disease, kidney disease, or other states where regulatory mechanisms are impaired.

NURSING ASSESSMENT OF CLIENT WITH FLUID VOLUME EXCESS

- Look for pitting edema, taut shiny skin (pale and cool to the touch), weight gain, increased pulse rate, bounding pulse, distended neck and hand veins, dyspnea, moist rales or crackles, noticeable swelling, or tightening of rings, shoes, or clothes, use of over-the-counter or prescribed medications such as diuretics, antacids, laxatives, and morphine, high levels of sodium in the diet, skeletal muscle weakness, paresthesis, increased GI motility.

- Signs of hypotonic overhydration: polyuria, diarrhea, nonpitting edema, cardiac dysrhythmias associated with electrolyte dilution, projectile vomiting, anxiety, restlessness

NURSING INTERVENTIONS FOR CLIENT WITH FLUID VOLUME EXCESS

- If the overhydration is isotonic and mild to moderate, the treatment will be to decrease intake and allow the kidneys to rid the body of the extra fluid.

- Dietary intake should be evaluated and salt intake discouraged.

- Drug therapy may be required for moderate-to-severe overhydration, provided renal failure is not the cause of the problem. Osmotic diuretics may be used to avoid initiating or exacerbating electrolyte disturbances although some experts feel osmotic diuretics may increase vascular volume and induce pitting edema. High-ceiling (loop) diuretics may be required if osmotic diuretics are not effective.

- Medical treatment will center around treating the underlying cause of the overhydration: digoxin, amrinone, or deslanoside address poor cardiac output. Dexamethosone, mannitol, or urea is used to treat cerebral edema. If there is pulmonary edema, bronchodilators, oxygen, vasodilators, and a semi-Fowler's position will be indicated.

- Careful monitoring of intake and output is required, along with frequent assessment of specific gravity, and other clinical signs.

- Establish goals and expected outcomes for the client, including education and discharge planning.

REFERENCES

Barta MA. Correcting electrolyte imbalances. RN 1987 February; 30–33.

Burns D. Working up a thirst. Nursing Times 1992; 88 (26).

Calloway C. When the problem involves magnesium, calcium, or phosphate. RN 1987; May: 30–35.

Carpenito LJ. Handbook of nursing diagnosis. 4th ed. Philadelphia: JB Lippincott, 1991.

Chenevey B. Overview of fluids and electrolytes. Nursing Clinics of North America 1987; 22(4).

Collier L and Lewis S. Medical-surgical nursing: assessment and management of clinical problems. St. Louis: Mosby, 1992.

Ignatavicius D and Bayne M. Medical-surgical nursing: a nursing process approach. Philadelphia: WB Saunders, 1991.

LaGrange K. Fluid and electrolytes. Stanford, CA: Stanford University Hospital Nursing Continuing Education, 1990.

CHAPTER 6

INTRAVENOUS THERAPY, PARENTERAL NUTRITION, AND BLOOD TRANSFUSION

The principal uses of IV therapy are:

- To maintain or restore body water, electrolytes, vitamins, proteins, calories, and nitrogen

- To restore acid–base balance

- To replenish blood volume or needed blood components

- To give quick access for drug administration

The type, amount, and flow rate of IV fluids administered are determined by the physician on the basis of the client's laboratory evaluation, clinical condition and weight. Generally, the bigger the client, the more fluid will be required and the faster it will be used. Elderly, frail, and smaller clients will usually require a slower rate, to avoid circulatory overload. Primary nursing responsibilities in IV therapy are:

- Selection of appropriate IV site
- Starting the IV using careful therapeutic technique
- Maintenance of appropriate flow rates
- Constant clinical assessment of client's fluid and electrolyte status
- Prevention and treatment of complications
- Monitoring of urine output (should be 30–60 ml/hr)
- Accurate recording of intravenous and other fluid intake and output

6-1 THE IV INSERTION SITE

Peripheral Veins

CHOOSING THE SITE

- Choose veins of the upper extremities if at all possible, as IV insertion in the lower extremities carries a high risk of thromboembolism.

- Avoid veins on the inner aspect of the arm.

- Using upper arm veins before hand veins may cause damage to the vein and prohibit use of the hand veins. Therefore start with distal branches of larger veins such as those in the back of the hand. The basilic or cephalic veins are good, especially for KVO (keep vein open) IVs. Save larger veins above the hand for rapid infusions and blood or medications regularly added by piggyback (Figure 6-1).

- The antecubital vein is generally reserved for laboratory blood work if possible.

- Alternative sites include: the great saphenous and femoral veins in the thigh, the great saphenous vein in the ankle, the venous plexus of the dorsum, the dorsal venous arch, and the medial marginal veins of the foot. Use these only if there is no other alternative. Check with the physician first.

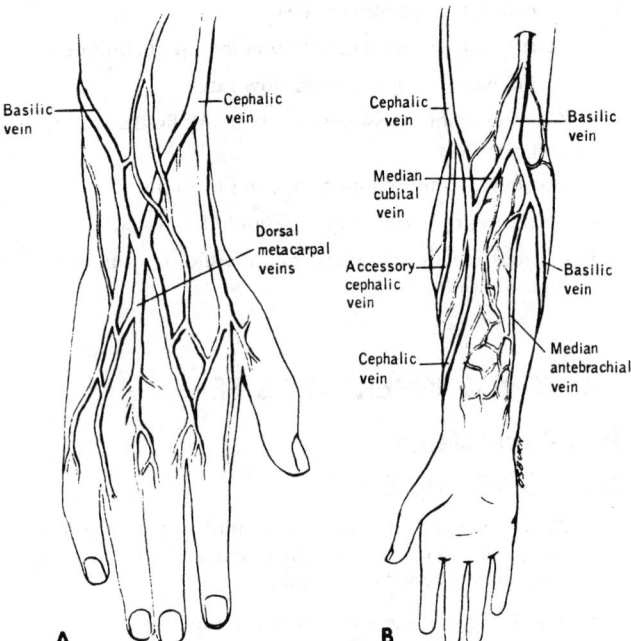

Figure 6–1. (A) Superficial veins of the dorsal aspect of the hand. (B) Superficial veins of the forearm. (From Sutton AL. Bedside nursing techniques in medicine and surgery. Philadelphia: WB Saunders, 1969: 85. Reprinted with permission.)

STARTING A PERIPHERAL IV

- Complete Table 10-7, Checklist of Guidelines for Therapeutic Nursing Procedures, including checking orders and client/family instruction.

- Carefully set up all your equipment at bedside; select catheter and needle based on expected duration of therapy, type of IV solution, vein size, etc. (Table 6-1, Figure 6-2). Use large-bore needles (No. 18, 19) for blood, parenteral nutrition, viscous fluids, and long-term therapy; smaller needles for short-term therapy, and KVO lines.

TABLE 6–1. TYPES OF INTRAVENOUS ADMINISTRATION UNITS

METAL NEEDLES	PLASTIC CATHETERS
Straight needles Winged infusion set (butterfly) Heparin lock	Over-the-needle catheter (angiocath) Over-the-needle catheter with resealable cap Through-the-needle catheter (intracath) In-lying (cut down) catheter (requires MD)
• Easy to insert but prone to infiltrate • Less likely to cause phlebitis • Indicated for short-term therapy • Indicated for 5% DW, KVO IVs, nonviscous solutions	• Harder to insert, but easier to secure • More prone to becoming infected • Indicated for longer-term therapy • Indicated for blood, total parenteral nutrition, viscous IV solutions

Needle gauge sizes: 14, 16, 18, 19, 20, 21, 22, 24, 25, 28, 32

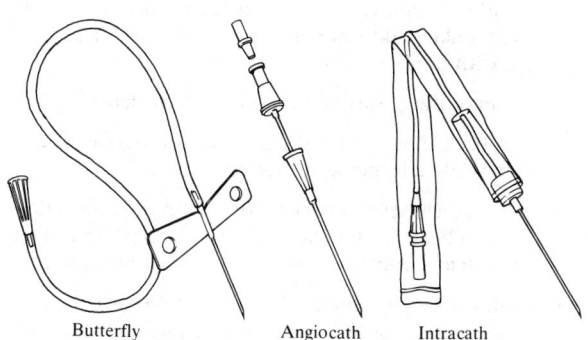

Butterfly   Angiocath   Intracath

Figure 6–2. Types of intravenous administration units.

- Mark appropriate times on bottle according to flow rate, or use preprinted labels. Mark tubing with time and date IV is started and your initials.

- Check bottle or bag for leaks, impurities, or anything that suggests insterility. Discard if there is a question.

- Use strict aseptic technique to connect tubing to bottle and flush air out of tubing.

- Wear gloves for protection when performing actual venipuncture (see Section 9-2 or Universal Precautions and Guidelines for Handling Blood or Body Fluids).

- Apply constricting band above IV site.

- To distend the veins for identification after applying the tourniquet:

  - Manually compress the vein above the insertion site

  - Have the client clench and unclench fist

  - Lightly tap the vein (gently, to avoid injury or vasospasm)

  - Allow extremity to be dependent a few minutes (loosen tourniquet) and/or

  - Wrap the arm in warm towels for 15–20 min, or use well-covered hot water bottle or heating pad.

- After careful cleansing of the IV site with alcohol or povidone iodine, use an outward circular motion, anchor skin, and insert the needle at a 45-degree angle with the bevel up into the vein.

- Observe the flashback of blood into catheter.

- Pull back inner stylet slightly to prevent shearing of vein while advancing catheter.

- Advance catheter upwards (direction of venous flow back to heart), while keeping the skin taut to reduce friction and enhance easy advancement of catheter.

- Connect tubing filled with fluid or heparin lock to catheter making sure no air enters line.

- Apply antiseptic ointment and secure in place with sterile gauze and tape. Transparent dressings may also be used. Avoid ointment. Dressings on peripheral IV sites should be changed every 24–48 hr. Mark with time, date, and your initials.

- Check client frequently for patency of IV site, correct flow rate, and complications of IV therapy.

- Change IV site every 48–72 hr.

EXTENDED PERIPHERAL CATHETERS

An extended peripheral catheter is a long catheter, usually 6 inches in length, and is also often referred to as a midarm catheter. It can be made of polyurethane, silicone rubber, or Aquavene. An alternative to a short peripheral catheter, this catheter is useful for short-term intermittent therapies. It is placed by a certified RN in the antecubital area in the basilic or cephalic vein and is then advanced toward the upper arm. Generally, if there is no leakage, blockage, or other complications, the catheter can remain for the course of therapy.

Central Veins

Central veins are used when medications are hypertonic or highly irritating (i.e., protein hydrosylate, hypertonic NaCl, chemotherapeutic agents) or during shock or cardiac arrest or other times when peripheral blood flow is diminished. These are also indicated for long-term therapy. The physician usually places the catheter in the superior vena cava via the left or right subclavian vein or the internal or external jugular vein. There are various types of central venous catheters (Table 6-2).

MANAGEMENT OF SHORT-TERM MULTILUMEN CATHETERS

When multiple IV lines are needed, such as when a client needs CVP monitoring, repeated blood tests, parenteral nutrition, and IV medications, multilumen catheters are indicated. The physician inserts this type of catheter the same way a single-lumen central venous catheter is placed. At the proximal end of the catheter, each lumen has a color-coded

Text continued on page 237

TABLE 6–2. CENTRAL VENOUS (CV) CATHETERS

Listed here are several types of central venous catheters. Catheter choice is dependent on the client, type of infusion therapy, and length of therapy.

TYPE	DESCRIPTION	USES	NURSING CONSIDERATIONS
Short-term (sutured)			
Silicone rubber	Single lumen. Flexible. Usually sutured in place. Easily inserted at bedside. Easily removed. Limited function.	Short-term CV access. Emergency access. Used for clients who need only one lumen.	• Assess frequently for signs of infection and clot formation.
Polyurethane	Dual or triple lumen. Less flexible, but not stiff. Allows infusion of multiple solutions through the same catheter—even incompatible solutions	Short-term CV access. Client with limited insertion site who needs multiple infusions.	• Know gauge and purpose of each lumen. • Use the same lumen for the same purpose, for example, blood drawing or antibiotics.
Hickman/ Broviac	Made of silicone rubber. May be single, dual, or triple lumen.	Long-term CV access. Home therapy. Multiple lumens used for clients needing multiple infusions.	• Two surgical sites require dressing after insertion. • Observe for kinks or tears.

TABLE 6–2. CENTRAL VENOUS (CV) CATHETERS *Continued*

TYPE	DESCRIPTION	USES	NURSING CONSIDERATIONS
			• Repair kit is available.
			• Use non-serrated clamp for disconnections or any time the catheter is open.
			• Know gauge and purpose of each lumen.
Groshong (sutured or tunneled)	Made of silicone rubber. Translucent with blue stripe. Single or double lumen. Tip has three-way valve which closes when line disconnects, preventing air from entering line or blood from coming out of line. Dacron cuff anchors catheter and prevents bacterial migration.	Long-term CV access. Client allergy to heparin.	• Flush with enough saline solution to clear catheter, especially after drawing or administering blood.
			• See sutured, tunneled, implanted-vascular access port, and peripherally inserted central catheters.

Table continued on following page

TABLE 6–2. CENTRAL VENOUS (CV) CATHETERS *Continued*

TYPE	DESCRIPTION	USES	NURSING CONSIDERATIONS
	Blunt end makes it difficult to clear substances from its tip.		
Implanted Vascular Access Port	Made of silicone rubber or silastic. Single or dual lumens. Port and catheter are not visible. Requires non-coring needle for access. Surgically implanted in a pocket in the subcutaneous tissue, using local anesthetic. Port produces lump under skin, usually on upper torso. Port has self-sealing septum. Some made with Groshong tip. Usually top entry; some double lu-	Long-term CV access. Often inserted for chemotherapy.	• Non-coring needle needs to be changed weekly • Assess need for topical anesthetic prior to insertion of non-coring needle.

TABLE 6–2. CENTRAL VENOUS (CV) CATHETERS *Continued*

TYPE	DESCRIP-TION	USES	NURSING CONSID-ERATIONS
	men ports may have side entry or be accessed from any angle.		
Peripherally inserted central catheter (PICC)	Made of silicone rubber, very thin and flexible. Single or dual lumens. Peripherally inserted. Insertion site in or near the antecubital fossa. Easily inserted at bedside. May be inserted by RN in some states. Long path to CV insertion.	Long-term CV access. Clients at risk for fatal complications from other insertion sites. Clients who need CV access but face or have had head and neck surgery.	• Check for signs of phlebitis and thrombus formation. • Observe for catheter migration.

and labeled extension. At the distal end, each lumen exists through separate openings, 2.2 cm apart. After the catheter is inserted, the openings lie in the superior vena cava, just above the right side of the heart.

The nurse should assist with insertion of the catheter as follows:

• Complete Table 10-7, Checklist of Guidelines for Therapeutic Nursing Procedures.

- Check with physician before insertion as to whether lumen should be heparinized. Some catheters are already thrombus resistant.

- Assist physician during insertion of the catheter at bedside and the suturing of the catheter to client's skin in two places. Support the client.

- Dress the insertion site: Apply povidone-iodine and wrap a precut sterile gauze sponge around the catheter. Place one or two more gauze sponges over the site and cover them with nonallergenic tape. To apply the tape securely, have the client rotate arm away from the torso and turn the head away from the insertion site. A transparent dressing such as IV 3000 may also be used.

- Label the dressing with the date, time, and your initials.

- Gather the IV tubes up near the top of the dressing and secure temporarily to decrease tension at the insertion site.

- Slowly infuse IV fluids at a keep-open rate, until physician ensures correct catheter placement with a chest x-ray.

Key points for maintaining a multilumen catheter are as follows:

- Change dressings and IV tubing according to your hospital policy, usually every 24–48 hr or at the time a new IV is hung. Use strict aseptic technique and teach clients the importance of maintaining a clean, dry insertion site.

- Use luerlock tubing to prevent air embolism.

- Prevent the catheter from becoming kinked or dislodged by reminding client not to tug on or lie on the line and to call you immediately if a tube becomes disconnected or a hub breaks.

- Use color codings for standardized functions in your hospital. For example, if your hospital uses white for drawing blood, label it as such and use it only for that.

- While drawing blood, be sure to stop infusions through the other lines temporarily to avoid contamination of the blood sample.

- To keep lines patent, use a continuous IV infusion such as heparin in saline, or cover the extension opening with an injection cap and flush the line with heparin injections every 8 hr. Use the same flush procedure as for heparin locks.

- See insert directions when using self-sealing injection caps.

- Be particularly alert when giving multiple infusions for signs of fluid overload and/or electrolyte imbalance. If you see elevated cardiovascular or blood pressure readings, distended jugular veins, increased respiratory rate, dyspnea, rales, or general edema, slow the infusions and report immediately (see Table 6-6).

6-2 REGULATING IV FLOW RATES

Calculating Drip Rates

Physicians usually order IV rates in milliliter per hour. Nurses regulate flow rates using drops (gtt)/minute. To convert milliliter per hour to gtt/min the formula is

$$\text{gtt/min (flow rate)} = \text{gtt/ml (from calibration of set)} \times \frac{\text{ml/hr}}{60}$$

The size of the drop varies according to calibration of the set; refer to Table 6-3 for precalculated rates.

For example, the physician orders you to give 1000 ml of 5% dextrose in water over 10 hr using microdrip.

$$\text{gtt/min} = 60 \text{ (drip factor)} \times \frac{100 \text{ (ml/hr)}}{60 \text{ (min in 1 hr)}}$$

$$= \frac{6000}{60} = 100 \text{ gtt/min}$$

For this same problem, you could also look on Table 6-3 in the last column for number of hr/1000-ml bag, go down

TABLE 6–3. CALIBRATING IV DRIP RATES

| Prescription | ml/24 hrs | DROPS PER MINUTE | | | No. of hrs/1000 ml bag |
		Regular (15/ml)	Micro drip (60/ml)	Macro drip (10/ml)	
40 ml/hr	1000	10	40	7	24
50 ml/hr	1200	12	50	8	20
60 ml/hr	1500	15	60	10	16.6
80 ml/hr	2000	20	80	13	12.5
100 ml/hr	2500	25	100	16	10
125 ml/hr	3000	30	125	20	20
150 ml/hr	3600	38	150	25	25

to 10 (1000 ml over 10 hr) and carry over to the microdrip
(60/ml) column for the precalculated rate.

- A handy tip: remember that if using a 60 gtt/ml IV set
  (microdrip), the ml/min (flow rate) is the same as the
  gtt/min.

- A keep-open rate (KVO) is 50 ml/hr or less. Use a
  microdrip. Also use the smallest possible container
  because it must be discarded and a new one hung
  every 24 hr (or per hospital policy).

- Use microdrips for neonates, for critically ill clients,
  and when giving certain critical drugs such as insulin,
  morphine, heparin and certain cardiac drugs. Do not
  use when giving blood or parenteral nutrition, which
  require macrodrips and special administration sets.

Infusion Control Devices

An IV controller or pump may be used to accurately regulate the infusion rate. This is especially useful if fluid
administration must be watched very carefully, such as
when fluid is being infused to an infant, frail elderly person,
or when critical drugs are infused. Both IV controllers and
pumps can be volumetric or nonvolumetric.

- Volumetric devices deliver fluids at constant volume
  over long periods and are more accurate than nonvolumetric.

- Nonvolumetric infusion control devices may be used when short-term accuracy is needed.

- Most devices are volumetric.

Controllers depend on gravity to maintain a precise flow and are adequate for most infusions. Pumps use positive pressure to deliver the prescribed volume of fluid. Neonates, elderly clients, and clients with congestive heart failure or pulmonary edema may require a pump. Pumps regulate the flow of volume, whereas controllers sense the drops infusing. Most controllers and pumps can be electronically programmed. The nurse enters the amount of fluid that is hung (i.e., 1000 ml), and the rate at which it is to infuse per hour. The device displays how much fluid has infused and the amount remaining at any given time.

Most infusion control devices have alarms that indicate when fluid cannot be infused at the prescribed rate for any reason (e.g., the bottle is empty, there is air in the line, or an occlusion blocks the lumen). Infiltration does not necessarily trigger the alarm. The nurse must troubleshoot any identified problem and correct it to ensure proper infusion of fluids. Since there are many types and models of infusion devices it is important for nurses to become familiar with the models used in their institutions. Problems should be identified before the alarm is turned off. Pumps can be designed as peristaltic or syringe driven:

Peristaltic pumps A peristaltic device moves fluid by intermittently squeezing the IV tubing. Blood components cannot be infused through a peristaltic pump, as the pressure on the tubing will cause hemolysis of cells. These pumps are used mostly for enteral feeding.

Syringe pumps Syringe pumps provide precise infusion by controlling the rate by drive speed and syringe size. This will omit the drip-rate variables. Syringe pumps are useful for critical infusions of small doses of high-potency drugs.

The technology related to infusion devices is rapidly changing. Client needs have driven the production of the complicated systems now available. A few of these are described here:

Disposable elastomeric infusion system This system is a portable design with an elastomeric reservoir. When the reservoir is filled, it exerts positive pressure to deliver the medication with an integrated flow restrictor that controls the flow rate. This system does not require batteries or electronic programming. It is used for chemotherapy, antibiotics and pain medication.

Implantable pumps There are many different implantable infusion pumps because of their convenience and reliability. They are used to deliver morphine and other pain medications. These pumps deliver minute amounts of drugs each day.

Portable pumps Lightweight, compact infusion pumps have assisted in the management of long-term care. The pump can deliver medications in small doses set by the nurse. The client can wear this device in a belt or in a pocket. The pump may have a syringe, cassette, or mini-bag.

Multiple-channel pumps Clients requiring two, three, or four simultaneous infusions can be treated in the hospital or home with these devices. Multiple channel pumps provide accurate precise delivery while taking up little space and simplifying the client's environment. Multiple-channel pumps decrease drug compatibility issues.

Patient-Controlled Analgesia (PCA) These devices can be used at home or in the hospital to allow the client to administer narcotics intravenously as needed for pain control. A PCA device is programmed to deliver a set amount of narcotic. They have a remote control bolus mechanism. The client or nurse can deliver a bolus of medication at set intervals. These pumps can be ambulatory or pole-mounted.

Factors Affecting Flow Rates (Troubleshooting)

1. Height of the IV container: The container should be at least 3 ft above the insertion site.

2. Diameter of the tubing: The clamp controls the flow by affecting the diameter of the tubing. Flow will be faster through larger cannulas or needles.

3. Length of tubing: Extension tubing will decrease flow rate.

4. Viscosity of fluid: Blood, blood products, and parenteral nutrition require larger cannula than water or saline (no. 19 or larger, and the appropriate drip chamber size.)

5. Infiltration: Symptoms are edema, discomfort, and cool skin.

6. Displaced needle: Tip of needle or catheter may be lodged against vein wall. To correct, untape and gently pull back on needle.

7. Kinking: Lying on the tubing can cause blockage of flow.

8. Clot formation at catheter tip: Do not forcibly irrigate, as this may cause a pulmonary embolism.

6-3 COMMONLY USED IV SOLUTIONS

The main types of intravenous solutions are

1. Carbohydrate solutions (2.5%, 5%, 10%, 15%, 50% dextrose in water)

2. Electrolyte solutions containing sodium (0.2%, 0.45%, 0.9%, 3%, 5% sodium chloride)

3. Special-purpose electrolyte solutions (potassium solutions, Ringer's, Ringer's lactate)

4. Solutions combining dextrose and sodium (0.045% sodium chloride in 5% dextrose)

5. Protein hydrolysates (amino acid solutions)

6. Solutions containing alcohol (5% alcohol and 5% dextrose in water)

7. Colloidal solutions (plasma, plasma expanders)

8. Blood and blood products

9. Fat emulsions

Always know the tonicity of the solution you are giving, the indications for it, the fluid and electrolyte status of the client, and disease states/constitutional factors that may influence how the intravenous therapy will be received by the client (refer to Chapter 5, Fluid and Electrolyte Balance).

Note: Any IV solution that has additives in it must be clearly marked with red tape or per hospital policy and given with great care. This is particularly true of potassium, because severe cardiac arrhythmias can occur with rapid administration.

Refer to Table 6-4 for electrolyte compositions and indications for common IV solutions.

6-4 IV DRUG ADMINISTRATION

The IV push, piggyback, and heparin lock methods of drug administration require extra caution. It is critical that drugs be given slowly (in most cases), and that the client is carefully observed for allergic or adverse reactions. Also, drugs and IV solutions must be compatible. See Section 7-3 in Drug Administration Chapter for a more complete discussion of this topic, and Table 6-5 IV Drug Compatibility Chart for drug compatibilities.

6-5 COMPLICATIONS OF IV THERAPY

With vigilance and expertise, complications of IV therapy can be minimized. Refer to Table 6-6 for symptoms, prevention, and treatment.

6-6 PARENTERAL NUTRITION

In cases where oral intake or tube feedings are not tolerated or may be hazardous, parenteral nutrition can provide necessary calories, amino acids, and electrolytes via the intravenous route. Solutions that have a low concentration may be given through a peripheral vein but more highly concentrated solutions must be given via a central vein. The concentration depends on the components in the particular solution.

Text continued on page 252

TABLE 6—4. QUICK GLANCE CHART OF COMMON IV FLUIDS *Continued*

PRODUCT	OSMO-LARITY	pH	NONELECTROLYTE Dext.	NONELECTROLYTE Cal.	CATIONS/LITER Na	CATIONS/LITER K	CATIONS/LITER Ca	CATIONS/LITER Mg	ANIONS/LITER Cl	ANIONS/LITER Acetate	ANIONS/LITER Lactate	Uses
Dextrose Solutions												
5% dextrose and water	Iso	4.8	5	17								Supplies calories as carbohydrates; prevents dehydration; maintains water balance; promotes sodium diuresis
10% dextrose and water	Hyper	4.7	10	34								
20% dextrose and water	Hyper	4.8	20	68								
50% dextrose and water	Hyper	4.6	50	170								
Saline Solutions												
0.45% NaCl	Hypo	5.9			77				77			Treats alkalosis; corrects fluid loss; treats sodium depletion
0.9% NaCl	Iso	6.0			154				154			
3% NaCl	Hyper	6.0			513				513			

Table continued on following page

TABLE 6–4. QUICK GLANCE CHART OF COMMON IV FLUIDS

PRODUCT	OSMO-LARITY	pH	NONELEC-TROLYTE		CATIONS/LITER				ANIONS/LITER			Uses
			Dext.	Cal.	Na	K	Ca	Mg	Cl	Acetate	Lactate	
Dextrose and Saline Solutions												
5% dextrose/0.2% NaCl	Iso	4.6	5	17	34				34			Promotes diuresis; corrects moderate fluid loss; prevents alkalosis; provides calories and sodium chloride
5% dextrose/0.45% NaCl	Hyper	4.6	5	17	77				77			
5% dextrose/0.9% NaCl	Hyper	4.4	5	17	154				154			
10% dextrose/0.9% NaCl	Hyper	4.8	10	34	154				154			

Multiple Electrolyte Solutions

Solution	Tonicity												Comments
Ringer's solution	Iso	304	6.0		147	4	4	0	155	0	0	0	Replaces fluid lost through vomiting or gastrointestinal suctioning; treats dehydration; restores normal fluid balance
Lactated Ringer's	Iso	273	6.5		130	4	3	0	109	0	0	28	
Normosol R (Abbott)	Iso	295	6.4	18	140	5		3	98	27	0	0	
Plasma Lyte M with dextrose* (Baxter)	Hyper	383	5.2	18	40	16	5	3	40	12	12	12	

*The addition of dextrose to any multiple electrolyte solution renders the solution hypertonic.

From Phillips LD. Manual of IV therapeutics. Philadelphia: FA Davis, 1993. Reprinted with permission of F. A. Davis Company.

TABLE 6–5. IV DRUG COMPATIBILITY

KEY
C = Compatible
L = Compatible for a limited period of time
I = Incompatible
* = Conflicting data
– = Data unavailable
■ = Identical drug

	1. amikacin	2. aminophylline	3. amphotericin B	4. ampicillin	5. calcium chloride	6. calcium gluconate	7. cefamandole	8. cefazolin	9. cefoxitin	10. chloramphenicol	11. cimetidine	12. clindamycin	13. dexamethasone	14. diphenhydramine	15. gentamicin
1. amikacin	■	*	I	I	C	C	–	I	C	C	C	C	*	C	–
2. aminophylline	*	■	–	–	–	C	–	–	–	C	I	I	C	C	–
3. amphotericin B	I	–	■	I	I	I	–	–	–	–	I	–	–	I	I
4. ampicillin	I	–	I	■	–	I	–	–	–	–	*	*	–	–	I
5. calcium chloride	C	–	I	–	■	–	–	–	–	C	–	–	–	–	–
6. calcium gluconate	C	C	I	I	–	■	I	I	–	C	–	I	C	C	I
7. cefamandole	–	–	–	–	–	I	■	–	–	–	*	C	–	–	I
8. cefazolin	I	–	–	–	–	I	–	■	–	L	I	C	C	–	I
9. cefoxitin	C	–	–	–	–	–	–	–	■	–	C	C	–	–	I
10. chloramphenicol	C	C	–	–	C	C	–	L	–	■	–	–	C	C	I
11. cimetidine	C	I	I	*	–	–	*	*	C	–	■	C	C	–	C
12. clindamycin	C	I	–	*	–	I	C	C	C	–	C	■	–	–	C
13. dexamethasone	*	C	–	–	–	C	–	C	–	C	C	–	■	I	I
14. diphenhydramine	C	C	I	–	–	C	–	–	–	C	–	–	I	■	I
15. gentamicin	–	–	I	I	–	I	I	I	I	I	C	C	I	I	■
16. heparin	I	C	C	*	–	C	–	–	L	C	–	C	L	–	I
17. hydrocortisone	C	C	C	*	C	C	–	–	–	C	–	C	L	I	I
18. insulin, regular	–	I	–	–	–	–	–	–	C	–	C	–	–	–	I
19. lidocaine	–	C	–	*	C	C	C	–	–	C	C	–	C	C	C
20. methicillin	I	C	–	I	C	C	–	–	–	I	–	–	C	C	I
21. methylprednisolone	–	*	–	–	–	I	–	–	–	C	–	C	–	–	–
22. metoclopramide	–	–	–	–	–	I	–	–	–	–	C	C	C	–	–
23. metronidazole	C	C	–	*	–	–	*	C	*	C	–	C	–	–	C
24. mezlocillin	–	–	–	–	–	–	–	–	–	–	–	–	–	–	I
25. multivitamin infusion	–	–	–	–	–	–	–	C	–	–	–	–	–	–	–
26. nafcillin	–	*	–	–	–	–	–	–	–	C	–	–	C	C	–
27. oxacillin	*	–	–	–	–	–	–	–	–	C	–	–	–	–	–
28. oxytocin	–	–	–	–	–	–	–	–	–	C	–	–	–	–	–
29. penicillin G	*	I	I	–	C	C	–	–	–	C	C	C	–	C	*
30. piperacillin	–	–	–	–	–	–	–	–	–	–	–	C	–	–	–
31. potassium chloride	*	C	I	–	–	C	–	–	–	C	C	C	–	–	–
32. procainamide	–	–	–	–	–	–	–	–	–	–	–	–	–	–	–
33. ranitidine	C	–	I	*	–	–	–	*	–	C	–	I	C	–	C
34. ticarcillin	–	–	–	–	–	–	–	–	–	–	–	–	–	–	–
35. tobramycin	–	–	–	–	–	C	I	–	C	–	–	*	–	–	–
36. vancomycin	C	*	–	–	–	C	–	–	–	I	C	–	I	–	–
37. verapamil	C	C	I	*	C	C	C	C	C	C	C	C	C	–	C

TABLE 6–5. IV DRUG COMPATIBILITY (Continued)

	16. heparin	17. hydrocortisone	18. insulin, regular	19. lidocaine	20. methicillin	21. methylprednisolone	22. metoclopramide	23. metronidazole	24. mezlocillin	25. multivitamin infusion	26. nafcillin	27. oxacillin	28. oxytocin	29. penicillin G	30. piperacillin	31. potassium chloride	32. procainamide	33. ranitidine	34. ticarcillin	35. tobramycin	36. vancomycin	37. verapamil
1.	I	C	–	–	I	–	–	C	–	–	–	*	–	*	–	*	–	C	–	–	C	C
2.	C	C	I	C	C	*	–	C	–	–	*	–	I	–	C	–	–	–	–	–	*	C
3.	C	C	–	–	–	–	–	–	–	–	–	–	I	–	I	–	I	–	–	–	–	I
4.	*	*	–	*	I	–	–	*	–	–	–	–	–	–	–	–	–	*	–	–	–	*
5.	–	C	–	C	I	–	–	–	–	–	–	–	C	–	–	–	–	–	–	–	–	C
6.	C	L	–	C	C	I	I	–	–	–	–	–	C	–	C	–	–	–	–	C	C	C
7.	–	–	–	C	–	–	–	*	–	–	–	–	–	–	–	–	–	–	–	I	–	C
8.	–	–	–	–	–	–	C	–	–	–	–	–	–	–	–	–	*	–	–	–	–	C
9.	L	C	–	–	–	–	*	–	C	–	–	–	–	–	–	–	–	–	–	C	–	C
10.	C	C	–	C	I	C	–	C	–	–	C	C	C	C	–	C	–	C	–	–	I	C
11.	–	–	C	C	–	C	C	–	–	–	–	–	C	–	C	–	–	–	–	–	C	C
12.	C	C	–	–	–	C	C	C	–	–	–	–	–	C	C	C	–	I	–	*	–	C
13.	L	L	–	C	C	–	C	–	–	–	C	–	–	–	–	–	–	C	–	–	I	C
14.	–	I	–	C	C	–	–	–	–	–	C	–	–	C	–	–	–	–	–	–	–	–
15.	I	I	I	C	I	–	C	I	–	–	–	–	*	–	–	C	–	–	–	–	–	C
16.	■	*	I	C	*	C	–	C	–	–	C	–	–	*	–	C	–	–	–	–	I	C
17.	*	■	L	C	*	–	–	*	–	–	I	–	–	C	C	C	–	–	–	–	C	C
18.	I	L	■	C	–	I	–	–	–	–	–	–	–	–	–	–	–	–	–	–	–	C
19.	C	C	C	■	–	–	–	–	–	–	–	–	C	–	C	C	–	–	–	–	–	C
20.	*	*	–	–	■	–	–	–	–	–	I	–	–	C	–	C	–	–	–	–	I	C
21.	C	–	I	–	–	■	C	–	–	I	–	–	*	–	–	–	C	–	–	–	–	C
22.	–	–	–	–	–	C	■	–	C	–	–	–	C	–	–	–	C	–	–	–	–	–
23.	C	*	–	–	–	–	–	■	–	C	–	–	C	–	–	–	–	–	C	–	–	–
24.	–	–	–	–	–	–	–	–	■	–	–	–	–	–	–	–	–	–	–	–	–	*
25.	–	–	–	–	–	C	C	–	–	■	–	–	L	–	–	–	–	–	–	–	–	C
26.	C	I	–	–	–	I	–	–	–	–	■	–	–	C	–	–	–	C	–	–	–	*
27.	–	–	–	–	–	–	–	–	–	–	–	■	–	–	C	–	–	–	–	–	–	*
28.	–	–	–	–	–	–	–	–	–	–	–	–	■	–	–	–	–	–	–	–	–	C
29.	*	C	–	C	C	*	–	*	–	L	–	–	–	■	–	*	–	C	–	–	C	C
30.	–	C	–	–	–	–	–	–	–	–	–	–	–	–	■	C	–	–	–	–	–	C
31.	C	C	–	C	C	–	C	–	–	–	C	C	–	*	C	■	–	–	–	–	C	C
32.	–	–	–	C	–	–	–	–	–	–	–	–	–	–	–	–	■	–	–	–	–	C
33.	–	–	–	–	–	–	–	–	–	–	–	–	C	–	–	–	–	■	C	C	C	–
34.	–	–	–	–	–	–	–	–	–	–	–	–	–	–	–	–	–	C	■	C	–	C
35.	–	–	–	–	–	–	C	–	–	–	–	–	–	–	–	–	C	–	–	■	–	C
36.	I	C	–	–	I	–	–	–	–	–	–	–	–	–	–	–	C	–	C	–	■	C
37.	C	C	C	C	C	C	–	–	*	C	*	*	C	C	C	C	C	–	C	C	C	■

Data from Deglin JD, Vallerand AH. Davis's drug guide for nurses. 3rd ed. 1993:1258–1259, reprinted with permission.

TABLE 6–6. COMPLICATIONS OF IV THERAPY

COMPLICATION	PREVENTION	INTERVEN-TIONS
Circulatory Overload Overload of fluid that occurs with too rapid rate of infusion and more frequently in infants or the elderly. Congestive heart failure or pulmonary edema can ensue. *Symptoms:* Edema, rales, shortness of breath, distended neck veins, decreased urine output	Assess client history for presence of heart condition. Carefully monitor flow rate. Place client in semisitting position. Monitor urine output, fluid status q 1 hr.	Slow IV to keep-open rate. Report vital signs and all symptoms to MD. Raise to sitting position, if BP allows. Have resuscitative equipment ready. Assess breath sounds for rales and cardiac status.
Pyrogenic Reaction Generalized febrile reaction due to contaminated equipment. *Symptoms:* increased temp., chills, flushing, backache 30 min to 1 hr after start of IV	Check all IV equipment, site, and solutions for defects, exp dates. Use indwelling catheter only when necessary.	Slow infusion to keep-open rate, check vital signs, notify MD. Send all equipment to lab. Get blood cultures.
Infection Local infection can spread systemically. *Symptoms:* redness, swelling, pain	Use rigid aseptic technique. Frequently rotate IV site (q 48–72 hr or per hospital policy). Change dressing q 24–48 hr. Adequately anchor catheter.	Local: Apply warm compresses. Administer antibiotics if ordered.

TABLE 6–6. COMPLICATIONS OF IV THERAPY
Continued

COMPLICATION	PREVENTION	INTERVEN-TIONS
	Periodically apply antimicrobial ointment at infusion site.	
Infiltration Dislodging of needle causing edema, discomfort, cool skin	Fasten needle securely. Check tubing for kinks. Avoid looping of tubing below bed level. Check IV site and rate frequently.	Stop infusion. Limit arm movement. Apply 3 × 3 gauze pad and remove needle. Apply warm compresses. Restart infusion elsewhere.
Superficial Thrombo-phlebitis Caused by overuse of a vein, an irritating infusion solution, clot formation, or use of large-bore needles	Use aseptic technique. Change veins q 48–72 hr. Administer irritating solutions through large veins.	Apply cold compresses first to relieve pain and inflammation, followed with warm, moist compresses.
Air Embolism Air enters circulatory system, can cause death. *Symptoms:* increased BP, cyanosis, tachycardia, loss of consciousness	Replace initial bag or bottle before it is empty. Clamp the nearly empty bottle in Y-type sets. Allow fluid to flow through tubing and needle to force air out before infusing. Secure all connections.	Immediately turn client on left side with head down. Air will pass into right ventricle and allow blood to pass into lungs, where it will dissipate. Administer oxygen.
Drug Overload Toxic concentrations in heart can	Carefully monitor flow rate, drug	Related to specific drug,

Table continued on following page

TABLE 6–6. COMPLICATIONS OF IV THERAPY
Continued

COMPLICATION	PREVENTION	INTERVEN-TIONS
lead to dizziness, fainting, shock	dosages, serum levels.	antidote. Stop drug infusion, but KVO.
Nerve Damage Can result from splinting the arm too tightly. *Symptoms:* numbness of fingers or hand	Place padding where bandage is applied.	Massage arm, do range-of-motion exercises. Instruct client to open and close hand several times q hr. Physical therapy may be required.
Fluid and Electrolyte Imbalances	Control flow rate. Monitor lab values. Carefully assess (see Table 5-4, Fluid and Electrolyte Imbalances).	Intervene accordingly to correct imbalance.

Total parenteral nutrition (TPN) solutions provide all of the client's energy and nutrient requirements: protein, carbohydrates, fats, electrolytes, vitamins, trace elements, and water. The highly concentrated amino acid and glucose solutions need to be administered through a central vein. A client may receive TPN indefinitely.

Peripheral parenteral nutrition (PPN) provides a more limited nutritional therapy. These solutions contain fewer non-protein calories and lower amino acid concentrations, and may include fat. PPN is meant for short-term therapy to maintain nutritional status.

Clients receiving parenteral nutrition need to be monitored for changes in fluid and electrolyte status and in glucose, amino acid, mineral, and vitamin levels. They also need to be assessed for tolerance to the nutrient solution and early signs of complications (Table 6-7).

Text continued on page 257

TABLE 6–7. COMPLICATIONS OF PARENTERAL NUTRITION

COMPLICATION	SIGNS AND SYMPTOMS	INTERVENTIONS
Catheter-related complications		
Pneumothorax and hydrothorax	Tachypnea, respiratory distress, pain, decreased breath sounds, cyanosis. Rarely, a slow-leaking pneumothorax may present at a later stage with similar findings.	• Symptomatic treatment with oxygen. • Chest tube will be inserted.
Sepsis	Fever, lethargy, chills, erythema, or pus at insertion site, glucosuria.	• Remove catheter and culture tip. • Treat with appropriate antibiotic
Cracked or broken catheter	Fluid leading out of tubing or blood backing out.	• Apply nonserrated clamp above the break to prevent air from getting in the line or blood from coming out.
Extravasation of the infusate	Catheter out of the vein. Swelling, edema, pain, and coolness over catheter site or of head, neck, face; possible vesicle discoloration and/or sloughing of skin at the infusion site.	• Discontinue infusion. • Catheter removal. • Symptomatic management of skin as per institutional protocol.
Metabolic complications		
Hyperglycemia	Elevated blood and urine glucose levels, fatigue, rest-	• Identify the etiology of the hyperglycemia.

Table continued on following page

TABLE 6–7. COMPLICATIONS OF PARENTERAL NUTRITION *Continued*

COMPLICATION	SIGNS AND SYMPTOMS	INTERVENTIONS
	lessness, weakness, confusion, anxiety, delirium or coma, polyuria, dehydration	• Adjust PN flow rate. • Start insulin therapy.
Hypoglycemia	Muscle weakness, diaphoresis, nervous instability, trembling, faintness, headache, hunger, palpitations, diplopia, confusion	• Infuse dextrose 10%.
Hyperosmolar nonketotic syndrome	Confusion, dehydration, seizures, coma, hyperglycemia, glycosuria	• Stop dextrose. • Give insulin and rehydrate.
Hypernatremia	Excessive watery diarrhea; dry, sticky mucous membranes; oliguria; agitation; and firm, rubbery tissue turgor.	• Eliminate sources of sodium intake.
Hyponatremia	Diarrhea, apprehension, seizures, abdominal cramps	• Restore sodium concentration to normal without producing a fluid volume excess.
Hyperkalemia	Diarrhea, colic, nausea (all reflect GI hyperactivity), dizziness, paresthesia, muscle weakness, cramps, pain, ECG alterations	• Obtain laboratory confirmation. • Eliminate sources of potassium intake. • Client may need Kayexalate enemas; IV insulin plus dextrose administration;

TABLE 6–7. COMPLICATIONS OF PARENTERAL NUTRITION *Continued*

COMPLICATION	SIGNS AND SYMPTOMS	INTERVENTIONS
		extrarenal dialysis.
		• Monitor ECG pattern.
Hypokalemia	Arrhythmias, muscle weakness, paresthesia, paralysis Abdominal cramps, polyuria, tetany, twitching	• Increase potassium supplementation. • Increase calcium supplementation.
Hyperphosphatemia	Same as hypocalemia but less severe	• Obtain laboratory confirmation. • Eliminate sources of phosphate intake.
Hypophosphatemia	Muscular hypotonia, paresthesias, hyperventilation, respiratory distress, irritability, weakness, coma	• Increase phosphate supplementation.
Hypermagnesemia	Lethargy, hypotension, respiratory depression; ECG alterations	• Obtain laboratory confirmation. • Eliminate sources of magnesium intake.
Hypomagnesemia	Disorientation, agitation, CNS irritability, tremors, muscle cramps, paresthesia	• Increase magnesium supplementation.
Hepatic dysfunction	Increased bilirubin levels, increased serum transaminase, lactate dehydrogenase	• Decrease carbohydrate and add fat emulsion.
Metabolic acidosis	Decreased serum bicarbonate level,	• Use acetate or lactate salts of

Table continued on following page

TABLE 6–7. COMPLICATIONS OF PARENTERAL NUTRITION *Continued*

COMPLICATION	SIGNS AND SYMPTOMS	INTERVENTIONS
	increased serum chloride level	sodium or hydrogen.
Electrolyte or mineral imbalances		• Corrections of an electrolyte imbalance may require concomitant correction of another electrolyte because of their interdependence. Use of IV, IM, or oral route is determined by the client's condition and the severity of the situation.
Mechanical complications		
Air embolism	Respiratory difficulty, tachypnea, cyanosis, chest pain, loss of consciousness, seizure, hypertension	• Clamp catheter. • Place client in Trendelenburg position on the left side, administer oxygen.
Thrombosis	Swelling of arm, neck, and face; pain at the insertion site and along vein; malaise; fever	• Remove catheter. • Administer Heparin if ordered. • Venous flow studies may be done.
Clotted catheter	Interrupted flow rate, hypoglycemia	• Reposition catheter. Attempt to aspirate clot. • May need urokinase to clear catheter lumen.

TABLE 6–7. COMPLICATIONS OF PARENTERAL NUTRITION *Continued*

COMPLICATION	SIGNS AND SYMPTOMS	INTERVENTIONS
Too rapid an infusion	Headache, nausea, lethargy	• Check the rate of infusion. • Check infusion pump.
Phlebitis	Pain, tenderness, redness, and warmth	• Apply gentle heat to the insertion site. • Elevate the insertion site, if possible.

Nursing Functions in TPN Infusion

• Assure that each bag or bottle has a label listing the contents of the solution, total volume, expiration date, and time solution was hung.

• TPN solutions should not hang for more than 24 hr.

• Maintain the rate of infusion as prescribed. Never speed up or slow down rate.

• Change tubing every 24–48 hr per hospital policy. Make sure all tubing junctions are secure.

• Change dressing at the infusion site every 24–48 hr or per hospital policy. Use strict aseptic technique.

• Check infusion pump every 30 min.

• Record vital signs every 4–8 hr. Be alert for elevated temperature.

• Test for glycosuria. If glycosuria persists, finger-stick blood glucose testing will be necessary.

• Use TPN infusion line for TPN only. Fat emulsion is the only exception to this rule.

• Record accurate intake and output.

- Weigh client daily.

- Monitor results of routine laboratory tests, such as serum electrolytes, blood urea nitrogen, and glucose, and report abnormal findings to the physician so appropriate changes in the TPN solution can be made.

- Monitor the client for signs and symptoms of nutritional alteration.

- Provide emotional support.

- Provide frequent mouth care.

Fat Emulsions

Fat emulsions prevent and treat essential fatty acid deficiency and provide a major source of energy or an energy-calorie combination. Fat emulsions may be administered as part of a total parenteral nutrition solution, along with a peripheral parenteral nutrition solution, or separately through a central or peripheral line.

- Use a particulate filter according to the manufacturer's recommendations (a 1.2 micron filter is preferred).

- Check fat emulsion for separation or oily appearance. Do not infuse if these are noted.

- Never add anything to the fat emulsion solution.

- Discard any unused portion; a contaminated emulsion can support microbial growth. Guidelines from the CDC recommend not hanging these solutions more than 12 hr.

- Start the infusion at a flow rate of 1 ml/min for 30 min, then proceed as ordered.

- Observe closely for allergic reactions for the first 30 min.

6-7   BLOOD TRANSFUSIONS

Blood Grouping and Compatibility

Typing and cross-matching determine donor and recipient blood compatibility. Red cells from the donor are com-

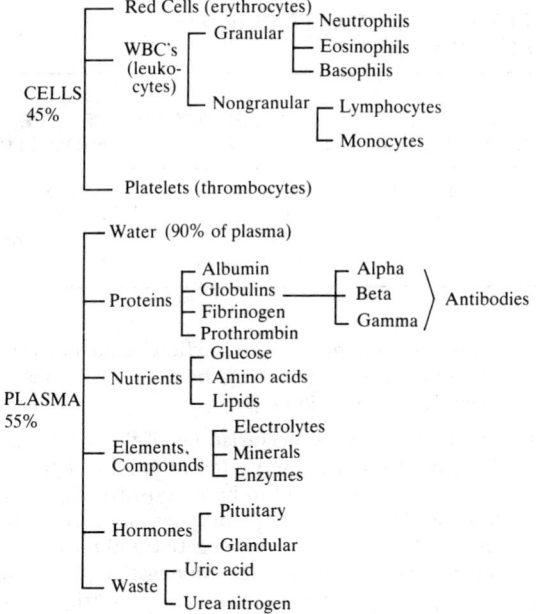

Figure 6–3. Blood composition.

bined with serum (plasma minus fibrinogen) from the recipient (Figure 6-3 serves as brief reminder of blood composition). If agglutination or hemolysis occurs, the blood is incompatible (Table 6-8). The test can take up to 45 min to complete in the laboratory.

UNIVERSAL DONOR, RECIPIENT

- Group O is the universal donor: It has both anti-A and anti-B antibodies and can therefore receive only type O blood, but can give to all other groups because it has neither A nor B antigens.

- Group AB is the universal recipient: It has neither anti-A nor anti-B antibodies, and could therefore receive blood from all other groups.

TABLE 6–8. BLOOD GROUPING AND COMPATIBILITY

BLOOD GROUP	% OF POPULATION	CAN BE DONOR TO TYPE	CAN RECEIVE FROM TYPE
A	41	A or AB	A or O
B	9	B or AB	B or O
AB	3	AB	A, B, AB, or O
O	47	A, B, AB, or O	O

- Except in emergency cases where availability is a problem, persons receiving blood transfusions are given their own blood type.

- Rh factor: If one of the variations of the many agglutinogens in the Rh group is found to be in a person's blood, he or she is said to be Rh-positive. Eighty-five percent of whites and 99% of other races are Rh-positive; 15% of whites are Rh-negative and must not receive Rh-positive blood. The Rh-negative person may develop anti-Rh antibodies, which could trigger a hemolytic reaction. Though this may not take place with the first transfusion, subsequent transfusions could result in agglutination.

Nursing Considerations for Administration of Blood and Blood Products

- Complete Table 6-9, Checklist for Blood Transfusions and Blood Products, before each blood transfusion you administer, making absolutely sure you do the positive ID check with another nurse.

- Wear gloves when performing actual venipuncture, complying with federal standards for handling blood and body fluids.

- Use only isotonic saline (0.9% NaCl) before or during the transfusion. *Never add drugs or other solutions to the line through which you are giving blood.*

TABLE 6–9. CHECKLIST FOR BLOOD AND BLOOD PRODUCT TRANSFUSIONS

Before Blood Arrives

I know:
- ☐ The overall condition of the client
- ☐ If there are predisposing factors to circulatory overload (e.g., congestive heart failure, old age)
- ☐ Why the client is receiving the particular blood product
- ☐ The client's pertinent lab values (CBC, blood chemistry, clotting times)
- ☐ If client has a history of allergy to blood or blood products

I have:
- ☐ Double checked the doctor's orders
- ☐ Gathered appropriate equipment for the particular blood product
- ☐ Started an IV with appropriate size needle and normal saline (do not give more than 50–60 ml)
- ☐ Given any ordered premedications (antihistamine, antipyretic)

When Blood Arrives

I have:
- ☐ Inspected it for gas bubbles or changes of color
- ☐ Taken baseline vitals
- ☐ Explained the procedure to the client
- ☐ Positively identified the client and the blood with another nurse for absolute certainty of blood type compatability (see below)
- ☐ Planned to stay with the client or check frequently for the first 10–20 min of transfusion to make sure the rate is slow (2 ml/min, 20 gtt/min) and that there are no untoward reactions

Client ID Check (Do not infuse unless information matches!)

1. Client's full name (armband and ask client)
2. Client's ID number
3. Blood unit number
4. Blood group and Rh factor
5. Expiration date
6. Type and cross-match number

- Start the saline using the appropriate administration set, filter, and needle before the blood arrives from the blood bank, at a very slow rate. Table 6-10 lists major blood products with important nursing considerations.

Text continued on page 268

TABLE 6–10. SUMMARY OF BLOOD COMPONENTS

BLOOD COMPONENT	VOLUME	ACTION AND USES	INFUSION GUIDE	SPECIAL CONSIDERATIONS
Whole blood	200 mL RBCs 300 mL plasma Total = 500 mL	Massive blood loss Restore blood volume Raise hemoglobin and hematocrit	0.9% sodium chloride primer Transfuse over 2–4 h Y blood set necessary Shelf life: 35 d (1,2) CPDA-1 ADSOL 49 d Filter	Always ABO and Rh Identical 1 unit whole blood raises the hemoglobin 1 g and hematocrit 3–4%
Red cells PRBCs	250 mL (same amount of hemoglobin and hematocrit as whole blood)	Acute anemia with hypoxia Chronic symptomatic anemia Aplastic anemia Bone marrow failure due to malignancy or chemotherapy	Same as whole blood Transfuse over 1½–2 h	May add 50 mL normal saline to RBCs to decrease viscosity ABO and Rh identical 1 U PRBCs raises the hemoglobin 1 g and hematocrit 3–4%

Washed red cells	200–250 mL	Provides leukocyte-poor RBCs for patient with recurrent allergic or febrile transfusion reactions	Same as whole blood 24 h expiration date	Lab needs advanced notice to prepare cells. This procedure is an open system: once ordered and the process of washing started, it must be used
Deglycerolized red cells (frozen)	200–250 mL	Prolonged storage of blood, especially rare blood types. Minimizes febrile or allergic reactions	Same as whole blood. Infuse over 1½–2 h. Expires in 24 h	Blood bank will not deglycerolize until requested, and takes about 1 hr. ABO/Rh compatible
Granulocytes Leukopheresis	300–400 mL. Note: Suspended in 200–200 mL of plasma	Clients with neutropenia, fever, or significant infection unresponsive to antibiotics	Usually administered for 4 consecutive days. Standard blood filter. Administer slowly over 2–4 hours. Administer as soon as collected or at least within 24 h	Reactions are common. Check vitals every 15 min. Note: Febrile reactions occur in about two thirds of clients. Chills, fever, and allergic reactions common

Table continued on following page

TABLE 6–10. SUMMARY OF BLOOD COMPONENTS *Continued*

BLOOD COMPONENT	VOLUME	ACTION AND USES	INFUSION GUIDE	SPECIAL CONSIDERATIONS
				Requires premedication to control reactions
Platelets Random	60–70 mL/U minimum Usual dose: 6–10 U	Control bleeding in platelet deficiencies Thrombocytopenia Bone marrow hypoplasia due to chemotherapy	Administer as rapidly as patient can tolerate; 1–2 mL/min Recommended 150–200 mL/h, platelet administration set (syringe push or Y type) Use a Y filter with saline as primer	Requires 20 min pooling time by laboratory ABO/Rh preferred but not necessary

Fresh frozen plasma (FFP)	200–250 mL	Replacement of coagulation factors Increases clotting factors Factor deficiencies (e.g., factor V or XI) Thrombotic thrombocytopenia purpura	Storage is at 18°C for 1 y Standard blood filter	Does not provide platelets 1 mL of FFP raises the level of clotting factor 2–3%
Cryoprecipitate (concentrated fibrinogen)	Each unit contains 150 mg fibrinogen/15 mL plasma (5–10 mL U) with 10 mL saline added. Usual order is for 6–10 U	Used to control bleeding associated with deficiency in coagulation factors Treatment of hemophilia A, von Willebrand's disease, hypofibrinogenemia, factor VIII deficiency, DIC associated with obstetric complications	Administer with filter provided with product Give as fast as client tolerates Monitor pulse while infusing	ABO compatible with patient's red cells If blood group unknown, use AB blood Rh match not required Must be used within 3 hr after reconstituted

Table continued on following page

TABLE 6–10. SUMMARY OF BLOOD COMPONENTS *Continued*

BLOOD COMPONENT	VOLUME	ACTION AND USES	INFUSION GUIDE	SPECIAL CONSIDERATIONS
Albumin 5% = 12.5 g/ 250 mL 25% = 12.5 g/ 50 mL	5% solution is in concentration of 250 mL or 500 mL; 25% solution is in 50–100 mL concentration	Plasma volume expander Hypovolemic shock Support blood pressure during hypotensive episodes Induce diuresis in fluid overload	May be administered as rapidly as tolerated if for reduced blood volume Normal rates: 2–4 mL/min for 5% solution; 1 mL/min for 25% solution Supplied in glass bottles with tubing for administration	25% albumin is hypertonic and is five times more concentrated than 5% solutions. Give with extreme caution; can cause circulatory overload No type or cross-match is necessary Store at room temperature
Plasma protein fraction (PPF)	Glass bottle with tubing, 250 mL	Same as albumin	Equivalent to 5% albumin	Has fewer purification steps

Intravenous serum globulin (IVIgG)	Lyophilized powder reconstituted with sterile water for injection following manufacturer directions	Primary immunodeficiency disorders Idiopathic thrombocytopenic purpura (ITP) Chronic B-cell lymphocytic leukemia Restores, strengthens, or modifies immunity	Do not need saline primer Standard administration set with vented airway Some manufacturers supply administration set Dose range: 200–400 mg/kg Rates of infusion are specific Rates are increased gradually	than albumin No type and cross-match necessary Has a high sodium content Severe reactions are rare No type and cross-match necessary Anaphylactic reaction can occur and is the greatest risk

Data from Phillips LD. Manual of IV therapeutics. Philadelphia: FA Davis, 1993. Reprinted with permission.

- Do not store blood on the nursing unit, only in carefully monitored refrigerators in the blood bank.

- Blood sent up to the units must be used within 30 min or returned to the blood bank because of the danger of bacterial proliferation.

- Be familiar with the complications of blood transfusion—the prevention, signs and symptoms, and nursing interventions (Table 6-11). If a blood reaction is suspected, stop the transfusion, keep the IV line open with normal saline, and report the signs and symptoms.

- See specific blood product for rates of infusion (see Table 6-10).

- Change tubing after 2 units of blood have been administered.

- Slow infusion rates may cause whole blood or red cells to stop running. In this case, clamp the blood tubing and run saline through it for a minute before restarting blood. Do not repeat more than twice, to avoid increasing the sodium intake. Specially designed pressure cuffs may be used for slow-running blood.

Whole Blood and Specific Blood Products

INDICATIONS, ADMINISTRATION, AND MAJOR RISKS

Blood is living tissue. A transfusion can be regarded as a type of transplant. Knowledge of the wide variety of blood and blood products and attention to detail are essential. Whole blood is rarely used except in cases of massive blood loss. Risks of transfusion can be minimized when only the needed component is given. Refer to Figure 6-3 as a reminder of blood constituents. Use Table 6-10 whenever administering a blood or blood product transfusion, as each blood product requires particular specifications for administration.

Text continued on page 273

TABLE 6–11. COMPLICATIONS OF BLOOD TRANSFUSIONS

REACTION	PREVENTION	INTERVENTIONS
Hemolytic		
Causes ABO or Rh incompatibility; intradonor incompatibility; administering hemolyzed or fragile red blood cells due to the age of the blood; improper storage or coming in contact with incompatible IV solutions.	Before transfusion, check donor and recipient blood types to ensure blood compatibility; also identify client with another nurse. Transfuse blood slowly for first 15–20 min; closely observe client for the first 20 min of the transfusion.	• Stop transfusion immediately. • Monitor blood pressure. • Treat shock with intravenous colloids, oxygen, epinephrine, a diuretic, and vasopressor. • Obtain posttransfusion reaction blood and urine samples for evaluation. • Observe for signs of hemorrhage resulting from disseminated intravascular coagulation.
Signs and Symptoms Shaking, chills, fever; bursting feeling in the head; pain in the neck and lumbar area; nausea; vomiting; chest pain; shock and renal failure		
Allergic		
Cause Blood contains something to which the client is allergic.	Premedicate with antihistamine if client has a history of allergic reactions. Observe client closely for the first 20 min of the transfusion.	• Stop transfusion, keep IV open. • Administer antihistamines. • Monitor for anaphylactic reaction and administer epinephrine and steroids, if indicated.
Signs and Symptoms Urticaria, edema, wheezing, headache; infrequently, anaphylactic shock will occur		

Table continued on following page

TABLE 6–11. COMPLICATIONS OF BLOOD TRANSFUSIONS *Continued*

REACTION	PREVENTION	INTERVENTIONS
Circulatory Overload		
Causes Some clients with compromised cardiovascular systems will experience heart failure, shock, pulmonary edema, and cyanosis if too much blood is administered.	Give packed cells instead of whole blood; properly space transfusions; give at correct rate, monitor elderly, frail, or clients with congestive heart failure closely.	• Stop transfusion, keep IV open. • Administer diuretics, oxygen, digitalis, morphine, aminophylline as directed. • Assess breath sounds and vital signs frequently. • In severe cases, place client upright, feet down. • Rotate tourniquets to extremities. • Prepare for phlebotomy.
Signs and Symptoms Increase in venous pressure, distended neck veins, dyspnea, cough, frothy sputum, rales		
Febrile		
Causes Presence of bacterial lipopolysaccharides	Premedicate with antipyretic; use leukocyte-poor or washed red blood cells (RBCs)	• Stop transfusion, keep vein open; relieve symptoms with an antipyretic, antihistamine, or meperidine
Signs and Symptoms Sudden chilling, fever, headache, flank pain		
Plasma protein incompatibility		
Cause IgA incompatibility	Transfuse only IgA deficient blood or well-washed RBCs; stop transfusion, keep vein open; treat with broad-spectrum antibiotics and steroids.	• Treat for shock by administering oxygen, fluids, epinephrine, and possibly a steroid, as ordered.
Signs and Symptoms Flushing, abdominal pain, diarrhea, fever, dyspnea, hypotension, chills		

TABLE 6–11. COMPLICATIONS OF BLOOD TRANSFUSIONS *Continued*

REACTION	PREVENTION	INTERVENTIONS
Bacterial contamination *Cause* Presence of gram-negative organisms that can survive cod species of Pseudomonas *Signs and Symptoms* Rapid onset of chills; high fever, vomiting, diarrhea; marked hypotension; shock; signs of renal failure	Observe blood before transfusion for gas, clots, and dark purple color. Use air-free, touch-free method to draw and deliver blood. Maintain strict storage control. Transpose each unit of blood over 2–4 hr; terminate the transfusion if the time period exceeds 4 hr. Maintain sterile technique when administering blood products.	
Delayed transfusion reaction *Cause* Result of red blood cell antigen incompatibility other than the ABO Group. Rapid production of red blood cell antibody occurs shortly after transfusion of the corresponding antigen, as a result of sensitization during previous transfusions or pregnancies. Occurs over 2 or more days, or		• No acute treatment is usually required. • Monitor hematocrit, renal function, and coagulation profile routinely for all clients receiving transfusions. • Notify physician and transfusion services if delayed reaction is suspected.

Table continued on following page

TABLE 6–11. COMPLICATIONS OF BLOOD TRANSFUSIONS *Continued*

REACTION	PREVENTION	INTERVENTIONS
up to several weeks, after the transfusion. Most reactions of this type go unnoticed and are common. *Signs and Symptoms* Decrease in hemoglobin and hematocrit levels; persistent low-grade fever; malaise; indirect hyperbilirubinemia		
Potassium Intoxication *Cause* An abnormally high level of potassium in stored plasma caused by BC lysis *Signs and Symptoms* Immediate onset of hyperkalemia; slow, irregular heart beat; nausea and muscle weakness; intestinal colic, diarrhea; muscle twitching; ECG changes	Use fresh blood when administering massive transfusions.	• Obtain an ECG. • Administer Kayexalate orally or by enema.
Hypothermia *Cause* Rapid infusion of large amounts of cold blood, which decreases myocardial temperature	Warm blood to 95–98.6 degrees, especially before massive transfusions; slow or stop transfusion, de-	• Stop transfusion. • Warm client with blankets. • Obtain an ECG.

TABLE 6–11. COMPLICATIONS OF BLOOD TRANSFUSIONS *Continued*

REACTION	PREVENTION	INTERVENTIONS
Signs and Symptoms Shaking chills, hypotension, ventricular fibrillation; cardiac arrest, if core temperature falls below 86 degrees F	pending on reaction; expect a worse reaction in hypothermic client or clients with elevated potassium levels; slowly administer calcium gluconate IV.	
Hypocalcemia *Cause* A reaction to toxic proportions of citrate, which is used as a preservative in blood. The citrate ion can combine with calcium, causing a calcium deficiency, or normal citrate metabolism is hindered by the presence of liver disease. *Signs and Symptoms* Tingling sensation in fingers; muscle cramps; hypotension; tetany	Transfuse blood slowly. Monitor potassium and calcium levels. Use blood less than 2 days old if administering multiple units.	

REFERENCES

Atkins J. A nurse's guide to TPN. RN 1986; June: 20–24.

Craven RF. Fundamentals of nursing: human health and function. Philadelphia: JB Lippincott, 1992.

Holder C and Alexander J. Guide to IV therapy. Am J Nurs February 1990; 43–47.

Loeb S, et al. IV therapy: clinical skillbuilders. Springhouse, PA: Springhouse; 1990.

Lorenz BL. Are you using the right IV pump? RN 1990; May: 31–36.

Methany NM. Why worry about IV fluids? Am J Nurs 1990; June: 50–55.

Phillips LD. Manual of IV therapeutics. Philadelphia: FA Davis, 1993.

Querin JJ and Stahl LD. Twelve simple, sensible steps for successful blood transfusions. Nursing '90 1990; October: 68–81.

Stanford University Hospital, Department of Nursing. Nursing care manual, central venous catheters maintenance and care and blood drawing. April, 1993.

Thomason SS. Using a groshong central venous catheter. Nursing '91 1991; October: 58–60.

Ward L. Patient teaching for home IV therapy. RN 1990; April: 86–88.

CHAPTER 7

DRUG ADMINISTRATION

Administering medications is one of the most important and critical responsibilities you hold as a professional nurse. Absolute concentration while giving medications is key for the safety of your clients. If possible, work alone and without interruption; however always check with the physician, pharmacist, your client or another nurse if you have a question.

7-1 GUIDELINES FOR THE SAFE AND EFFECTIVE ADMINISTRATION OF DRUGS

Prior to Administration of Any Drug

- Be familiar with the following aspects of each medication administered:

1. **Drug name**

   - **Generic name:** nonproprietary name as designed by the United States Adopted Names (USAN) and United States Pharmacopeia (USP)

   - **Trade name:** proprietary (brand) name

   - Synonyms, abbreviations, and former names may also be used to designate a medication such as acetaminophen (paracetamol), INH (isoniazid), phenytoin (formerly diphenylhydantoin).

2. **Drug Action** (pharmacological activity and use)

3. **Dosage**

   - All dosages should be specified in metric units; apothecary units are outdated and subject to error.

   - Some drugs such as vitamins, penicillin, insulin, and heparin are measured in units of activity unique to that drug.

   - Electrolytes are measured in milliequivalents (mEq), except for phosphorus, which is measured in millimoles (mM).

   - If a client cannot swallow tablets or has a nasogastric (NG) tube, consult the pharmacist. Many medications are available as liquids but the dosing schedule may be different than the tablet form. Although many tablets can be crushed and capsules opened, some specially coated or sustained-release formulations cannot.

- Liquids should be measured in milliliters in an oral syringe or calibrated measuring cup.

- Use caution when measuring dosages in drops. While the USP defines a dropper as 20 drops water equal to 1 ml, each dropper must be individually calibrated because droplet size varies from one medication to another. It is preferable to specify the quantity in milliliters.

4. **Routes of Administration**

- Oral, including sublingual, buccal, nasogastric tube

- Rectal

- Vaginal

- Topical

- Intradermal

- Subcutaneous

- Intramuscular

- Intravenous

- Parenteral, via specific access devices (e.g., heparin lock, Hickman catheter, Portacath catheter, Mediport)

- Epidural

- Intrathecal

5. **Contraindications** (pregnancy, heart disease, allergies, etc.)

6. **Adverse Reactions** (nausea, vomiting, diarrhea, constipation, rash, cough, fever, etc.)

7. **Interaction** with other drugs, food, or laboratory tests

8. **Therapeutic Monitoring Parameters** (physical or laboratory tests to oversee drug action)

- Drug level monitoring is used to establish drug efficacy and minimize toxicity. Drug dosages are maintained or adjusted based upon the results. For maximal benefit, the sample should be drawn according to the times on Table 7-1. Resampling should follow the same procedure.

- If there is a question about any of the above information, check with the physician or pharmacist. An excellent reference book is the American Hospital Formulary Service published by the American Society of Hospital Pharmacists. The PDR is an advertising compendium of package inserts and is not a complete listing of drugs.

- Every client's medication orders should be clear, complete, and understood by the caregiver and, if possible, the client. If there is any doubt, contact the physician for clarification. When taking a verbal order, repeat the order back to the physician for verification.

- Check with the physician before withholding medication from a client who is going for a diagnostic test or to surgery and is NPO. It may be desirable to administer the drug in order to maintain a therapeutic blood level, or it may be the drug should be withheld because it interferes with a test or procedure.

- Always review the **Five Rights:** right client, right drug, right dose, right time, right route.

- Always read the label three times.

- Check the client's Adverse Drug Reaction Profile for any history of allergy or adverse drug reaction history.

Follow-up

- Make sure any medication left at the client's bedside (for example, nitroglycerin, topical cream or ointment, or ophthalmic medication) is there by physician order only. The medication should be properly labeled. Controlled substances and investigational drugs should not be left at the bedside.

TABLE 7–1. BLOOD LEVEL MONITORING

DRUG	THERA-PEUTIC RANGE	WHEN TO DRAW LEVELS
Carbamazepine	4–12mcg/ml	Just before next dose
Cyclosporine	Depending upon type of transplant 100–300ng/ml	Just before next dose
Digoxin	0.8–2ng/ml	IV >4 hr post dose PO >6 hr post dose
Gentamicin and tobramycin	Peak 4–10 mcg/ml Trough 0.5–2 mcg/ml	IV peak 30 min after 30 min infusion IV trough within 30 min before next dose IM peak 1 hr after IM injection IM trough within 30 min before next dose
Heparin	APTT 1.5–2.5 times control	4–6 hr post bolus dose and continuous infusion
Lidocaine	1–5mcg/ml	Anytime after 12 hr of infusion (steady state)
Lithium	0.6–1.2 mEq/L	12 hr after dose
Phenobarbital	15–40 mcg/ml	Trough level just before next dose
Phenytoin	10–20 mcg/ml	Trough level just before next dose
Procainamide	4–8mcg/ml 10–30mcg/ml total with NAPA	IV anytime after 12 hr of infusion PO trough just before next dose
Quinidine	1–5mcg/ml	Trough just before next dose
Theophylline	10–20 mcg/ml	IV anytime after 24 hr of infusion IV intermittent—

Table continued on following page

TABLE 7–1. BLOOD LEVEL MONITORING
Continued

DRUG	THERA-PEUTIC RANGE	WHEN TO DRAW LEVELS
		peak 30 min after dose or trough just before next dose
		PO liquid—peak 1 hr after dose or trough just before next dose
		PO sustained release formulations peak 4 hr after dose or trough just before next dose
Valproic acid	50–100 mcg/ml	Trough just before next dose
Vancomycin	Peak 30–40 mcg/ml	Peak 1 hr after 1 hr infusion
	Trough < 10mcg/ml	Trough within 30 min before next dose
Warfarin	Prophylaxis—PT 1.2–1.5 times control	Anytime after 24 hr of therapy or when other drugs or sensitizing factors are added or discontinued
	Therapeutic—PT 1.5–2.5 times control	

- Follow closely if drug level monitoring is being used. Make sure resampling is completed at the proper time. Be alert for signs of drug efficacy and/or drug toxicity. Document data carefully and report significant signs, symptoms, client statements, and laboratory results promptly to the physician. See also Table 3-11, Drug Toxicity Levels, p. 144.

- Chart *all* medications administered to the client as soon as possible *after* administration for accuracy, especially stat and prn doses, to avoid double dosing. When documenting drug administration or omission include the drug, dose, route of administration, time and person who gave the medication (nurse, physician, therapist, etc.), and reason for administration.

- Document the client's reaction to the medication (good pain relief, lower temperature, hypotension, etc.)

- **Adverse Drug Reaction Reporting**

  - Reporting adverse drug reactions is the most important mechanism for the FDA to monitor experiences with a drug after it has been approved. Moreover, each institution has a responsibility to review adverse reactions for continuous quality of care improvement.

  - An adverse drug reaction meets any of the following criteria:

    1. A reaction that is noxious, unexpected or unintended, and occurred at normal doses

    2. A hypersensitivity reaction

    3. A reaction not previously included in FDA labeling (package insert)

    4. A reaction that may prolong hospital stay

  - Follow your institution's policy and procedure for Adverse Drug Reaction reporting.

7-2 FACTORS AFFECTING DRUG ACTION

Age

The elderly may have diminished enzyme systems, chronic illnesses that can alter drug action, decreased blood flow to the kidneys and/or liver, metabolic changes, and other factors that may influence drug action. This group tends to take more medications on a regular basis than other populations and may be more susceptible to drug interactions.

Sex

Body weight, percentage of body fat, and hormonal changes can affect drug action.

Weight

Dosages are frequently calculated on the basis of the ratio of milligrams or micrograms of the drug to the client's weight in pounds or kilograms. Some drugs are dosed on the basis of lean body weight or body surface area.

Genetic Differences

The effects of enzymes may produce differences in drug metabolism.

Pathologic States

Pathology in the kidneys and liver particularly may affect drug action, as may congestive heart failure, acidosis, chronic obstructive pulmonary disease, diabetes, alcoholism, etc.

Route of Administration

Oral is the slowest, safest route, while parenteral is the fastest, least safe route.

Time of Administration

The body's biologic or diurnal rhythms may affect drug action. Whether or not there is food in the stomach is also a factor.

Immune System

A client's immune system may produce antibodies against a drug. This happens infrequently, but may present serious problems if the drug is subsequently readministered.

Tolerance

In some people, a decreased physiologic response develops with repeated administration of the drug.

Placebo Effect

Belief in the effectiveness of the drug can influence action.

Cumulation

A drug may be excreted more slowly than it is absorbed, which can lead to toxicity. Lithium and digoxin are examples of drugs that can accumulate to toxic levels.

Drug Interactions

Concurrent medications may interfere with drug actions. See Section 7-4 for more specific information.

7-3 PARENTERAL DRUG ADMINISTRATION

Many factors must be kept in mind when administering parental medications, since drugs are absorbed more quickly and directly via these routes than other routes. The client's age, size, cardiovascular status, disease process, fluid and electrolyte status, activity level, and the other factors listed in Section 7-2 must be considered. Listed here are nursing guidelines for giving these therapeutic medications.

Intradermal Drug Administration

- Inject into the dermal layer with medication forming a bleb under the epidermis.
- Skin tests are often given via this route.
- Use a 25–27 gauge, 1/2 to 1 inch needle.
- Inject at a 15-degree angle with the bevel of the needle upward.

Subcutaneous Drug Administration

- Inject into fat pad with the same type of needle as for intradermal injections.
- Inject no more than 1 ml of fluid into one site.
- Insulin and heparin are commonly given by this route.
- Rotate sites according to schedule to maintain skin integrity.

Intramuscular Drug Administration

- Do not mix incompatible drugs in the same syringe (Table 7-2).
- Inject no more than 3 ml of fluid into one site.
- Use a 19–23 gauge, 1- to 1 1/2-inch needle.
- Help client to relax and remain still.
- Use the ventrogluteal site when possible in adults (as it is farther away from the sciatic nerve).
- Grasp injection site firmly.
- Rotate sites and always chart the site used (dorsal, gluteal, deltoid muscle, vastus lateralis). See Figure 7-1.
- Inject at a 90-degree angle.
- Insert the needle quickly, stabilize the syringe, inject the medication slowly, and withdraw the needle quickly.
- *Do not give IM medications to clients receiving anticoagulants or thrombocytopenics.*

Intravenous Drug Administration

- Always check the IV diluent, concentration, and infusion rate before administering any drug intravenously. Many medications have compatibility, volume, and rate of administration limitations. Although charts are helpful, consult a pharmacist for any questions regarding drug delivery.
- When giving multiple IV medications, always flush the line with IV fluid or saline in between doses, since

TABLE 7–2. COMPATIBILITY OF DRUGS COMBINED IN A SYRINGE

Atropine sulphate
C | Benadryl (diphenhydramine)
C* C* | Codeine
C* C* | | Compazine
C C* C* C* | Demerol (meperidine)
| C* C* C* Cd | Dilaudid (hydromorphone)
C* C C* C* Cd | | Droperidol/Fentanyl
C* C | | | – – | Morphine
C* C* C* C* | | | Cd | Nubain (nalbuphine)
C* C C* C* C* | C* C C | Phenergan (promethazine)
C* C C* C* C* | C* C C C | Reglan (metoclopramide)
C* C C* C* C* | C* C* | C C | Robinul (glycopyrrolate)
C* C* C* C* | | C* | C* C C C* | Stadol (butorphanol)
C* C* C* C* | C* C* | C* C* C* | C* | Scopolamine
C* C C* C* C* | C* C C C C C C* C* | Talwin (pentazocine)
C* C* C* C* C* | C* C* C* C* C* C* C* C* C* | Thorazine (chlorpromazine)
| C* C* C* C* | C* | C* C* C* C* | C* C* C* | Versed (midazolam)
C* C C* C* C C C C C C C C C C C C* C | Vistaril (hydroxyzine)

Note: Diazepam (Valium), and most barbiturates are incompatible with many medications. Consult specialized sources.

Key: C = Compatible
C* = Compatible only for a limited time (may become unstable after 5–15 minutes)
I = Incompatible
Cd = Conflicting data
– = Data unavailable

Data from Hodgson BB, Kizior RJ, Kingdon RT. Nurse's drug handbook. Philadelphia: WB Saunders, 1993. Loeb S et al. Nursing '94 drug handbook. Springhouse, PA: Springhouse Corp., 1994. Phillips LD. Manual of IV therapeutics. Philadelphia: FA Davis, 1993.

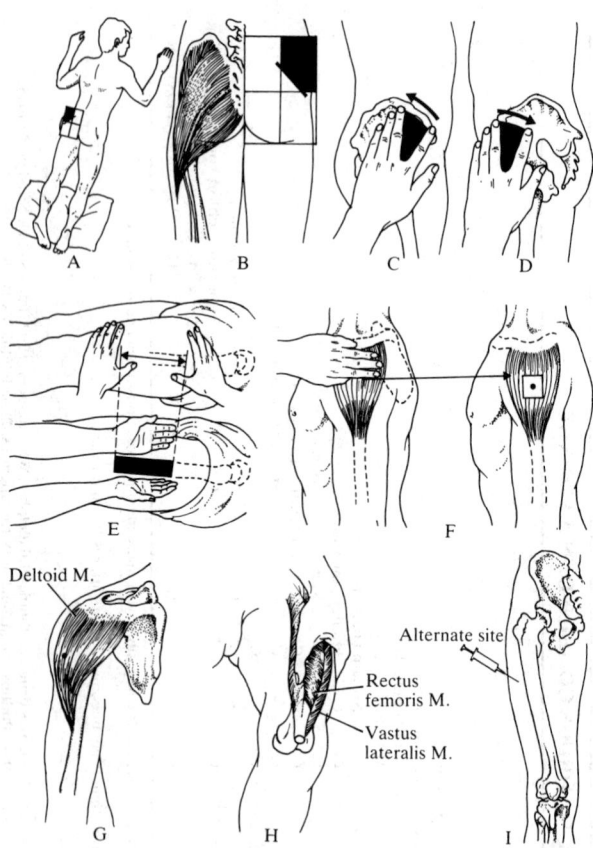

Figure 7–1. Intramuscular injection sites. A. Position for IM injection (some nurses prefer client on side with upper knee bent when injecting in the ventrogluteal site) B. The gluteus medius site C. Right ventrogluteal area D. Left ventrogluteal area E. Vastus lateralis F. Deltoid G. Pediatric injection site—deltoid H. Pediatric injection site—anterior surface of midlateral thigh I. Pediatric injection site—anterolateral surface of upper thigh

medications may be incompatible. Refer to Table 6-5 on page 248 or check with your pharmacist to ensure IV mixture compatibility. Some medications, such as Valium, cannot be mixed with any other drug.

- When administering antimicrobial therapy, see Table 7-3 for preparation and administration guidelines.

- Prevent vein irritation and extravasation when giving IV medications; always verify the patency of an IV before administering any additive.

- Vein irritation can be minimized by diluting the drug and administering the drug slowly.

Calculating IV Administration Rates

- Administer IV push medication over a *minimum* of one minute.

- For intermittent IV administration:

  1. Note the drop rate of the IV set (15, 20, 60 drops/ ml), for example 20 gtts/ml.
  2. Note the infusion volume, for example 60 ml.
  3. Note the infusion rate:

  $$\frac{60 \text{ ml}}{30 \text{ min}} = \frac{2 \text{ ml}}{\text{min}} \times \frac{20 \text{ gtts}}{\text{ml}} = \frac{40 \text{ gtts}}{\text{min}}$$

- Calculating rates of infusion for drugs dosed as mg or mcg/kg/minute

  1. Calculate dose to be infused per minute:

     rate per minute $\times$ kg = mcg/mg per minute

     For example: 3 mcg/kg/min $\times$ 80 kg = 240 mcg/min

  2. Divide dose rate by concentration of IV:

     $$\frac{\text{dopamine}}{\text{IV volume}} = \frac{200 \text{ mg}}{250 \text{ ml}} = \frac{800 \text{ mcg}}{\text{ml}}$$

     $$\frac{240 \text{ mcg/min}}{80 \text{ mcg/ml}} = \frac{0.3 \text{ ml}}{\text{min}}$$

  3. To convert dose/min to dose/hr, multiple by 60.

Text continued on page 291

TABLE 7–3. ANTIMICROBIAL AGENTS PREPARATION AND ADMINISTRATION GUIDELINES*

DRUG	DOSE	FLUID	VOLUME	INFU-SION RATE	COMMENT
Acyclovir (Zovirax)	500 mg	D5W or NS	100 ml	1 hr	Max concentration = 7 mg/ml
Amikacin (Amikin)	500 mg	D5W or NS	100 ml	30 min	
Amphotericin B (Fungizone)	50 mg	D5W	500 ml	2–4 hr	Central line: max conc = 0.25 mg/ml Peripheral line: max conc = 0.1 mg/ml
Ampicillin (Omnipen-N)	1 gm	NS	50 ml	30 min	
	2 gm	NS	100 ml	30 min	
Aztreonam (Azactam)	1 gm	D5W or NS	50 ml	30 min	Max concentration = 20 mg/ml
	2 gm	D5W or NS	100 ml	30 min	
Cefamandole (Mandol)	1 gm	D5W or NS	50 ml	30 min	
	2 gm	D5W or NS	100 ml	30 min	
Cefazolin (Kefzol)	1 gm	D5W or NS	50 ml	30 min	
	2 gm	D5W or NS	100 ml	30 min	
Cefotaxime (Claforan)	1 gm	D5W or NS	50 ml	30 min	
	2 gm	D5W or NS	100 ml	30 min	
Cefotetan (Cefotan)	1 gm	D5W or NS	50 ml	30 min	
	2 gm	D5W or NS	100 ml	30 min	
Ceftazidime (Tazidime)	1 gm	D5W or NS	50 ml	30 min	
	2 gm	D5W or NS	100 ml	30 min	
Ceftriaxone	1 gm	D5W or	50 ml	30	

**TABLE 7–3. ANTIMICROBIAL AGENTS
PREPARATION AND ADMINISTRATION
GUIDELINES*** *Continued*

DRUG	DOSE	FLUID	VOLUME	INFU-SION RATE	COMMENT
(Rocephin)		NS		min	
	2 gm	D5W or	100 ml	30	
		NS		min	
Cefuroxime	0.75	D5W or	50 ml	30	
(Kefurox)	gm	NS		min	
	1.5	D5W or	100 ml	30	
	gm	NS		min	
Ciprofloxacin	200	D5W or	100 ml	60	
(Cipro)	mg	NS		min	
	400	D5W or	250 ml	60	
	mg	NS		min	
Clindamycin	300	D5W or	50 ml	30	
	mg	NS		min	
	600	D5W or	100 ml	30	
	mg	NS		min	
	900	D5W or	100 ml	30	
	mg	NS		min	
Doxycycline	100	D5W or	100 ml	60	Protect from
	mg	NS		min	light
	200	D5W or	250 ml	60	
	mg	NS		min	
Erythromycin	0.5	NS	100 ml	60	
	gm			min	
	1 gm	NS	250 ml	60	
				min	
Fluconazole	200		100 ml	60	Administer
(Diflucan)	mg			min	undiluted.
	400		200 ml	120	Administer
	mg			min	undiluted.
Forscarnet		D5W or		60–	Central line:
(Foscavir)		NS		120	administer
				min	undiluted.
		D5W or		60–	Peripheral
		NS		120	line: dilute to
				min	less than 12
					mg/ml
					Rate of infu-sion not to exceed 1 mg/ kg/min
Ganciclovir	500	D5W or	100 ml	60	Follow guide-lines of cy-toxic agents
(DHPG)	mg	NS		min	

Table continued on following page

TABLE 7–3. ANTIMICROBIAL AGENTS PREPARATION AND ADMINISTRATION GUIDELINES* *Continued*

DRUG	DOSE	FLUID	VOLUME	INFU-SION RATE	COMMENT
					for proper handling and disposal of unused portions
Gentamicin	< 80 mg	D5W or NS	50 ml	30 min	
	> 80 mg	D5W or NS	100 ml	30 min	
Imipenem-Cilastin (Primaxin)	0.5 gm	NS	100 ml	30 min	1 gram should be infused
	1 gm	NS	250 ml	60 min	over a minimum of 60 min Infusion-related side effects: hypotension, flushing
Metronidazole (Flagyl)	500 mg		100 ml	60 min	Administer undiluted.
Miconazole (Monistat)	200 mg	D5W or NS	250 ml	120 min	Use glass container
Minocycline (Minocin)	100 mg	D5W or NS	500 ml	6 hr	
	200 mg	D5W or NS	1000 ml	6 hr	
Nafcillin (Nafcil)	1 gm	D5W or NS	50 ml	30 min	Extravasation may cause tissue sloughing
	2 gm	D5W or NS	100 ml	30 min	and necrosis.
Penicillin G	< 2 MU	D5W or NS	50 ml	30 min	Each 1 MU of penicillin G
	> 2 MU	D5W or NS	100 ml	30 min	potassium contains 1.7 mEq of potassium and 0.3 mEq of sodium. Each 1 MU of penicillin G sodium contains 2

**TABLE 7–3. ANTIMICROBIAL AGENTS
PREPARATION AND ADMINISTRATION
GUIDELINES*** *Continued*

DRUG	DOSE	FLUID	VOLUME	INFU-SION RATE	COMMENT
Ticarcillin-Clavulanate (Timentin)	3.1 gm	D5W or NS	100 ml	30 min	mEq of sodium. Each gram of ticarcillin contains 5.2–6.5 mEq of sodium.
Tobramycin (Nebcin)	< 80 mg	D5W or NS	50 ml	30 min	
	> 80 mg	D5W or NS	100 ml	30 min	
Trimetho-prim-Sulfa-methoxazole (Septra) 5ml vial	TMP 80 mg SMZ 400	D5W D5W	100 ml	60–90 min	Max conc = TMP 80 mg in 75 ml D5W
Vancomycin (Vancocin)	0.5 gm	D5W or NS	100 ml	60 min	Administer over less than 60 min is associated with "red-man/red-neck" syndrome
	1 gm	D5W or NS	250 ml	60 min	

References: 1. American Hospital Formulary Services Drug Information 1991. 2. Trissel LA. Handbook on injectable drugs. 6th Edition.
   *Approved by the Antibiotic Subcommittee 5/92
   From Janet Lau and Janice Tam. Blood level monitoring is used to establish drug efficacy and minimize. Stanford, CA. Prepared for Stanford University Hospital, 1993.

- Typical starting doses:

  - Inotropes (dopamine dolbutamine) = 5 mcg/kg/min

  - Vasodilators (nitroglycerin, nitroprusside) 0.5 mcg/kg/min

  - Vasopressors (epinephrine, norepinephrine, phenylephrine) 0.05 mcg/kg/min

- For a list of IV drug infusion concentrations and rates for adults, see Table 7-4.

- If the bottle or bag used was not a commercial pre-mixed IV or pharmacy-prepared admixture, be sure to label the container clearly with the IV solution, additive, date and time of preparation, and initials.

- Chart IV fluid in totaling intake records.

Vesicants

- While many drugs, especially if not well diluted, can cause pain and irritation upon infusion, the following drugs are among those that cause tissue necrosis if they extravasate into the tissues during IV administration:

> Amphotericin B (Fungizone)
> Antibiotics such as cephalosporins, erythromycin, nafcillin, vancomycin
> Calcium
> Carmustine
> Decarbazine (DTIC)
> Dactinomycin
> Daunorubicin
> Doxorubicin (Adriamycin)
> Mechlorethamine (Mustargen)
> Mitomycin C
> Plicamycin
> Potassium
> Sodium bicarbonate
> Streptozocin
> Vasopressors such as dopamine, epinephrine, norepinephrine
> Vinblastine (Velban)
> Vincristine (Oncovin)

NURSING ACTIONS WHEN ADMINISTERING VESICANTS

- Dilute the drug in the appropriate diluent to avoid high concentrations.

- Use a large vein and test for patency before administering.

TABLE 7–4. IV DRIP MEDICATION INFUSION RATES AND CONCENTRATIONS FOR ADULTS

DRUG	AMOUNT	SOLN-D5W	CONCEN-TRATION	70 KG PATIENT	DROPS/MIN (20 DROPS/ML)
AMINOCAPROIC ACID	25 GMS	250 ML	100 MG/ML	10–12.5 ML/HR	3–4 DROPS/MIN
AMINOPHYLLINE	1000 MG	500 ML	2 MG/ML	17.5–35 ML/HR	6–12 DROP/MIN
BRETYLIUM	500 MG	500 ML	4 MG/ML	15–45 ML/HR	5–15 DROPS/MIN
DOBUTAMINE	250 MG	250 ML	1000 MCG/ML	21–63 ML/HR	7–21 DROPS/MIN
DOPAMINE	400 MG	250 ML	1600 MCG/ML	5–40 ML/HR	2–13 DROPS/MIN
EPINEPHRINE	2 MG	250 ML	8000 NG/ML	7.7–30 ML/HR	2–10 DROPS/MIN
ESMOLOL	2.5 G	250 ML	10,000 MCG/ML	42–84 ML/HR	14–28 DROPS/MIN
FUROSEMIDE	100 MG	100 ML	1MG/ML	2–10 ML/HR	1–3 DROPS/MIN
HEPARIN	25,000 UNITS	250 ML	100 UN/ML	5–15 ML/HR	2–5 DROPS/MIN

Table continued on following page

TABLE 7–4. IV DRIP MEDICATION INFUSION RATES AND CONCENTRATIONS FOR ADULTS
Continued

DRUG	AMOUNT	SOLN-D5W	CONCEN-TRATION	70 KG PATIENT	DROPS/MIN (20 DROPS/ML)
ISOPROTERENOL	1 MG	250 ML	4 MCG/ML	75 ML/HR	25 DROPS/MIN
LIDOCAINE	2 G	250 ML	8 MCG/ML	7.5–30 ML/HR	2.5–10 DROPS/MIN
MIDAZOLAM	50 MG	100 ML	0.5 MG/ML	1–4 ML/HR	0.3–1.3 DROPS/MIN
NITROGLYCERIN	50 MG	250 ML	200 MCG/ML	1.5 ML/HR INITIALLY	0.5 DROPS/MIN
NITROPRUSSIDE	50 MG	250 ML	200 MCG/ML	6.3–210 ML/HR	2–70 DROPS/MIN
NOREPINEPHRINE	4 MG	250 ML	16,000 NG/ML	30 ML/HR INITIALLY	10 DROPS/MIN
PHENYLEPHRINE	20 MG	250 ML	80 MCG/ML	30 ML/HR INITIALLY	10 DROPS/MIN
PROCAINAMIDE	2 G	250 ML	8 MG/ML	7.5–30 ML/HR	2.5–10 DROPS/MIN
SUCCINYLCHOLINE	500 MG	250 ML	2 MG/ML	15–150 ML/HR	5–50 DROPS/MIN
TRIMETHAPHAN	500 MG	500 ML	1 MG/ML	18–180 ML/HR	6–60 DROPS/MIN

For general purposes by Steven R. Miller, Pharm. D. Stanford, CA. Prepared for Stanford University Hospital, 1993.

- If client complains of burning or pain, slow down the rate of infusion.

- If there is evidence of extravasation, stop drug immediately.

- Be knowledgeable of any specific antidotes that can be administered.

- Apply ice packs (heat for vinblastine and vincristine), and keep arm elevated.

- Evaluate lesion daily for signs of induration, inflammation, and tissue necrosis.

- A plastic surgery consult may be necessary for excision and debridement.

7-4 DRUG INTERACTIONS

With the increase in both the number of drugs available and the increasing complexity of drug regimes, the interactive potential of medications becomes more probable. A drug interaction is the pharmacological or clinical response to the administration of a drug combination. This response may be antagonistic (drug actions cancel each other), synergistic (drug effects are additive) or idiosyncratic (unpredictable). Drug interactions also occur with food, endogenous substances such as hormones, environmental chemicals such as insecticides or industrial solvents, and with laboratory studies such as thyroid tests.

However, not all drug interactions are undesirable. Sometimes drug synergy in a therapeutic response may allow for a lower dosage and thereby decrease potential toxicity. For example, the use of more than one anti-Parkinson drug may be indicated or a combination of anti-arrhythmics.

Table 7-5 is intended to be an advisory overview of significant drug interactions. There is a constant influx of new drug information especially as more is learned from clinical applications and widespread usage. Refer to a sourcebook such as *Drug Interaction Facts* for more extensive information and nursing implications. Refer to Table 7-6 when a client is taking an antacid with other medications.

Text continued on page 302

TABLE 7–5. SIGNIFICANT DRUG INTERACTIONS

DRUG OR DRUG CLASS	INTER-ACTING DRUG OR DRUG CLASS	PHARMACO-LOGICAL EFFECT
ACE (angiotension converting enzyme) inhibitors	Allopurinol	Higher potential for skin rash
ACE (angiotension converting enzyme) inhibitors	Potassium sparing diuretics	Hyperkalemia
ACE (angiotension converting enzyme) inhibitors	Lithium	Increased lithium levels
Acetaminophen	Sulfinpyra-zone	Increased risk of liver damage
Adenosine	Dipyrida-mole	Bradycardia
Alcohol	Acetamino-phen	Increased risk of liver damage
Alcohol	Sedatives	CNS depression
Alcohol	Disulfiram	Antabuse reaction
Alcohol	Vasodilators	Hypotension
Allopurinol	Ampicillin	Higher potential for skin rash
Aminoglycosides	Loop diuretics	Auditory toxicity resulting in hearing loss
Antihistamines, non-sedating	Azole antifungal agents	Cardiotoxicity and arrhythmias
Antihistamines, non-sedating	Macrolide antibiotics	Cardiotoxicity and arrhythmias
Beta blocker	Haloperidol	Hypotension
Beta blocker	Rifampin	Deterioration of blood pressure control
Beta blocker	Calcium channel blocker	Untoward cardiovascular effects
Bromocriptine	Sympathomimetics	Headache, tachycardia
Carbamazepine	Macrolide antibiotics	Carbamazepine toxicity

**TABLE 7–5. SIGNIFICANT DRUG
INTERACTIONS** *Continued*

DRUG OR DRUG CLASS	INTER-ACTING DRUG OR DRUG CLASS	PHARMACO-LOGICAL EFFECT
Cimetidine	Carmustin	Potential for increased bone marrow suppression
Clonidine	Tricyclic antidepressants	Hypertension
Corticosteroids	Barbiturates	Decreased pharmacological effect of corticosteroid therapy
Corticosteroids	Diuretics	Hypokalemia
Cyclosporine	Phenytoin	Decreased immunosuppressive activity
Cyclosporine	Lovastatin	Potential myopathy
Cyclosporine	Diltiazem	Increased cyclosporine toxicity
Cyclosporine	Fluconazole	Increased cyclosporine toxicity
Cyclosporine	Imipenem/cilastin	CNS toxicity
Cyclosporine	Macrolide antibiotics	Increased cyclosporine toxicity
Cyclosporine	Rifampin	Decreased immunosuppressive activity
Cyclosporine	Sulfonamides	Decreased immunosuppressive activity
Cyclosporine	Digoxin	Increased digoxin toxicity
Digoxin	Diuretics	Increased digoxin toxicity
Digoxin	Aminodarone	Increased digoxin toxicity
Digoxin	Erythromycin	Increased digoxin toxicity
Digoxin	Quinidine	Increased digoxin toxicity
Digoxin	Propafenone	Increased digoxin toxicity

Table continued on following page

TABLE 7–5. SIGNIFICANT DRUG INTERACTIONS *Continued*

DRUG OR DRUG CLASS	INTER-ACTING DRUG OR DRUG CLASS	PHARMACO-LOGICAL EFFECT
Digoxin	Verapamil	Increased digoxin toxicity
Dopamine	Phenytoin	Hypotension
Ganciclovir	Zidovudine	Hematological toxicity
Gembibrozil	HMG Co-A Reductase Inhibitors (cholesterol lowering agents)	Myopathy
Heparin	Aspirin	Increased potential for bleeding
Insulin	Beta blockers	Mask symptoms of hypoglycemia
Insulin	Alcohol	Hypoglycemia
Isoniazid	Rifampin	Potential for hepatotoxicity
Lithium	Nonsteroidal anti-inflammatory drugs (NSAIDS)	Increased lithium levels
Lithium	Thiazide diuretics	Increased lithium levels
Meperidine	Phenothiazine	Excessive sedation, hypotension
Methotrexate	Nonsteroidal anti-inflammatory drugs (NSAIDS)	Increased methotrexate toxicity
Methotrexate	Probenecid	Increased methotrexate toxicity
Methotrexate	Salicylates	Increased methotrexate toxicity

TABLE 7–5. SIGNIFICANT DRUG INTERACTIONS *Continued*

DRUG OR DRUG CLASS	INTER-ACTING DRUG OR DRUG CLASS	PHARMACO-LOGICAL EFFECT
Methotrexate	Sulfonamides	Increased methotrexate toxicity
Metronidazole	Alcohol	Antabuse reaction
Metronidazole	Barbiturates	Therapeutic failure of metronidazole
Monoamine oxidase inhibitor (MAOI) antidepressants	Levodopa	Hypertensive crisis
Monoamine oxidase inhibitor (MAOI) antidepressants	Meperidine	Coadministration may produce agitation, seizures, fever, coma, apnea, death
Monoamine oxidase inhibitor (MAOI) antidepressants	Sympathomimetics	Hypertension, fever
Monoamine oxidase inhibitor (MAOI) antidepressants	Tricyclic antidepressants	Fever, seizures, death
Monoamine oxidase inhibitor (MAOI) antidepressants	Foods high in tyramine	Hypertensive crisis
Monoamine oxidase inhibitor (MAOI) antidepressants	Anorexiants	Hypertensive crisis
Oral contraceptives	Phenytoin	Decreased contraceptive effectiveness
Oral contraceptives	Rifampin	Decreased contraceptive effectiveness
Oral contraceptives	Penicillins	Possible decreased contraceptive effectiveness
Penicillin	Tetracycline	Therapeutic failure of penicillin
Phenytoin	Acetaminophen	Increased risk of liver damage
Phenytoin	Isoniazid	Increased phenytoin levels

Table continued on following page

TABLE 7–5. SIGNIFICANT DRUG INTERACTIONS *Continued*

DRUG OR DRUG CLASS	INTERACTING DRUG OR DRUG CLASS	PHARMACOLOGICAL EFFECT
Phenytoin	Rifampin	Decreased phenytoin levels
Potassium	Potassium sparing diuretics	Hyperkalemia
Quinidine	Verapamil	Increased quinidine levels, arrhythmias, hypotension, heart block
Quinidine	Amiodarone	Increased quinidine levels, potential for fatal arrhythmias
Sucralfate	Oral drugs	Decreased absorption of drug
Sulfonylureas (oral antidiabetic agents)	Alcohol	Hypoglycemia, antabuse reaction
Sulfonylureas (oral antidiabetic agents)	Salicylates	Hypoglycemia
Sulfonylureas (oral antidiabetic agents)	Thiazide diuretics	Hyperglycemia
Sulfonylureas (oral antidiabetic agents)	Beta blockers	Mask symptoms of hypoglycemia
Sulfonylureas (oral antidiabetic agents)	Sulfonamides	Hypoglycemia
Terfenadine	Erythromycin	Cardiotoxicity
Tetracycline	Aluminum, bismuth, calcium, iron, magnesium, zinc salts	Decreased absorption of tetracycline
Theophylline	Adenosine	Decreased efficacy of adenosine
Theophylline	Barbiturates	Decreased theophylline level

TABLE 7–5. SIGNIFICANT DRUG INTERACTIONS *Continued*

DRUG OR DRUG CLASS	INTER-ACTING DRUG OR DRUG CLASS	PHARMACO-LOGICAL EFFECT
Theophylline	Beta blockers	Increased theophylline level; pharmacological antagonism
Theophylline	Cimetidine	Increased theophylline level
Theophylline	Phenytoin	Decreased pharmacological effect of both drugs
Theophylline	Erythromycin	Increased theophylline level and decreased erythromycin level
Theophylline	Quinolones	Increased theophylline level
Theophylline	Rifampin	Decreased theophylline level
Thiopurines	Allopurinol	Increased thiopurine toxicity
Tricyclic antidepressants	Sympathomimetics	Hypertension, arrhythmias
Valproic acid	Carbamazepine	Decreased valproic acid level
Valproic acid	Salicylates	Increased valproic acid level
Verapamil	Calcium	Decreased verapamil activity
Warfarin	Amiodarone	Potential for bleeding
Warfarin	Vitamin K, Vitamin E	Decreased anticoagulation effect
Warfarin	Barbiturates	Decreased effect of warfarin, upon D/C of barbiturate potential for bleeding
Warfarin	Erythromycin	Potential for bleeding
Warfarin	Cimetidine	Potential for bleeding
Warfarin	Nonsteroidal anti-	Potential for bleeding and adverse effects of

Table continued on following page

TABLE 7–5. SIGNIFICANT DRUG INTERACTIONS *Continued*

DRUG OR DRUG CLASS	INTER-ACTING DRUG OR DRUG CLASS	PHARMACO-LOGICAL EFFECT
	inflamma-tory drugs (NSAIDS) including aspirin	NSAIDS on platelet function
Warfarin	Metronida-zole	Potential for bleeding
Warfarin	Rifampin	Decreased anticoagula-tion effect
Warfarin	Sulfameth-oxazole/tri-methoprim	Potential for bleeding
Warfarin	Sulfinpyra-zone	Potential for bleeding
Warfarin	Carbamaze-pine	Decreased anticoagula-tion effect
Warfarin	Cephalo-sporins	Potential for bleeding
Warfarin	Quinine/quinidine	Potential for bleeding
Warfarin	Thyroid hormones	Potential for bleeding

Types of Drug Interactions

- Pharmacokinetic (one drug alters the rate or extent of the absorption, distribution, metabolism, or excretion of another drug). Examples of these pharmacokinetic mechanisms include:

  Altered GI absorption
  Altered pH of GI tract
  Altered intestinal microorganisms

TABLE 7–6. ANTACID DRUG INTERACTIONS

DRUG	ALUMINUM SALTS	CALCIUM SALTS	MAGNESIUM SALTS	MAGNESIUM ALUMINUM COMBINATIONS
Allopurinol	↓			
Benzodiazepines	↑		↓	↓
Calcitriol			x*	x*
Captopril				↓
Cimetidine				↓
Corticosteroids	↓		↓	↓
Dicumarol			↑	
Diffunisal	↓			
Digoxin	↓		↓	
Iron	↓	↓	↓	
Isoniazid	↓			
Ketoconazole				↓
Levodopa				↑
Nitrofurantoin			↓	
Penicillamine	↓		↓	↓
Phenothiazines	↓		↓	↓
Phenytoin		↓		↓
Quinidine		↑	↑	↑
Quinolones				↓
Ranitidine	↓			↓
Salicylates		↓		↓
Sodium polystyrene sulfonate	x†		x†	x†

Table continued on following page

TABLE 7–6. ANTACID DRUG INTERACTIONS
Continued

	ANTACID			
DRUG	ALU-MINUM SALTS	CALCIUM SALTS	MAGNE-SIUM SALTS	MAGNE-SIUM ALUMI-NUM COMBINA-TIONS
Tetracy-clines	↓	↓	↓	↓
Valproic acid				↑

Pharmacologic effect increased (↑) or decreased (↓) by antacids.

*Concomitant use in patients on chronic renal dialysis may lead to hypermagnesemia.

†Concomitant use may cause metabolic alkalosis in patients with renal failure.

From Takemoto C (ed). Pediatric dosing handbook and formulary. 94th ed. Children's Hospital/Los Angeles; Lexi-Comp, Inc. 1100 Terex Road, Hudson, OH: p. 59/1993.

Complexation or chelation
Damage to GI mucosa
Altered GI motility
Displaced protein binding
Altered drug metabolism by enzyme induction or enzyme inhibition (for example, liver enzymes)
Change in renal excretion

- Pharmacodynamic (the synergistic or antagonist effect of two drugs). Examples of these pharmacodynamic mechanisms include:

Change at drug receptor site
Additive CNS depression
Additive anticholinergic effect
Additive cardiovascular effects
Changes in the coagulation cascade
Changes in blood glucose concentration

7-5 SELECTED DRUG THERAPIES

These therapies have been selected to highlight here because the drug's potent effects make attention to detail and careful administration highly critical. The physician, client, nurse, and other members of the health care team must work together to control disease processes and make the therapy effective.

Cardiovascular Drug Therapies
DRUGS TO CONTROL HYPERTENSION

Hypertension is an important risk factor in cardiovascular disease, therefore long term blood pressure control is desirable for health maintenance. Nonpharmacological therapy for hypertension consists of sodium restriction with possible potassium and calcium supplementation, weight reduction, exercise training, smoking cessation, controlled alcohol intake, limited caffeine intake and stress management. Nurses must assist in educating clients in these areas, helping clients set achievable goals and form new habits. Pharmacological therapies include:

Diuretics

Diuretics (thiazides, such as chorothizide [Diuril], loop diuretics such as furosemide [Lasix], or potassium sparing diuretics such as spironolactone [Aldactone]) are used to reduce intravascular volume and counteract the fluid retention of other antihypertensives.

- Monitor electrolytes, especially potassium, uric acid, glucose, cholesterol, and triglyceride levels of clients on diuretics.
- Record accurate vital signs, particularly BP, and intake and output.

Drugs with Peripheral Sympatholytic Action

Drugs (such as reserpine, guanethidine, guanadrel, prazocin, doxzocin, terazosin) inhibit catecholamine activity at the receptor site.

- Monitor the client for orthostatic hypotension, nasal congestion, sedation, bradycardia, bronchospasm, depression.
- Titrate rather than discontinue the drug abruptly.

Drugs with Central Sympatholytic Action

Drugs (such as methyldopa, clonidine, guanabenz, guanfacine) decrease sympathetic outflow to the cardiovascular system.

- Monitor for sedation, dry mouth, postural hypotension, sexual dysfunction.
- Clonidine patch may cause dermatitis.
- Withdrawal from these agents may cause rebound hypertension.

Angiotension-Converting Enzyme Inhibitors (ACE)

These agents (such as catopril [Capoten], benazepril hydrochloride [Lotensin]) reduce the body's production of angiotensin II (a potent vasoconstrictor).

- Monitor for hyperkalemia, cough, loss of taste, angioderma, and renal insufficiency.
- Use cautiously in impaired renal function or serious autoimmune disease (i.e., systemic lupus erythamatosus).
- May cause dizziness or fainting, especially during initiation of therapy. Advise client to avoid sudden postural changes.

Calcium Channel Blockers

These agents (such as nifedipine [Procardia], verapimil [Calan], diltiazem HCl [Cardizem]) impair the transport of calcium, which decreases vascular smooth muscle tone.

- Monitor for excessive vasodilation (headaches, flushing) and conduction disturbances (palpitations).

Vasodilators

These agents (such as hydralazine [Apresoline], minoxidil [Loniten]) directly relax anteriolar smooth muscle and decrease peripheral vascular resistance.

- Monitor for headache, postural hypotension, tachycardia, or lupus-like syndrome (with hydralazine).

ANTIARRYTHMIC THERAPY

Drug selection for a particular arrthymia is based on a knowledge of cardiac anatomy and electrophysiology as well as the pharmacology of the agent. These drugs have serious adverse effects, therefore the benefit of drug therapy should be compared to the morbidity associated with the arrhythmia. Refer to Table 7-7 for a listing of agents. Also remember these drugs have many drug interactions. Refer to a drug interaction source book, such as *Drug Interaction Facts* published by Facts and Comparisons, St. Louis, MO, which is updated quarterly.

Nursing Considerations
- Assess client frequently and monitor carefully for fluid and electrolyte balance, neurostatus, cardiovascular status, and adverse effects of therapy (listed in Table 7-7).

- Drug level monitoring may be used, requiring careful timing of specimens and client observation.

- Teach clients and significant others important principles of disease management strategies, based on individual diagnosis and therapeutic regimen.

DRUGS USED TO TREAT CONGESTIVE HEART FAILURE

Congestive heart failure is characterized by congestion in both the pulmonary and systemic circulations. Pharmacological therapies include:

Digoxin
Digoxin's mechanism of action is to increase the force and decrease the rate of myocardial contraction.

Nursing Considerations
- Before giving drug, always check apical pulse for rate and rhythm for a full 60 seconds (client and/or caregivers should be taught this technique).

Text continued on page 312

TABLE 7–7. ANTIARRHYTHMIC AGENTS

DRUG	DOSAGE	INDICA-TION	ADVERSE EFFECT
Quinidine	Sulfate 200–400 mg q4–6h gluco-nate 324–648 mg q8–12h	Atrial fibril-lation, pre-mature atrial or ventricu-lar contrac-tions, ven-tricular tachycardia, Wolff-Parkin-son–White syndrome	Hypoten-sion, GI up-set, cin-shonism, thrombocy-topenia, other ar-rhythmias
Procainamide (Pronestyl)	50–100 mg/kg/day in divided doses q3–4h or q6 for sustained release IV loading dose 100 mg q 5 min to 1 gm Infusion 2–4 mg/min	Same as quinidine	Hyopoten-sion, lupus-like syn-drome, GI symptoms, blood dys-crasia, other ar-rhythmias
Disopyram-ide (Nor-pace)	PO 100–200 mg q6–8h	Atrial fibril-lation, pre-mature atrial or ventricu-lar com-plexes, ven-tricular tachycardia	Anticholin-ergic ef-fects (dry mouth, uri-nary reten-tion), heart failure, other ar-rhythmias
Lidocaine (Xylocaine)	IV loading 1–2 mg/kg may be repeated Infusion 1–4 mg/min	Ventricular tachyar-rhythmias including fi-brillation	Seizures, other CNS effects—drowsiness, agitation, paresthe-sias, other arrhyth-mias
Phenytoin (Dilantin)	PO loading 14 mg/kg PO maintenance	Arrhythmias resulting from digoxin	Ataxia, drowsiness, too-rapid

TABLE 7–7. ANTIARRHYTHMIC AGENTS *Continued*

DRUG	DOSAGE	INDICA-TION	ADVERSE EFFECT
	200–400 mg/day IV loading 50 mg q 5 min until 1 gm IV maintenance 200–400 mg/day	toxicity	injection may result in death
Mexiletine (Mexitil)	PO initial 100–200 mg q8h taken with food PO maintenance 100–300 mg q6–12h to max 1200 mg/day	Ventricular arrhythmias	CNS toxicities similar to lidocaine
Tocainide (Tonocard)	PO initial 200–400 mg q8h PO maintenance 200–600 mg q8h to a max of 2400 mg/day	Ventricular arrhythmias	CNS toxicities similar to lidocaine
Flecainide (Tambocor)	PO initial 100 mg q12h PO maintenance a maximum of 400 mg/day	Sustained ventricular tachycardia	Dizziness, flush, tremor, altered taste, other arrhythmias
Encainide (Enkaid) withdrawn from market; available only on a limited basis	PO initial 25 mg q8 PO maintenance a maximum of 200 mg/day	Life-threatening ventricular tachycardia	Other arrhythmias including heat block and ventricular fibrillation, heart failure, dizziness
Propafenone (Rhythmol)	PO initial 150 mg q8 PO maintenance	Supraventricular and ventricular	Other arrhythmias including

Table continued on following page

TABLE 7–7. ANTIARRHYTHMIC AGENTS *Continued*

DRUG	DOSAGE	INDICA-TION	ADVERSE EFFECT
	150–300 mg q8h	tachyar-rhythmias	heart block and ven-tricular fi-brillation, dizziness, metallic taste, bron-chospasm
Moricizine (Ethmozine)	PO initial 200 mg q8h PO maintenance 200–300 mg q8h	Supraven-tricular and ventricular tachyar-rhythmias	Bradycar-dia, heart failure, other ar-rhythmias, dizziness
Propranolol (Inderal)	PO 10–80 mg q6h long acting formu-lation available IV 1–5 mg	Supraven-tricular and ventricular tachyar-rhythmias	Hyopten-sion, heart block, heart fail-ure, bron-chospasm
Acebutolol	200 mg bid to a maximum of 1200 mg/day	Premature ventricular complexes	Hypoten-sion, brady-cardia, broncho-spasm, lu-pus-like syndrome
Esmolol (Brevibloc)	IV loading 500 mcg/kg IV maintenance a maximum of 300 mcg/kg/minute	Supraven-tricular tachycardias	Hypoten-sion, heart block, heart fail-ure, bron-chospasm, pain at in-jection site
Sotalol (Beta-pace)	PO initial 80 mg bid PO maintenance 160–320 mg PO maximum 640 mg qd	Life-threat-ening ven-tricular tachyar-rhythmias	Other ar-rhythmias

TABLE 7–7. ANTIARRHYTHMIC AGENTS *Continued*

DRUG	DOSAGE	INDICA-TION	ADVERSE EFFECT
Amiodarone (Cordarone)	PO initial 800–1600 mg/day PO maintenance 100–400 mg/day	Life-threatening ventricular tachyarrhythmias	Pulmonary toxicity, other arrhythmias, peripheral neuropathy, ataxia, photosensitivity, corneal deposits, thyroid abnormalities, skin discoloration
Bretylium (Bretylol)	IV initial 5 mg/kg IV infusion 1–2 mg/minute	Ventricular tachycardia, ventricular fibrillation	Nausea and vomiting, orthostatic hypotension, increased sensitivity to catecholamines, other arrhythmias
Verapamil (Isoptin, Calan)	IV initial 5–10 mg PO 40–120 mg tid, sustained release formulations available	Supraventricular tachycardias, rate control of atrial flutter or fibrillation	Hypotension, bradycardia, GI symptoms
Adenosine (Adenocard)	IV 6 mg may repeat with 12 mg	Paroxysmal supraventricular tachycardia	Transient dyspnea, chest discomfort,

Table continued on following page

TABLE 7–7. ANTIARRHYTHMIC AGENTS *Continued*

DRUG	DOSAGE	INDICA-TION	ADVERSE EFFECT
		including Wolff-Parkin-son–White	hypoten-sion
Digoxin (Lanoxin)	IV PO 0.125–0.5 mg/day	Atrial flutter, atrial fibrilla-tion, parox-ysmal atrial tachycardia	GI symp-toms, ab-normal vision, bradycar-dia, other arrhyth-mias

- Frequently assess pulmonary status, cardiovascular status, and neurological status, note changes.

- Dosing is based upon pharmacokinetic equations using client's lean body weight and creatinine clearance.

- Drug level monitoring may be implemented.

- Digoxin has a narrow therapeutic range and high potential for toxicity.

- Client teaching is imperative.

- Monitor frequently for signs of digitalis toxicity: anorexia, nausea, vomiting, diarrhea, fatigue, irritability, blurred vision, agitation, hallucinations.

- Signs of serious toxicity include lethargy, serious cardiac arrhythmias including heart block, bradyarrhythmias, and tachyarrhythmias.

- If symptoms of toxicity occur:

  - Send for stat serum potassium, magnesium and digoxin level

  - Treat arrhythmia

  - In serious overdosages Digibind, a digoxin specific antibody antidote, may be utilized.

Diuretics
Diuretics are used to reduce intravascular volume.

Nursing Considerations
- A low sodium diet may be recommended.
- Clients should be instructed about high potassium foods and taking potassium supplements (see Chapter 8, Table 8-8).
- Monitor serum electrolyte levels especially with loop diuretics such as furosemide (Lasix).

Vasodilators
Vasodilators are used to increase vascular capacity and decrease peripheral resistance.

- Isosorbide dinitrate is a venous vasodilator used in treatment of CHF. Monitor for adverse effects which include flushing, headache, postural hypotension.
- Hydralazine is an arteriolar vasodilator whose adverse effects include headache, postural hypotension, palpitations, lupus-like syndrome, myocardial ischemia.
- ACE inhibitors are balanced vasodilators whose adverse effects include dizziness and hypotension.

DRUGS USED TO TREAT ANGINA PECTORIS

Angina pectoris is characterized by substernal discomfort caused by myocardial ischemia. Pharmacological therapies include:

Nitroglycerin
- **Sublingual** route has a rapid onset of action
  - Dissolve one tablet under the tongue at first signs of substernal chest pain.
  - Do not exceed 3 tablets in 15 min. If pain is not relieved, immediate emergency treatment is needed.
  - Drug should be stored in original container, tightly closed and away from heat, light, and moisture.

- **Ointment**
  - Onset of action is 30 min, duration is 3–8 hr.
  - Measure onto paper applicator, spread over a 6-inch by 6-inch area of skin, cover with occlusive wrap.
- **Transdermal Patches**
  - Duration of action is 24 hr.
  - Client may become tolerant to nitrates so patches may be used for intermittent therapy.
  - Apply to hair-free, scar-free skin. Rotate sites.
- **IV Nitroglycerin**
  - Used in acute care settings to control unstable angina.

Isosorbide Dinitrate
  - Similar to nitroglycerin.
  - It is possible for client to become nitrate tolerant with continuous therapy.

Beta-Adrenergic Blocking Agents
  - These drugs decrease myocardial oxygen requirements but may increase coronary vasospasm.

Calcium Channel Blocking Agents
  - Cause systemic arterial dilation and improve coronary blood flow.

MYOCARDIAL INFARCTION

For drugs used in an MI, emergency assessment, CPR and interventions, see Sections 13-2 and 13-6 in Chapter 13, Emergency Assessment and Intervention.

Anticoagulant Therapy

Heparin and warfarin are used to prevent the formation of new blood clots in venous thromboembolism, pulmonary embolism, and the thromboembolic potential of such cardiac diseases as myocardial infarction, atrial fibrillation, and disorders of the heart valves. Heparin inactivates thrombin and prevents formation of fibrin; warfarin inhibits vitamin K and clotting factors formed in the liver. Heparin is also used prophylactically to prevent clot formation after major surgery, in the treatment of disseminated intravascular coagulation, and before oral anticoagulant therapy. Warfarin prevents clot formation long term.

Thrombolytic enzymes, such as streptokinase, urokinase, and alteplase (tissue plasminogen activator, t-PA), are also used to treat deep vein thrombosis, pulmonary embolism, and acute MI; however in contrast to the anticoagulants, they play an active role in the dissolution of clots rather than prevent clot formation.

Antiplatelet agents are sometimes used in conjunction with warfarin to inhibit platelet adhesion in prosthetic heart valves, and to prevent platelet aggregation in the treatment of thromboembolic disorders, and in clients with history of MI and/or stroke.

HEPARIN SODIUM (IV INFUSION)

Before Beginning Heparin Therapy

- Check for contraindications, such as hypersensitivity to the drug. Conditionally contraindicated in active bleeding, blood dyscrasias, or bleeding tendencies such as hemophilia, thrombocytopenia, or hepatic disease, suspected intracranial hemorrhage, suppurative thrombophlebitis, inaccessible ulcerative lesions (especially of GI tract), during or after brain, eye, or spinal cord surgery, during spinal tap or anesthesia, severe hypertension, and other conditions. Although the use of heparin is clearly hazardous in these conditions, a decision to use it depends on the comparative risk in failure to treat the coexisting risk thromboembolic disorder.

- Obtain a STAT activated partial thromboplastin time (APTT), prothrombin time (PT), and platelet count.

- Review current medication orders:

  - Any drugs given IM must be ordered by a different route, discontinued, or an alternative medication prescribed.

- Client must avoid meds that affect platelet function such as aspirin, nonsteroidal antiinflammatory drugs and dipyridamole.

- Note drugs which interact with heparin or warfarin (see Table 7-5), and do not administer if contraindicated. Check with physician.

Beginning Heparin Therapy

- Administer loading dose (typically 70–100 units/kg rounded to nearest 1000 units).

- Begin maintenance infusion (typically 10–15 units/kg/hr for DVT and 25 units/kg/hr for pulmonary emboli). It is advisable to use a standardized concentration of heparin such as 25,000 units in D5W 250ml which is 100 units/ml and deliver dose via an infusion device.

- Obtain APTT 6 hours after start of infusion.

Maintenance Heparin Therapy

- Infusion rate may be adjusted by the following conditions:

  1. Increase rate in the event of a massive embolism or APTT value <1.5 times control.

  2. Decrease rate in the event of a recent bleeding history such as GI bleed, age > 70 years, in the case of hematological disorders that result in increased bleeding or if there has been prior anticoagulation therapy or surgery within past 10 days.

- Obtain lab studies: repeat APTT 6 hr after any change in dose. Take APTT every day when stable. Obtain CBC, platelets, urinalysis as ordered.

- Examine all sites for bleeding daily: skin, nose, throat, urine, stool, emesis. Symptoms include: dark, tarry, or red stools, blood in urine or emesis, nose bleeds, wound bleeding, severe vaginal bleeding, gum bleeding, symptoms of hypovolemia such as low blood pressure.

- Begin teaching program as soon as appropriate for client (see Warfarin section below).

INTERMITTENT HEPARIN THERAPY (LOW DOSE, SQ)

This therapy is used for prophylaxis of venous thrombosis and pulmonary embolus. There is small risk of bleeding.

- Dosage: 5,000–10,000 units SQ 12 to 2 hr pre-op and 5,000–10,000 units q 8–12 hr post-op usually until client is ambulatory

- Give injections in the preferred site of the lower abdominal fat pad since this site is not involved in muscle activity and there will be less risk of capillary bleeding.

- Rotate sites of injection.

- Do not aspirate to check for blood return since this can cause bleeding into the tissue.

- Do not massage area, as it can cause bruising.

- Enoxaprin (Lovenox) is a low molecular weight heparin used to prevent deep vein thrombosis after hip replacement surgery. Normal dose: 30 mg SQ bid for 7–14 days.

ORAL ANTI-COAGULANT THERAPY (WARFARIN)

- Contraindicated in bleeding or hemorrhagic tendencies resulting from open wounds, visceral cancer, GI ulcers, severe hepatic or renal disease, severe uncontrolled hypertension, subacute bacterial endocarditis polycythemia vera, Vitamin K deficiency, after recent operations in eye, brain, or spinal cord. Use cautiously in diverticulitis, colitis, mild or moderate hypertension, mild or moderate hepatic or renal disease, lactation with drainage tubes in any orifice, with regional or lumbar block anesthesia, or in any condition increasing risk of hemorrhage.

- Dose is based upon PT (1.5–2.5 times control).

- There may be a loading dose or concurrent warfarin therapy with heparin.

- There are many determinants of warfarin response: diet (amount of Vitamin K), Vitamin K (antagonizes warfarin), concurrent drug therapy (many drug interactions), liver function, hypermetabolic state, hereditary resistance.

- Education is *essential* for clients on warfarin therapy. Emphasize the following points:

  - Client must avoid situations that could cause injury or bleeding (use of razors in shaving, vigorous toothbrushing, hard nose blowing, contact sports).

  - Client should consult with the physician or pharmacist before taking any drugs including any over-the-counter (OTC) analgesics or cold remedies.

  - Client must inform other health care providers (dentist, therapist) that client is on anticoagulant therapy.

  - Client should wear an ID band or carry a card indicating drug regime.

  - Client must know the signs and symptoms of bleeding and what to do in each situation.

  - Client is to take medication at the same time every day. Doses must not be skipped or changed without medical advice.

  - Client must comply with recommendations for medical visits and laboratory testing.

FIBRINOLYTIC AGENTS

These agents include streptokinase, urokinase, and tissue type plasminogen activator (tPA), used in the treatment of deep vein thrombosis, pulmonary edema, acute MI with life threatening symptoms. They actively dissolve clots rather than prevent new clot formation. Special hospital protocols are used for client selection and drug administration. The most serious adverse reaction is hemorrhage.

ANTIPLATELET THERAPY

These agents include aspirin, dypyridamole, sulfinpyra-zone, ticlopidine. Indications for use include: to maintain graft patency after CABG, as an adjunct to warfarin in clients with atrial fibrillation or mechanical heart valves, management of clients with unstable angina, to try to prevent reinfarction after MI and used in clients with a history of stroke. These agents may interact with many drugs. Be familiar with particular drug before administering.

Insulin Therapy

Insulin stimulates carbohydrate metabolism and has a direct effect on protein and fat metabolism. Exogenous insulin is necessary for the management of Type I diabetes (Insulin Dependent Diabetes Mellitus) and for some Type II (Non-Insulin Dependent Diabetes Mellitus) disease when glucose control by other means (diet, exercise, stress management, and oral hypoglycemic agents) fails, or during times of extreme stress (illness or surgery). The goal of insulin therapy is *hyperglycemic control.*

NURSING CONSIDERATIONS

- Insulin therapy will be in conjunction with the medical treatment plan which must become a part of the client's daily lifestyle. The individualized plan will include capillary blood glucose monitoring, urine testing, diet (see Diabetic Exchange Lists, Table 8-7) exercise, stress management, and medications. Thorough client teaching is essential.

- The American Diabetes Association, at Two Park Avenue, New York, New York, 10016, (212) 947-9707, has an array of educational materials.

- Current therapy stresses teaching clients to monitor their own blood glucose levels in order to determine insulin dosage. Urine testing of glucose is not always an accurate reflection of blood glucose; finger stick testing is preferred. However, urine testing for ketones and protein should still be performed.

- Many different types of insulin are available, however, they can be categorized into three main groups: short-acting, intermediate-acting, and long-acting (Table 7-8). Insulin strength is U-100 but U-40 is still available, especially in foreign countries. Human insulin from biotechnology is the least antigenic insulin, but animal source insulin is still available.

- Methods of insulin administration have become varied, but subcutaneous injection by needle and syringe is still the most common method.

TABLE 7–8. INSULIN PREPARATIONS

INSULIN PREPARATION	ONSET	PEAK	DURATION	COMPATIBILITY WITH REGULAR INSULIN
Regular Insulin (Humulin R, Novolin R)	0.5–1 hr	2.5–5 hr	6–8 hr	—
Isophane Insulin Suspension (NPH Insulin, Humulin N, Novolin N)	1–1.5 hr	4–12 hr	24 hr	yes
Insulin Zinc Suspension Prompt (Semilente)	1–1.5 hr	5–10 hr	12–16 hr	no
Insulin Zinc Suspension (Lente, Humulin L, Novolin L)	1–2.5 hr	7–15 hr	24 hr	yes
Insulin Zinc Suspension Extended (Ultralente)	4–8 hr	10–30 hr	>36 hr	yes

- Client should wear an ID bracelet indicating diabetic status.

INSULIN DOSAGES

- Subcutaneous treatment with insulin will vary according to absorbtion factors (i.e., whether a client has exercised or not, the injection site used, whether a client is dehydrated or cold, etc.), individual metabolism, and other factors. Decisions to divide the insulin and administer it in doses proportionate to individual needs are based on laboratory data, self-monitoring of blood glucose levels, and clinical observations.

- Dosing regimes for SQ insulin include:

  1. A single dose of intermediate-acting insulin
  2. Two daily injections of intermediate-acting insulin or a mixture of short-acting and intermediate-acting insulin
  3. One daily injection of an intermediate-acting insulin and 3–4 injections of a short-acting insulin
  4. Sliding-scale insulin with multiple daily injections of a short-acting insulin based on client's blood glucose level
  5. Continuous subcutaneous infusion of insulin

- For diabetic ketoacidosis, use regular insulin only: 25–150 units IV immediately, then additional doses may be given q 1 hr based on blood sugar level, until client is out of acidosis.

ADMINISTRATION GUIDELINES

- Use only regular insulin in clients with circulatory collapse, diabetic ketoacidosis, coma, hyperkalemia, or other emergencies requiring rapid drug action.

- Use cautiously in surgery (double check orders with physician), and in clients with high fever, thyroid, disease, severe infections, trauma, impaired hepatic or renal function, eating disorders, nausea, vomiting, or diarrhea.

- Check orders carefully and make sure measurement is absolutely accurate.

- Due to improved purity, insulins are stable and can be stored at room temperature for one–three months, unless drug package information states that refrigeration is needed.

- Check bottle for type of insulin and expiration date. Roll gently between the palms of your hands, never shake.

- When mixing other insulins with regular insulin (except semi-lente), draw the regular insulin into the syringe first.

- Consult a pharmacist for the stability of various admixtures.

- Rotate sites within anatomic regions (Figure 7-2) to avoid overuse of one area.

- Press but do not rub site after injection.

- Know the signs and symptoms and treatment of the complications of diabetes (Table 7-9). Ketoacidosis is a life-threatening condition that occurs secondary to insulin deficit. Inadequate insulin therapy and/or infection or stress (including surgery) can precipitate this condition. Treatment with insulin infusion and fluid and electrolyte therapy should be immediate.

- Cigarette smoking decreases the absorption of subcutaneously administered insulin. Advise clients not to smoke within 30 minutes of insulin injection.

- Some clients may develop insulin resistance and require large amounts of insulin to control diabetic symptoms. U-500 insulin is available for these clients although it may not be routinely stocked in every pharmacy. Give pharmacists two to three days notice before a prescription must be refilled. Never store U-500 insulin in the same area with other insulin preparations, as a precaution against possible overdose to other clients. U-500 insulin must be given with a U-100 syringe, as syringes for this drug are not available.

- Review and reinforce client teaching often.

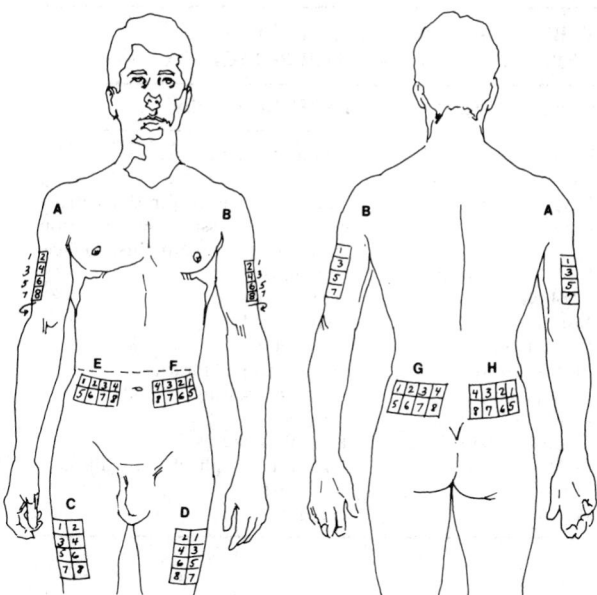

Figure 7–2. Insulin injection sites. (Adapted from Thatcher G. Where can you give your insulin? *American Journal of Nursing* 1985;85:836, with permission.)

ALTERNATIVE DELIVERY METHODS

Insulin pumps are at present the most sophisticated method of delivering insulin, however, they require a high level of client participation, are costly, and carry the potential for administering an excessive dose of insulin at a time. Screening of the client, both psychological and procedural, is necessary. The machine automatically administers a small amount of insulin or a dose infused at the basal rate (often equal to about half of the 24 hr total) every few seconds. Bolus doses can then be administered by activating a pre-entered program or pressing a button before any large food intake or when increased blood glucose levels occur (i.e., during illness).

- Pumps are battery operated and must be checked frequently. Insulin supply must be frequently replaced.

TABLE 7–9. CLINICAL SIGNS OF HYPOGLYCEMIA AND HYPERGLYCEMIA

HYPOGLYCEMIA	HYPERGLYCEMIA
Decreased temperature	Elevated temperature
Rapid strong pulse	Rapid, thready pulse
Unchanged respirations	Deep and rapid respirations, may progress to Kussmaul's respiration; fruity odor to breath, flushed face
Initially hypertensive	Hypotensive
Cool clammy skin	Warm, dry skin
Not dehydrated	Dehydrated
Dilated pupils	Soft globes
Profuse perspiration	Decreased perspiration
Alert progressing to coma	Alert progressing to coma
Possible seizures	Possible seizures
Weak, shaky, anxious	Polyuria, polyphagia, polydipsia, weakness
Hunger	Hunger

Sexual activity, swimming, and contact sports necessitate the removal of the pump.

- Though the infusion pump has many advantages, educating and supporting the person who is using the machine requires special training. Many infusion pump companies provide nurse educators and 24 hour toll-free numbers to assist clients with their pumps.

- Implantable infusion pumps and the artificial pancreas are experimental means of insulin delivery. Implantable infusion pumps are implanted surgically and still require external blood glucose testing. The artificial pancreas is a large machine that delivers insulin during surgery, labor and delivery, and dialysis procedures. Availability is limited at this time.

ORAL HYPOGLYCEMIC AGENTS

Oral hypoglycemic agents can only be used for noninsulin dependent diabetics (Type II). Their mechanism of action is to sensitize the cells to glucose and indirectly cause an increase in insulin production.

Nursing Considerations

- Contraindicated for treating Type I diabetics (insulin dependent), diabetes adequately controlled by diet, and Type II diabetes complicated by ketosis, acidosis, diabetic coma, Raynaud's disease, gangrene, renal or hepatic impairment, or thyroid or other endocrine dysfunction. Also contraindicated during pregnancy or breast-feeding.
- See Table 7-10 for a list of oral hypoglycemic agents.

TABLE 7–10. ORAL HYPOGLYCEMIC AGENTS

DRUG	TOTAL DAILY DOSE	ONSET OF ACTION	DURA-TION OF ACTION	COMMENTS
Acetohex-amide (Dymelor)	250–1500mg	1 hr	12–18hr	Avoid in patients with renal failure
Chlorprop-amide (Diabenese)	100–500mg	1hr	24–72hr	Highest incidence of hypoglycemia, potential antabuse-like reaction with alcohol
Tolazamide (Tolinase)	100–1000mg	4–6hr	16–24hr	Slow absorption
Tolbutam-ide (Orinase)	500–3000mg	1hr	6–12hr	Least potent with short half-life
Glipizide (Glucotrol)	2.5–40mg	1hr	16–24hr	Take on empty stomach
Glyburide (micronase, Diabeta)	1.25–20mg	1.5hr	18–24hr	Adjust dose in renal failure

- See also Tables G and H in Section 7-6 for a list of drugs that may cause hyperglycemia or hypoglycemia.

- Elderly clients may be more sensitive to these drugs' adverse reactions, i.e., hyperglycemia, hypersensitivity reactions, dilutional hyponatremia, skin rash.

- Client may require hospitalization during transition from insulin therapy to an oral antidiabetic. Careful monitoring is required.

- Reinforce client teaching regarding diet, exercise, foot care, infection control, and self-monitoring of glucose. Emphasize that client must not take OTC drugs or change drug dosage without doctor's approval. Reiterate recognition and interventions for hypoglycemia and hyperglycemia. Client should wear an ID card or bracelet to identify diabetic status.

Chemotherapy

Chemotherapeutic (anticancer) drugs represent a wide range of compounds with various mechanisms of action, such as alkylating agents, antimetabolites, hormones, antibiotic type drugs, mitotic inhibitors, radioactive labelled agents, and the bioengineered agents such as monoclonal antibodies. Because of the complexities and toxicities of drug administration, handling of these drugs should be restricted to specially trained personnel.

Aseptic and safe handling of parenteral chemotherapeutic drugs is essential because of their carcinogenic, mutogenic, and teratogenic potential. Drugs should be prepared in a vertical laminar flow hood and packaged for safe handling, transportation, administration, and disposal. Drugs should be clearly labeled as cytotoxic agents. The National Institutes of Health Division of Safety publishes a brochure containing recommendations for handling these agents.

The exact mechanism of action of these drugs is not fully understood but there are proposed ways in which these drugs affect tumor cells.

NURSING CONSIDERATIONS

One of the major client discomforts of chemotherapy is nausea and vomiting. Client comfort can be maximized by the following recommendations.

- To optimize therapy, start antiemetics before chemotherapy. Administer antiemetics on a schedule (not PRN) for highly and moderately emetogenic chemotherapy regimes.

- Antiemetics should be scheduled for delayed nausea and vomiting associated with cisplatin, carboplatin, cyclophosphamide, and doxorubicin.

- Nausea and emesis are better controlled when dexamethasone is added to ondansetron or metoclopramide.

- Increasing the dose of ondansetron above the maximum recommended daily dose does not improve efficacy.

- Lorazepam may be useful for anticipatory nausea and vomiting.

- Antiemetic regimes should be designed to meet the needs of the client. If a specific regime provides good control, it should be used in successive courses.

- Proper documentation of effective therapy is essential for continued successful treatment on subsequent courses of chemotherapy.

- See Table 7-11 for Emetogenic Potential of Chemotherapeutic Drugs.

- Combination drug regimes are used to increase the response rate by using agents with different mechanisms of action and to minimize the development of tumor resistance. These protocols are often known by their acronyms.

- See also Chapter 11, The Client with Cancer, for more information on cancer and chemotherapy.

Glucocorticoid Therapy

Glucocorticoids have anti-inflammatory, antiallergenic, antipyretic, and antistress effects. They are used to replace endogenous compounds and to treat immunosuppression and inflammation. Disease states in which glucocorticoids are used include: acute spinal cord injury, allergic condi-

TABLE 7–11. EMETOGENIC POTENTIAL OF CHEMOTHERAPEUTIC DRUGS*

HIGH** ($>$ 80%)	MODERATE*** (50%–80%)	LOWER EMETOGENIC POTENTIAL	
		(25%–50%)	(0–25%)
Cisplatin [$\geq$ 40 mg/m^2]	Actinomycin D	Asparaginase	Bleomycin
Cyclophos-phamide† [$>$ 1 gm/m^2]	Carmustine	Carboplatin†	Busulfan
Cytarabine [ARA-C] [$\geq$ 500 mg/m^2]	IV Cyclophos-phamide† [$<$ 1 gm/m^2]	Cytarabine [ARA-C] [$<$ 500 mg/m^2]	Etoposide [VP-16]
Dacarba-zine	Daunorubicin bolus [$\geq$ 30 mg/m^2]	Ifosfamide [low dose]	5-Fluorouracil
Nitrogen Mustard	Doxorubicin bolus† [$\geq$ 40 mg/m^2]	Mitomycin	Melphalan
Streptozo-cin	Idarubicin	Taxol	Methotrexate [low dose]
	Ifosfamide [$\geq$ 1 gm/m^2]		6-Thioguanine
	Methotrexate [$\geq$ 200 mg/m^2]		Vinblastine
	Plicamycin		Vincristine

*Dose, route and infusion rate all affect emetogenic potential.
** Also includes any combination regimen causing $>$ 80% incidence of N,V.
*** Also includes any regimen causing a $>$ 50% incidence of N, V.
†Peak emesis occurs 8–12 hours following administration.
  Prepared by Patrice Krstenzansky for general purposes at Stanford University Medical Center.

tions, cancers, cerebral edema, dermatological diseases, gastrointestinal diseases, hepatic diseases, organ transplants, primary or secondary adrenocortical insufficiency, renal diseases, respiratory diseases, rheumatic disorders, and collagen diseases.

NURSING CONSIDERATIONS

Dosage and Administration

- Dosages are highly individualized.

- See Table 7-12 for a comparison of glucocorticoid medications.

- Check for drug interactions before administering.

- Administer drug early in morning (between 6 a.m. and 9 a.m.) when the body's own production of steroids is highest, in order to reduce chances of adverse effects. Best administration time for prolonged, continuous therapy is between 7 a.m. and 8 a.m.

- Administer oral medication with food or an antacid to avoid gastric irritation.

- Insulin dosages may require adjustment while client is receiving glucocorticoid therapy.

- Do not omit dosages. If client is on long-term therapy (1 wk or longer), always gradually taper doses to wean the client from the drug before discontinuing.

- Prevent infection: some steroids suppress the immune system. Prevent client contact with contagious

TABLE 7–12. COMPARISON OF GLUCOCORTICOID MEDICATIONS

NAME	DURATION OF ACTION	EQUIVALENT DOSE
Cortisone acetate (Cortone)	8–12 hr	25 mg
Cortisol (hydrocortisone) (Cortef)	8–12 hr	20 mg
Prednisone (Deltasone)	18–36 hr	5 mg
Prednisolone (Delta-Cortef)	18–36 hr	5 mg
Methylprednisolone (Medrol)	18–36 hr	4 mg
Triamcinolone (Kenalog, Artistocort)	18–36 hr	4 mg
Dexamethasone (Decadron)	36–54 hr	0.75 mg
Betamethasone (Celestone)	36–54 hr	0.60 mg

visitors, observe CDC guidelines. Report any early signs of infection.

- Assess for adverse effects such as Cushing-type symptoms (e.g., moon face, buffalo hump, hirsutism, edema), nausea, vomiting, thirst, dizziness upon standing, abdominal pain, hematemesis, hypertension, hypokalemia, glaucoma, osteoporosis, pathologic fractures, delayed wound healing, amenorrhea, reduced resistance to infection, headache, hyperglycemia, mood changes (i.e., euphoria, depression, insomnia). Long-term therapy may result in adrenal suppression of hormones, cataracts, glaucoma, and damage to the optic nerve.

- Some clients may require lifelong therapy (i.e., adrenalectomy or hypophysectomy clients).

- Instruct clients on long-term therapy to wear an identification band. IV steroids may be necessary in times of stress, such as accident or trauma. Teach clients/families important dosage, administration, and assessment facts for their individual therapy plan.

7-6 DRUG REFERENCE LISTS

TABLE A. DRUGS ASSOCIATED WITH CNS EFFECTS*

The following are lists of some drugs that may affect your client's condition in the indicated ways. These lists are not all-inclusive. Always look up the nursing implications of the medications you are giving in the American Hospital Formulary, PDR, or other reliable source.

INSOMNIA	DROWSINESS	CONFUSION
Acyclovir	Anticholinergics	ACE inhibitors
Albuterol	Antihistamines	Alcohol
Amphetamines	Barbiturates	Acyclovir
Buproprion	Benzodiazepines	Amantadine
Caffeine	Beta blockers	Aminocaproic
Dapsone	Cimetidine	acid

TABLE A. DRUGS ASSOCIATED WITH CNS EFFECTS* *Continued*

INSOMNIA	DROWSINESS	CONFUSION
Fluoxetine	Narcotics	Amiodarone
Lidocaine	Neuroleptics	Amphotericin B
Metaproterenol	Nonsteroidal anti-	Anticholinergics
Phenylephrine	inflammatory	Anticonvulsants
Pseudoephedrine	drugs	Antihistamines
Theophylline	Skeletal muscle	Barbiturates
Thyroid hormones	relaxants	Benzodiazepines
	Tricyclic anti-	Bromocriptine
	depressants	Cephalosporins
		Ciprofloxacin
		Clonidine
		Corticosteroids
		Cyclosporin
		Digoxin
		H_2 antagonists
		Isoniazid
		Levodopa
		Metoclopramide
		Metronidazole
		Phenothiazines
		Salicylates
		Tamoxifen
		Vincristine

*This is not a complete list. Any drug may produce an idiosyncratic effect.

TABLE B. DRUGS THAT MAY CAUSE CONSTIPATION*

Aluminum containing antacids
Anticholinergics
Antihistamines
Antipsychotics
Barium compounds
Binding resins
Bismuth compounds
Calcium
Calcium channel blockers

Table continued on following page

TABLE B. DRUGS THAT MAY CAUSE CONSTIPATION* *Continued*

Clonidine
Diphenoxylate
Disopyramide
Diuretics
Iron
Levodopa
Loperamide
MAO inhibitors
Opiates
Phenothiazines
Tricyclic antidepressants
Vincristine

*This is only a partial list. Any drug may cause an idiosyncratic reaction.

TABLE C. DRUGS THAT MAY CAUSE DIARRHEA*

ACE inhibitors
Antibiotics
Beta blockers
Calcotonin
Cimetidine
Guanethidine
High doses of Vitamin C
Iron
Lactose
Laxatives
Magnesium antacids
Methyldopa
Non-steroidal anti-inflammatory drugs
Potassium
Quinine
Quinidine
Sorbitol
Theophylline

*This is only a partial list. Any drug may cause an idiosyncratic reaction.

TABLE D. DRUGS THAT SHOULD OR SHOULD NOT BE TAKEN WITH FOOD OR WATER

For proper swallowing of tablets and capsules, have clients take with a full 8 oz glass of water, not just a sip to get it down. Advise clients not to lie flat immediately after taking the medication in order to minimize irritation to the esophagus.

DRUGS THAT SHOULD BE TAKEN WITH PLENTY OF WATER*

These drugs should be taken with at least one 8 oz glass of water to enhance their action or to minimize their potential adverse reactions.

Antidiarrheals	Norfloxacin
Cathartics	Penicillamine
Cephalosporins	Potassium salts
Expectorants (guiafenisen, iodinated glycerol)	Stool bulking agents
	Stool softeners
Lithium	Sulfonamides
Naladixic acid	Tetracyclines
Nonsteroidal anti-inflammatory drugs	Tiopronon

DRUGS THAT SHOULD BE TAKEN ON AN EMPTY STOMACH*

These drugs should be taken on an empty stomach to maximize absorption. Check with a pharmacist for specific drug information.

Ampicillin	Penicillamine
Captopril	Penicillin
Dipyridamole	Sucralfate
Glypizide	Tetracycline
Nitrates (isosorbide dinitrate, NTG)	Tiopronin
Norfloxacin	Trientine

DRUGS THAT SHOULD BE TAKEN WITH FOOD*

Some drugs can be taken with food or a large glass of water to lessen stomach irritation. Check with a pharmacist for specific drug information.

Table continued on following page

TABLE D. DRUGS THAT SHOULD OR SHOULD NOT BE TAKEN WITH FOOD OR WATER
Continued

DRUGS THAT SHOULD BE TAKEN WITH FOOD*

Altretamine
Azathioprine
Bethanecol
Carbamazepine
Chenodiol
Estrogens
Etretinate
Griseofulvin
Lithium
Misoprotol
Nitrofurantoin
Nonsteroidal anti-inflammatory
  drugs
Opiates
Chloroquine
Citrates
Clofazimine
Clofibrate
Corticosteroids
Pancreatic enzymes
Pentoxifylline
Phenazopyridine
Phosphates
Quinacrine
Quinine
Salicylates
Ticlopidine

*This list is not all-inclusive

TABLE E. DISCOLORATION OF URINE DUE TO DRUGS

Pink	Dark	Black	Yellow-Brown
Amino-pyrine	Cascara	Cascara	Cascara
Anthraqui-none dyes	Levodopa	Ferrous salts	Chloroquine
Danthron	Metronida-zole	Iron dex-tran	DeWitt's pills
Deferox-amine	Nitrites	Levodopa	Methylene blue
Merbromin	P-aminosali-cylic acid	Methocar-bamol	Metronidazole
Phenol-phthalein	Phenacetin	Methyldopa	Nitrofurantoin
Phenolthia-zines	Phenol	Naphtha-lene	Primaquine
Phenytoin	Primaquine	Phenacetin	Quinacrine
Salicylates	Quinine	Phenols	Senna
	Resorcinol	Quinine	Sulfonamides
	Riboflavin	Sulfon-amides	**Rust**
	Senna		Cascara
			Chloroquine
			Metronidazole
			Nitrofurantoin
			Phenacetin

TABLE E. DISCOLORATION OF URINE DUE TO DRUGS *Continued*

Red
Anthraquinone
Cascara
Daunorubicin
Dimethylsulfoxide
DMSO
Doxorubicin
Heparin
Ibuprofen
Methyldopa
Oxyphenbutazone
Phenacetin
Phenazopyridine
Phenolphthalein
Phenolthiazines
Phensuximide
Phenylbutazone
Phenytoin
Rifampin
Senna

Red-Brown
Cascara
Methyldopa
Oxyphenbutazone
Phenacetin
Phenolphthalein
Phenothiazines
Phenylbutazone

Green
Anthraquinone
DeWitt's pills
Indigo blue
Indigo carmine
Indomethacin
Methocarbamol
Methylene blue
Nitrofurans
Phenols
Resorcinol
Suprofen

Green-Yellow
DeWitt's pills
Methylene blue

Milky
Phosphates

Orange
Chlorzoxazone
Dihydroergotamine mesylate
Heparin sodium
Phenazopyridine
Rifampin
Sulfasalazine
Warfarin

Orange-Red
Chlorzoxazone
Doxidan

Blue
Anthraquinone
Indigo blue
Indigo carmine
Methocarbamol
Methylene blue
Nitrofurans
Resorcinol
Triamterene

Blue-Green
Amitriptyline
Anthraquinone
DeWitt's pills
Doan's® pills
Indigo blue
Indigo carmine
Methylene blue

Brown
Anthraquinone dyes
Cascara
Levodopa
Methocarbamol
Methyldopa
Metronidazole
Nitrofurans

Riboflavin
Senna
Sulfonamides

Yellow
Nitrofurantoin
Phenacetin
Riboflavin
Sulfasalazine

Yellow-Pink
Cascara
Senna

Table continued on following page

TABLE E. DISCOLORATION OF URINE DUE TO DRUGS *Continued*

Phenytoin	Phenazopyri-	Nitrofuran-	**Brown-**
Quinine	dine	toin	**Black**
Red-	Rifampin	Phenacetin	Quinine
Purple	**Orange-**	Primaquine	
Chlorzoxa-	**Yellow**	Quinine	
zone	Fluorescein	Rifampin	
Ibuprofen	sodium	Senna	
Phenacetin	Rifampin	Sodium dia-	
Senna	Sulfasalazine	trizoate	
		Sulfon-	
		amides	

Data from Drugdex-Drug Consults, Micromedex, vol. 62. Rocky Mountain Drug Consultation Center, Denver, CO: November, 1989.

TABLE F. DISCOLORATION OF FECES DUE TO DRUGS

Pink	Black
Anticoagulants	Acetazolamide
Aspirin	Alcohols
Heparin	Alkalies
Oxyphenbutazone	Aminophylline
Phenylbutazone	Amphetamine
Salicylates	Amphotericin
Red	Antacids
Anticoagulants	Anticoagulants
Aspirin	Aspirin
Heparin	Betamethasone
Oxyphenbutazone	Charcoal
Phenolphthalein	Chloramphenicol
Phenylbutazone	Chlorpropamide
Pyrvinium	Clindamycin
Salicylates	Corticosteroids
Tetracycline syrup	Cortisone
Orange-Red	Cyclophosphamide
Phenazopyridine	Cytarabine
Rifampin	Dicumarol
	Ethacrynic acid
	Ferrous salts

TABLE F. DISCOLORATION OF FECES DUE TO DRUGS *Continued*

Red-Brown
Oxyphenbutazone
Phenylbutazone
Rifampin

Light Brown
Anticoagulants

Dark Brown
Dexamethasone

Gray
Colchicine

Green
Indomethacin
Iron
Medroxyprogesterone

Greenish Gray
Oral antibiotics
Oxyphenbutazone
Phenylbutazone

Yellow
Senna

Yellow-Green
Senna

Blue
Chloramphenicol
Methylene blue

Tarry
Ergot preparations
Ibuprofen
Salicylates
Warfarin

Black (*cont*)
Floxuridine
Fluorouracil
Halothane
Heparin
Hydralazine
Hydrocortisone
Ibuprofen
Indomethacin
Iodine drugs
Iron salts
Levarterenol
Levodopa
Manganese
Melphalan
Methylprednisolone
Methotrexate
Methylene blue
Oxyphenbutazone
Paraldehyde
Phenacetin
Phenolphthalein
Phenylbutazone
Phenylephrine
Phosphorous
Potassium salts
Prednisolone
Procarbazine
Pyrvinium
Reserpine
Salicylates
Sulfonamides
Tetracycline
Theophylline
Thiotepa
Triamcinolone
Warfarin

White/Speckling
Aluminum hydroxide
Antibiotics (oral)
Indocyanine green

Data from Drugdex-Drug Consults, Microdex, vol. 62. Rocky Mountain Drug Consultation Center, Denver, CO: November, 1989.

TABLE G. DRUGS THAT MAY CAUSE HYPERGLYCEMIA*

Adrenergic drugs	Corticosteroids	Oral contraceptives
Alcohol	Diazoxide	Phenothiazines
Amphetamines	Epinephrine	Phenytoin
Barbiturates	Glucocorticoids	Sympathomimetics
Beta blockers	Marijuana	Thiazide diuretics

*This is not a complete list.

TABLE H. DRUGS THAT MAY CAUSE HYPOGLYCEMIA*

Acetaminophen
Allopurinol
Anabolic steroids
Beta blockers
Dicumarol
Disopyramide
Ethanol
Insulin
MAO inhibitors
Pentamidine
Propranolol
Oral anti-diabetic agents
Salicylates

*This is not a complete list.

TABLE I. CONTROLLED SUBSTANCES

The Drug Enforcement Administration (DEA) together with the Department of Justice is the chief federal agency responsible for enforcing The Controlled Substances Act of 1970 that regulates the manufacture, distribution, and dispensing of drugs that have potential for abuse. In many cases state laws have additional restrictions, such as the requirement for triplicate prescription forms.

Drugs are placed into five DEA schedules based upon their potential for abuse and their potential for psychological and

TABLE I. CONTROLLED SUBSTANCES *Continued*

physical dependence. It is essential that all health-care professionals be knowledgeable and compliant with all regulations regarding controlled substances.

SCHEDULE	DESCRIPTION	EXAMPLES
Schedule I (C-I)	High abuse potential, no accepted medical use	Heroin, marijuana, LSD
Schedule II (C-II)	High abuse potential with severe dependence liability	Opiates, amphetamines, some barbiturates
Schedule III (C-III)	Less abuse potential than C-II, moderate dependence liability	Nonamphetamine stimulants, nonbarbiturate sedatives, limited amounts of some narcotics
Schedule IV (C-IV)	Less abuse potential than C-III, some dependence liability	Anti-anxiety agents, sedatives
Schedule V (C-V)	Limited abuse potential	Antitussives and antidiarrheals containing small amounts of narcotics

TABLE J. FDA PREGNANCY CATEGORIES

These categories were devised by the FDA to estimate the potential for a drug to cause birth defects. Assignment of a drug to a category is based upon the reliability of previously published reports and the assessment of the potential benefits of the drug outweighing the potential risks of taking the drug. Pregnancy Category X means that there is data implicating the drug as a teratogen, or the risk/benefit ratio does not warrant the drug's use in pregnancy and thus the drug is contraindicated. Regardless of the assigned category, no drug should be used during pregnancy without a clear demonstration of need and a determination of the risk/benefit ratio.

Table continued on following page

TABLE J. FDA PREGNANCY CATEGORIES
Continued

PREGNANCY CATEGORY	EXPLANATION
A	Studies in pregnant women do not demonstrate a risk to the fetus in the first trimester of pregnancy, with little risk in later trimesters.
B	Animal studies do not demonstrate a risk to the fetus but there are no controlled studies in pregnant women or animal studies have shown an adverse effect that was not confirmed in controlled studies in pregnant women in the first trimester and there is no evidence of risk in second and third trimesters.
C	Animal studies have revealed adverse effects but there were no adequate studies in pregnant women. Drug should be given only if the risk/benefit ratio justifies its use.
D	There is evidence of human fetal risk but the potential benefit of using the drug for the treatment of a serious disease or life-threatening situation may be acceptable despite the risk.
X	Studies in animals or humans demonstrate fetal abnormalities or evidence of fetal risk. The use of the drug by pregnant women outweighs the potential benefit and is contraindicated in pregnant women.

REFERENCES

Goodman and Gilman, eds. The pharmacological basis of therapeutics. 8th ed. New York: Pergamon Press, 1990.

Herfindal, Gourley, Hart, eds. Clinical pharmacy and therapeutics. 5th ed. Baltimore, MD: Williams & Wilkins, 1992.

Hodgson BB, Kizior RJ, Kingdon RT. Nurse's drug handbook. Philadelphia: WB Saunders, 1993.

Knoben JE, ed. Handbook of clinical drug data. 7th ed. Hamilton, IL: Drug Intelligence Publications, 1993.

Loeb S et al. Nursing '94 drug handbook. Springhouse, PA: Springhouse Corp., 1994.

McEvoy G, ed. American hospital formulatory service. Bethesda, MD: ASHP, 1993.

Taketomo C, ed. Pediatric dosing handbook and formulary. 1993; 94 ed. Children's Hospital/Los Angeles, Lexi-Comp Inc, Hudson, OH.

Tatro DS, ed. Drug interaction facts. St. Louis: Facts & Comparisons, 1993.

Trissel LA. Handbook on injectable drugs. Bethesda, MD: ASHP, 1992.

USPDI. 13th ed. 1993 Vol. I Drug Information for the Health Care Professional. Vol. II Advice for the Patient.

Young LY, Koda-Kimble MA, eds. Applied therapeutics the clinical use of drugs. 5th ed. Applied Therapeutics Inc. PO Box 5077, Vancouver, WA.

NUTRITION AND MEDICAL NUTRITION THERAPY

Nutrition is concerned with the body of scientific knowledge related to the food and fluid requirements of man for growth, activity, reproduction, and maintenance of health. In health care, registered dieticians have primary responsibility for the application of nutritional science to man in various conditions of health and disease. Nurses work with registered or licensed dieticians, dietetic technicians, physicians, and other members of the health care team to assess, prevent, and correct nutritional problems.

Within the scientific, nutrition, and medical communities, there has been an increased focus on the relationship of nutrition to chronic diseases. Although this interest derives to some extent from the increase and longevity of the elderly population, it is also prompted by the desire to prevent premature deaths from cancer and cardiovascular disease. Chronic diseases account for 65% of the deaths in the United States annually. Of the ten leading causes of death, five are associated with nutrition: heart disease, stroke, atherosclerosis, diabetes, and some kinds of cancer. The impact of proper nutrition on morbidity and mortality usually remains unacknowledged until adulthood. However, it now appears that prevention of the degenerative diseases manifested later in life should begin in childhood.

8-1 UNITED STATES AND CANADIAN NUTRITION POLICY

The United States nutrition policy has been guided by the Recommended Dietary Allowances (RDAs) found in Table 8-1. Canadian Nutrition Policy Guidelines are found in Table 8-2, Recommended Nutrient Intakes.

RDAs have been a part of the nutrition program of governmental agencies for fifty years. A turning point for dietary guidance occurred in 1977 with the issuance of the Dietary Goals that define nutrition goals appropriate to health and the prevention of degenerative diseases. The current Dietary Guidelines are:

- Eat a variety of foods.
- Maintain a healthy weight.
- Choose a diet low in fat, saturated fat, and cholesterol.
- Choose a diet with plenty of vegetables, fruits, and grain products.
- Use sugars only in moderation.
- Use salt and sodium only in moderation.
- If you drink alcoholic beverages, do so in moderation.

The Food Guide Pyramid

To help people put the Dietary Guidelines into practice, the USDA developed the Food Guide Pyramid (Figure 8-1). A food guide translates recommendations of nutrient intake into recommendations for food intake. It provides a conceptual framework for selecting the kinds and amounts of foods of various types that together provide a nutritionally satisfactory diet. The food guide pyramid emphasizes foods from the five major food groups shown graphically in the

Text continued on page 350

TABLE 8–1. RECOMMENDED DAILY DIETARY ALLOWANCES[a]

Category	Age (years) or Condition	Weight (kg)	Weight (lb)	Height (cm)	Height (in)	Protein (g)	Vita-min A (µg RE)[b]	Vita-min D (µg)[c]	Vita-min E (mg α-TE)[d]	Vita-min K (µg)
Infants	0.0–0.5	6	13	60	24	13	375	7.5	3	5
	0.5–1.0	9	20	71	28	14	375	10	4	10
Children	1–3	13	29	90	35	16	400	10	6	15
	4–6	20	44	112	44	24	500	10	7	20
	7–10	28	62	132	52	28	700	10	7	30
Males	11–14	45	99	157	62	45	1,000	10	10	45
	15–18	66	145	176	69	59	1,000	10	10	65
	19–24	72	160	177	70	58	1,000	10	10	70
	25–50	79	174	176	70	63	1,000	5	10	80
	51+	77	170	173	68	63	1,000	5	10	80
Females	11–14	46	101	157	62	46	800	10	8	45
	15–18	55	120	163	64	44	800	10	8	55
	19–24	58	128	164	65	46	800	10	8	60
	25–50	63	138	163	64	50	800	5	8	65
	51+	65	143	160	63	50	800	5	8	65
Pregnant						60	800	10	10	65
Lactating	1st 6 months					65	1,300	10	12	65
	2nd 6 months					62	1,200	10	11	65

[a]The allowances, expressed as average daily intakes over time, are intended to provide for individual variations among most normal persons as they live in the United States under usual environmental stresses. Diets should be based on a variety of common foods in order to provide other nutrients for which human requirements have been less well defined.
[b]Retinol equivalents. 1 retinol equivalent = 1 µg retinol or 6 µg β-carotene. See text for calculation of vitamin A activity of diets as retinol equivalents.
[c]As cholecalciferol, 10 µg cholecalciferol = 400 IU of vitamin D.
[d]α-Tocopherol equivalents. 1 mg d-α tocopherol = 1 α-TE. See text for variation in allowances and calculation of vitamin E activity of the diet as α-tocopherol equivalents.

		WATER-SOLUBLE VITAMINS							MINERALS						
Category	Age (years) or Condition	Vita-min C (mg)	Thia-min (mg)	Ribo-flavin (mg)	Niacin (mg NE)[e]	Vita-min B$_6$ (µg)	Fo-late (µg)	Vita-min B$_{12}$ (µg)	Cal-cium (mg)	Phos-phorus (mg)	Mag-nesium (mg)	Iron (mg)	Zinc (mg)	Iodine (µg)	Sele-nium (µg)
Infants	0.0–0.5	30	0.3	0.4	5	0.3	25	0.3	400	300	40	6	5	40	10
	0.5–1.0	35	0.4	0.5	6	0.6	35	0.5	600	500	60	10	5	50	15
Children	1–3	40	0.7	0.8	9	1.0	50	0.7	800	800	80	10	10	70	20
	4–6	45	0.9	1.1	12	1.1	75	1.0	800	800	120	10	10	90	20
	7–10	45	1.0	1.2	13	1.4	100	1.4	800	800	170	10	10	120	30
Male	11–14	50	1.3	1.5	17	1.7	150	2.0	1,200	1,200	270	12	15	150	40
	15–18	60	1.5	1.8	20	2.0	200	2.0	1,200	1,200	400	12	15	150	50
	19–20	60	1.5	1.7	19	2.0	200	2.0	1,200	1,200	350	10	15	150	70
	25–50	60	1.5	1.7	19	2.0	200	2.0	800	800	350	10	15	150	70
	51+	60	1.2	1.4	15	2.0	200	2.0	800	800	350	10	15	150	70
Females	11–14	50	1.1	1.3	15	1.4	150	2.0	1,200	1,200	280	15	12	150	45
	15–18	60	1.1	1.3	15	1.5	180	2.0	1,200	1,200	300	15	12	150	50
	19–24	60	1.1	1.3	15	1.6	180	2.0	1,200	1,200	280	15	12	150	55
	25–50	60	1.1	1.3	15	1.6	180	2.0	800	800	280	15	12	150	55
	51+	60	1.0	1.2	13	1.6	180	2.0	800	800	280	10	12	150	55
Pregnant		70	1.5	1.6	17	2.2	400	2.2	1,200	1,200	320	30	15	175	65
Lactating	1st 6 months	95	1.6	1.8	20	2.1	280	2.6	1,200	1,200	355	15	19	200	75
	2nd 6 months	90	1.6	1.7	20	2.1	260	2.6	1,200	1,200	340	15	16	200	75

[e] 1 NE (niacin equivalent) is equal to 1 mg of niacin or 60 mg of dietary tryptophan. (Modified from Food and Nutrition Board, National Research Council, 1989.)

Reprinted with permission from Recommended Dietary Allowances. 10th ed. Copyright 1989 by the National Academy of Sciences. Courtesy of the National Academy Press, Washington, D.C.

TABLE 8–2. RECOMMENDED NUTRIENT INTAKES (RNI), CANADA, 1990, BASED ON AGE, ENERGY, AND BODY WEIGHT EXPRESSED AS DAILY RATES*

AGE	SEX	ENERGY (kcal)	WEIGHT (kg)	THIAMIN (mg)	RIBOFLAVIN (mg)	NIACIN (NE)†	n-3 PUFA‡ (g)	n-6 PUFA (g)	PROTEIN (g)
Months									
0–4	Both	600	6.0	0.3	0.3	4	0.5	3	12
5–12	Both	900	9.0	0.4	0.5	7	0.5	3	12
Years									
1	Both	1100	11	0.5	0.6	8	0.6	4	19
2–3	Both	1300	14	0.6	0.7	9	0.7	4	22
4–6	Both	1800	18	0.7	0.9	13	1.0	6	26
7–9	Male	2200	25	0.9	1.1	16	1.2	7	30
	Female	1900	25	0.8	1.0	14	1.0	6	30
10–12	Male	2500	34	1.0	1.3	18	1.4	8	38
	Female	2200	36	0.9	1.1	16	1.1	7	40

13–15	Male	2800	50	1.1	1.4	20	1.4	9	50
	Female	2200	48	0.9	1.1	16	1.2	7	42
16–18	Male	3200	62	1.3	1.6	23	1.8	11	55
	Female	2100	53	0.8	1.1	15	1.2	7	43
19–24	Male	3000	71	1.2	1.5	22	1.6	10	58
	Female	2100	58	0.8	1.1	15	1.2	7	43
25–49	Male	2700	74	1.1	1.4	19	1.5	9	61
	Female	2000	59	0.8	1.0	14	1.1	7	44
50–74	Male	2300	73	0.9	1.3	16	1.3	8	60
	Female	1800	63	0.8‡‡	1.0‡‡	14‡‡	1.1‡‡	7‡‡	47
75+	Male	2000	69	0.8	1.0	14	1.0	7	57
	Female§§	1700	64	0.8‡‡	1.0‡‡	14‡‡	1.1‡‡	7‡‡	47
Pregnancy (additional)									
1st Trimester		100		0.1	0.1	0.1	0.05	0.3	5
2nd Trimester		300		0.1	0.3	0.2	0.16	0.9	20
3rd Trimester		300		0.1	0.3	0.2	0.16	0.9	24
Lactation (additional)		450		0.2	0.4	0.3	0.25	1.5	20

Table continued on following page

TABLE 8–2. RECOMMENDED NUTRIENT INTAKES (RNI), CANADA, 1990, BASED ON AGE, ENERGY, AND BODY WEIGHT EXPRESSED AS DAILY RATES* *Continued*

AGE	SEX	VITA-MIN A (RE)§	VITA-MIN D (µg)	VITA-MIN E (mg)	VITA-MIN C (mg)	FOLATE (µg)	VITA-MIN B$_{12}$ (µg)	CAL-CIUM (mg)	PHOS-PHORUS (mg)	MAGNE-SIUM (mg)	IRON (mg)	IODINE (µg)	ZINC (mg)
Months													
0–4	Both	400	10	3	20	50	0.3	250¶	150	20	0.3**	30	2**
5–12	Both	400	10	3	20	50	0.3	400	200	32	7	40	3
Years													
1	Both	400	10	3	20	65	0.3	500	300	40	6	55	4
2–3	Both	400	5	4	20	80	0.4	550	350	50	6	65	4
4–6	Both	500	5	5	25	90	0.5	600	400	65	8	85	5
7–9	Male	700	2.5	7	25	125	0.8	700	500	100	8	110	7
	Female	700	2.5	6	25	125	0.8	700	500	100	8	95	7
10–12	Male	800	2.5	8	25	170	1.0	900	700	130	8	125	9
	Female	800	5	7	25	180	1.0	1100	800	135	8	110	9
13–15	Male	900	5	9	30	150	1.5	1100	900	185	10	160	12
	Female	800	5	7	30	145	1.5	1000	850	180	13	160	9
16–18	Male	1000	5	10	40††	185	1.9	900	1000	230	10	160	12
	Female	800	2.5	7	30††	160	1.9	700	850	200	12	160	9
19–24	Male	1000	2.5	10	40††	210	2.0	800	1000	240	9	160	12
	Female	800	2.5	7	30††	175	2.0	700	850	200	13	160	9
25–49	Male	1000	2.5	9	40††	220	2.0	800	1000	250	9	160	12
	Female	800	2.5	6	30††	175	2.0	700	850	200	13	160	9

50–74	Male	1000	5	7	40††	220	2.0	800	1000	250	9	160	12
	Female	800	5	6	30††	190	2.0	800	850	210	8	160	9
75+	Male	1000	5	6	40‡‡	205	2.0	800	1000	230	9	160	12
	Female§§	800	5	5	30††	190	2.0	800	850	210	8	160	9
Pregnancy (additional)													
1st Trimester		100	2.5	2	0	300	1.0	500	200	15	0	25	6
2nd Trimester		100	2.5	2	10	300	1.0	500	200	45	5	25	6
3rd Trimester		100	2.5	2	10	300	1.0	500	200	45	10	25	6
Lactation (additional)		400	2.5	3	25	100	0.5	500	200	65	0	50	6

*From Recommended Nutrient Intakes for Canadians. Bureau of Nutritional Sciences, Ottawa, 1990.

†NE = niacin equivalents.

‡PUFA = polyunsaturated fatty acids.

§RE = retinol equivalents.

||Protein is assumed to be from breast milk and must be adjusted for infant formula.

¶Infant formula with high phosphorus should contain 375 mg calcium.

**Breast milk is assumed to be the source of the mineral.

††Smokers should increase vitamin C by 50%.

‡‡Level below which intake should not fall.

§§Assumes moderate physical activity.

Reproduced with permission of the Minister of Supply and Services, Canada, 1993.

three lower levels, namely, breads and starches, vegetables, fruits, meat and meat alternates, and milk. Each of these food groups provides some, but not all, of the nutrients required for health. Food in one group cannot replace those in another, nor is one food group more important than another. For good health, all five groups are needed. The tip of the pyramid shows fats, oils, and sweets. These are foods such as salad dressings and oils, cream, butter, margarine, sugars, soft drinks, candies, and sweet desserts. These foods provide calories and little else nutritionally. Most people should use them sparingly.

A frequently asked question is "what counts as a serving?" For the bread, cereal, rice and pasta, a serving is 1 slice of bread, 1 oz of ready-to-eat cereal, and 1/2 c. of

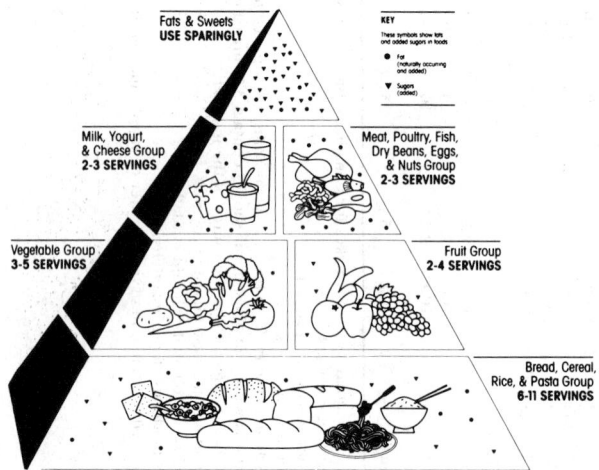

Figure 8–1. The food guide pyramid. (US Department of Agriculture. The food guide pyramid. Home and garden bulletin: No. 252. Washington, D.C. Government Printing Office, 1992.)

cooked cereal, rice, or pasta. In the vegetable group, a serving is 1 c. of raw leafy vegetables, 1/2 c. cooked or chopped raw vegetables. In the fruit group, 1 medium apple, banana, orange, or 1/2 c. chopped, cooked, or canned fruit, or 6 oz. fruit juice are a serving. A serving of milk, yogurt or cheese is 1 c. milk or yogurt or 1 1/2 oz of natural or 2 oz of processed cheese. In the meat, poultry, fish, dry beans, eggs, and nuts group, one serving is 2–3 oz cooked lean meat, poultry, or fish. The following are meat alternates: 1/2 c. cooked dry beans, 1 egg, or 2 T. nut butter count as 1 oz of lean meat.

8-2 ESSENTIAL NUTRIENTS

Food guides like the pyramid work because foods serve as important vehicles for taking nutrients into the body. About 40 essential nutrients have been identified and possibly others are yet to be discovered. The known nutrients include macronutrients (carbohydrates, proteins, and fats) whose constituent substances supply energy and build tissue, and micronutrients (vitamins and minerals) that the body uses in much smaller amounts to regulate and control body processes. Lastly, water is also essential for normal body function.

Carbohydrates, Protein, Fats

Carbohydrates are either complex (starches) or simple (sugars). Carbohydrates should provide 50–65% of total calories. They have 4 cal/g. Complex carbohydrates such as whole grain breads, cereals, and crackers are stabilizing in terms of blood sugar. Simple sugars such as dextrose and sucrose cause a rapid rise in blood sugar and increased demand for insulin. Proteins are either complete (e.g., meat, milk, eggs) or incomplete (need multiple raw ingredients to have all of the eight essential amino acids). Proteins should provide 15–20% of the total calories. They have 4 cal/g. Examples of incomplete proteins that can be used together to provide all the amino acids are rice and beans, beans and cheese, rice and cheese, or cornmeal and beans. Fats are either saturated (primarily animal sources) or polyunsaturated (vegetable sources). It is recommended that fats should be no more than 25–30% of total calories. Fats have 9 cal/g.

Vitamins, Minerals

Vitamins are organic compounds that cannot be synthesized in the body and are essential for specific metabolic reactions. A well balanced diet is the best source of all the vitamins and minerals. If deficiencies exists, they are usually multiple. Conditions where deficiencies are to be suspected are anorexia, bulimia, alcoholism, prolonged diarrhea, biliary obstruction, intestinal disease, thyrotoxicosis, prolonged infection, cancer, and mental illness. In pregnancy, the requirement for vitamins is increased and supplements are suggested.

Analysis of the human body reveals the presence of a wide variety of minerals. However, the function and requirements of only a few are known. By weight, calcium accounts for 50% of total minerals in our body and phosphorus for 25%. The additional 25% is divided among magnesium, sodium, chloride, potassium, sulfur, iron, zinc, copper iodide, manganese, fluoride, molybdenum, cobalt, selenium, chromium, tin, nickel, vanadium, and silicon.

Water

Water is an essential solvent for cell function. It is essential to the physiologic processes of digestion, absorption, and excretion of metabolic end products and indigestible substances. In healthy individuals water intake is controlled mainly by thirst. Thirst is stimulated when blood osmolality increases with a change in volume or when extracellular volume decreases. With advancing age, the sensation of thirst declines, thus when caring for the elderly, special attention must be given to adequate fluid intake. Water or fluids enter the body through liquids and in association with foods, especially fruits and vegetables. About 30% of our fluid requirements are fulfilled in association with foods.

There is no provision for water storage in the body; therefore, the amount lost every day must be replaced.

Fluid requirements can be estimated by several different techniques. One technique suggests that 1 mL of water be provided for every calorie required. Another suggests that adults require 1,500 mL per meter square of surface area, or on average 32 mL per kilogram of body weight. For infants, 100–150 mL per kilogram body weight provides a good estimate of fluid requirements. Additional fluid requirements are created during the use of oxygen masks, or respirators without humidifiers. Fever increases fluid needs by 13% for every degree centigrade above normal. Fluid requirements are summarized in Table 8-3 (see also Chapter 5).

TABLE 8–3. BASELINE FLUID REQUIREMENTS

Method 1
Based on standard body weight for height, sex, and age for obese clients and on actual body weight for others, except infants weighing less than 5 kg:
- First 10 kg of body weight: 100 cc/kg/day
- Second 10 kg of body weight: 50 cc/kg/day
- All weight above 20 kg: 20 cc/kg/day if <50 years; 15 cc/kg/day if >50 years

Example: For a 30-year-old person weighing 50 kg, the calculation is as follows.

$$10 \text{ kg} \times 100 \text{ cc/kg/day} = 1{,}000 \text{ cc}$$
$$10 \text{ kg} \times 50 \text{ cc/kg/day} = 500 \text{ cc}$$
$$30 \text{ kg} \times 20 \text{ cc/kg/day} = 600 \text{ cc}$$
$$\text{Total fluid requirement} = 2{,}100 \text{ cc}$$

Method 2
Based on standard body weight for height, sex, and age for obese clients and on actual body weight for others:
- Children over 20 kg: 1,500 cc + 30 cc/kg each kg over 20 kg
- Previously vigorous young adults with large muscle mass: 40 cc/kg/day
- Adults aged 18–55 years: 35 cc/kg/day
- Older clients with no major cardiac or renal disease: 30 cc/kg/day

---

American Dietetic Association. Handbook of clinical dietetics. New Haven: Yale University Press, 1992; p. 33. Reprinted with permission.

8-3 BODY WEIGHT AND CALORIC REQUIREMENTS

One of the most controversial issues in nutrition is selecting the best technique of describing adequate or ideal body weight. An alternative to the Metropolitan weight tables (Table 8-4) is the calculation of body mass index (BMI), which evaluates body weight for height, kg/m². This index is calculated by dividing body weight in kilograms by height in square meters. The nomogram (Figure 8-2) can be used as a quick method for calculating BMI. With this technique, individuals can be quickly assessed for appropriateness of body weight. A BMI between 19 and 24 kg/m² for women and between 20 and 25 kg/m² for men is considered ideal weight range. BMI greater than 30 kg/m² defines obesity and less than 15 kg/m² defines severe underweight.

Another controversial area is selecting the best method to estimate caloric requirement for adults. A preferred method is using the Harris-Benedict equation. Estimate Basal Energy Expenditure (BEE). Then add an activity factor to estimate the total caloric requirement for maintenance of current body weight. This equation takes into consideration sex, age, height, and weight.

Women: BEE (kcal/day) = 655.1 + (9.6 × wt. kg) + (1.8 × ht. cm) − (4.7 × age yr)
Men: BEE (kcal/day) = 66.5 + (13.8 × wt. kg) + (5.0 × ht. cm) − (6.8 × age yr)
Total caloric requirement (kcal/day) = BEE × activity factor × injury factor.

For most adults who are going about their usual activities, an activity factor of 1.5 will estimate caloric requirement. If a person is confined to a wheelchair or to bed the activity factor decreases to 1.3 or 1.2. Caloric requirements increase for severe injuries (injury factor). Surgery, mild to moderate infection, skeletal trauma, and burns over less than 20% of body surface area require caloric estimates to increase from 1.1 to 1.4. For severe infection, blunt or head trauma, and burns over more than 20% of body surface

TABLE 8–4. RECOMMENDED WEIGHTS FOR MEN AND WOMEN

Desirable weights, ages 25–59. Weight in pounds according to frame (in indoor clothing weighing 5 lb for men and 3 lb for women; shoes with 1-in. heels).

Height Feet	Inches	MEN Small Frame	MEN Medium Frame	MEN Large Frame	Height Feet	Inches	WOMEN Small Frame	WOMEN Medium Frame	WOMEN Large Frame
5	2	128–134	131–141	138–150	4	10	102–111	109–121	118–131
5	3	130–136	133–143	140–153	4	11	103–113	111–123	120–134
5	4	132–138	135–145	142–156	5	0	104–115	113–126	122–137
5	5	134–140	137–148	144–160	5	1	106–118	115–129	125–140
5	6	136–142	139–151	146–164	5	2	108–121	118–132	128–143
5	7	138–145	142–154	149–168	5	3	111–124	121–135	131–147
5	8	140–148	142–157	152–172	5	4	114–127	124–138	134–151
5	9	142–151	148–160	155–176	5	5	117–130	127–141	137–155
5	10	144–154	151–163	158–180	5	6	120–133	130–144	140–159
5	11	146–157	154–166	161–184	5	7	123–136	133–147	143–163
6	0	149–160	157–170	164–188	5	8	126–139	136–150	146–167
6	1	152–164	160–174	168–192	5	9	129–142	139–153	149–170
6	2	155–168	164–178	172–197	5	10	132–145	142–156	152–173
6	3	158–172	167–182	176–202	5	11	135–148	145–159	155–176
6	4	162–176	171–187	181–207	6	0	138–151	148–162	158–179

From Statistical Bulletin, Metropolitan Life Insurance Company, 1983. Reprinted with permission.

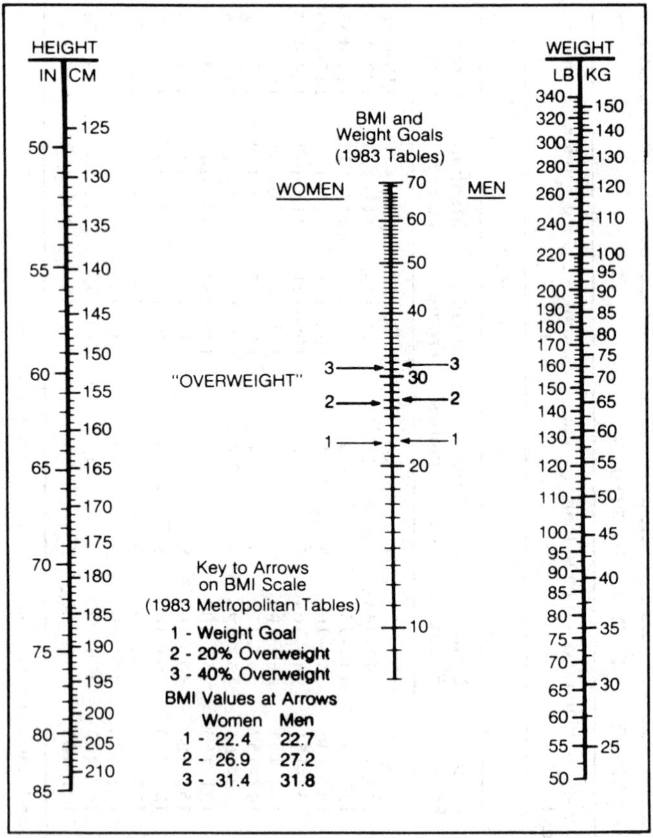

Figure 8–2. Nomograph for body mass index (kg/m²). (Thomas AE, McKay DA, Cutlip MB. A nomograph method for assessing body weight. Am J Clin Nutr 1976; 29:302–304. Reprinted with permission.)

area, caloric requirement increases by 1.4 to 1.8. When food is consumed orally, it is difficult to overfeed; however, when nutrients are being supplied by parenteral routes, the body cannot tolerate a total caloric intake greater than twice BEE.

8-4 NUTRITIONAL ASSESSMENT

Nutritional status expresses the degree to which physiologic needs for nutrients are being met. It has become customary in most medical settings for the registered dietician to screen every admission for basic nutritional needs, following up with a more detailed nutritional assessment if needed, and to recommend specific medical nutrition therapy when poor nutritional status is identified or the client is at risk for nutritional decline. A complete nutritional assessment includes examination of clinical, anthropomorphic, laboratory, and dietary information. The summation of the nutritional status report frequently includes recommendations to the physician for medical nutrition therapy.

Nurses must help establish successful therapy designed to meet the individual treatment needs of the client based on thorough assessment. Using the following assessment data will help you determine if a client is at risk for developing poor nutritional status or is malnourished. When appropriate call the registered dietician responsible for the medical nutrition of the client to confirm your findings.

- An inadequately nourished person can be underweight, overweight, or obese. A client whose weight is 20% greater than ideal or 10% less than ideal and who has had an unintentional weight gain or loss of 10% is considered at risk for poor nutritional status.

- Use the triceps skin-fold measurement to determine the body's energy stores or body fat. Average ranges of TSF are 10 to 12 mm in men and 21 to 25 mm in women, however, wide variations occur.

- Assess biochemical data: hemoglobin, red blood cell indices, hematocrit, serum albumin concentration, transferrin levels, total lymphocyte count, BUN, and urine creatinine levels.

- Clinical signs of poor nutrition include dull, dry patchy hair; dry, scaly, rough, skin; dry reddened eyes; swollen, reddened tongue; reddened, dry, cracked mucous membranes; rapid heart rate; soft, underdeveloped muscles; irritability; inattentiveness; confusion; apathy; lethargy; and sleep disturbances.

- Identify the client at risk for nutritional problems. Included are those with chewing or swallowing difficulties, inadequate food intake, restricted or fad diets, intravenous fluids (other than total parenteral nutrition for 10 or more days), inadequate food budget, inadequate food preparation facilities, inadequate food storage facilities, physical disabilities, or those who are elderly and living and eating alone.

- Based on your assessment, set goals for improving client's nutritional status in collaboration with the physician and registered dietician.

8-5 SELECTED MEDICAL NUTRITION THERAPIES

Alterations in nutrient composition, consistency, and content form the backbone of most medical nutrition therapeutic diets. In this section, the most common therapies are reviewed and outlined for your use in working with clients. When you are faced with a medical nutrition therapy that goes beyond the scope of this chapter or calls for more in-depth clarification, contact the registered dietician assigned to your client. Every facility that meets requirements for accreditation will have a diet manual or nutrition care manual that contains specific information about each medical nutrition therapy used in that facility as well.

Planning the medical nutrition therapy required for an individual client begins with the physician order for nutrition therapy. Usually the physician will prescribe a specific therapy, but often the physician may request the opinion of the registered dietician for the therapeutic nutrition treatment.

Clear Liquid Diets

Clear liquid diets include only foods that are clear and liquid at body temperature. A clear liquid diet is used as a transitional diet from intravenous feeding to resumption of regular oral intake or to temporarily prevent dehydration. It is a useful short-term measure in the recovery phase of conditions that can result in paralytic ileus. When followed over a 48-hr period clear liquid diets reduce colonic residue to a minimum, as necessary in preparation for bowel surgery or gastrointestinal examination procedures.

- The only foods that meet the clear liquid diet are bouillon, fat-free broth, coffee, tea, strained fruit juice, flavored gelatin, carbonated beverages, Popsicles, fruit ices, and hard candy.

- This diet should be used for a minimal period of time since nutrient requirements cannot be met with such a limited food list.

- If the diet is required for more than 24 hr, a nutrition supplement that meets the parameters of clear liquid diets should be added.

- A diet order for clear liquids should be evaluated and reordered every 24 hr to prevent a decrease in the client's nutritional status.

Modified Fluid Diets

Modified fluid diets vary in consistency of foods from liquids to soft and are designed primarily for use in conditions of impaired chewing or swallowing. The most restrictive modified fluid diets include only foods that are liquid at body temperature. These diets are used to provide oral nourishment and fluid for the client with alterations in pharyngeal function, postoperative diet for the client too weak to chew, or in the nutritional management of dysphagia.

DYSPHAGIA

- The client with dysphagia has the inability to transfer liquid or solid foods from the oral cavity to the stomach.

- Dysphagia may be caused by an underlying central neurologic or isolated mechanical dysfunction.

- In the nutritional management of dysphagia, treatment plans must be individualized.

- Factors to be evaluated are bolus consistencies, position of the client, rate of feeding, and specific swallowing technique.

- The use of this diet is determined by client tolerance and specific disease conditions.

- Food choices must prevent aspiration and nasal regurgitation.

- Initially the nutrition plan involves the speech pathologist or occupational therapist for swallowing evaluation, the dietician to recommend appropriate foods, and the nurse for observation at all oral intake episodes.

When the client is restricted to foods of liquid consistency only, adequate variety must be included to meet nutrient requirements.

Enteral Feeding by Tube

Generally the term "tube feeding" is used to describe a diet of liquid formula or blenderized foods of a consistency that will flow through a tube. Tube feedings deliver essential nutrients in liquid form into a functional gastrointestinal tract for the client who has an impaired ability to ingest food. Tube feedings can also be used as transitional feedings when parenteral nutrition is being discontinued or as a supplement to oral intake when nutritional needs are not being met. Tube feedings come in a variety of formulations and, today, most are commercially produced, ready-to-serve, and easy to administer. Rarely does a facility provide blenderized tube feedings produced in the facility.

Types of tube-feeding formulas vary according to concentration of nutrients, carbohydrate, protein, and fat; need for digestion, intact nutrients, partially digested, or monomeric nutrients; and a variety of other specifications. The registered dietician determines from the physician order, medical history, and nutritional assessment the most appropriate formula, amount, and rate of delivery. Formula may be delivered in bolus feedings or continuous feeding controlled by a pump. The choice of method is determined by the medical nutrition team for each client.

- For successful tube feeding, the head of the bed should be elevated 30–45 degrees during intermittent or bolus feeding and for two hr following.

- Gastric residuals should be measured every 4 hr or prior to each bolus feeding.

- Feeding should be stopped if the residual exceeds 100 ml for bolus feeding or 115% of the hourly rate for continuous feeding.

- Microbial contamination is a hazard of enteral nutrition solutions. Sanitary handling and administration techniques must be followed.

- Once opened, formulas should be kept refrigerated until used and should be allowed to hang no more than 8 hr.

- Feeding administration sets should be changed daily.

- Possible complications of tube feedings and management strategies are summarized in Table 8-5.

Parenteral Nutrition

Parenteral nutrition is the technique of delivering adequate nutrients into large-diameter veins, i.e., subclavian, to avoid damage to the vein from hypertonic solutions. Advances in the techniques of delivering nutrients by vein permit the delivery of some solutions via smaller, peripheral veins. Parenteral nutrition is used when the gastrointestinal tract is dysfunctional due to obstruction or ileus following surgery, trauma, disease, and infection. This method of supplying nutrition is usually temporary; however, parenteral nutrition can be used for long-term nutritional management of the client with severe malabsorption because of intestinal resection. Parenteral nutrition solutions are a combination of glucose, amino acids, electrolytes, minerals, and vitamins. Lipids are delivered from a separate bottle. Table 8-6 contains a suggested monitoring

Text continued on page 366

TABLE 8–5. POSSIBLE ADVERSE REACTIONS TO TUBE FEEDINGS

PROBLEM	POSSIBLE CAUSES	MANAGEMENT STRATEGY
Mechanical Complications		
Tube displacement	Coughing, vomiting	Replace tube and confirm placement.
	Dislodgment by patient	Replace tube; restrain patient if necessary; consider alternate feeding route.
	Inadequate taping of tube	Position tube properly and tape correctly.
Tube obstruction or clogging	Improperly crushed medications	Use liquid medications when possible.
	Medications mixed with incompatible formulas	Follow drug nutrient interaction guidelines, and flush tube before and after addition of medications.
	Formula residue adhering to tube; failure to irrigate properly	Flush tube with 20 to 50 mL water before starting and after stopping feeding. Flush tube at least every 4 hours during continuous infusion.
Gastric retention; aspiration pneumonia	Delayed gastric emptying	Re-position tube into small intestine.
	Patient lying flat during infusion	Elevate head of bed to 30° or more during and for 2 hours after infusion.
	Displaced feeding tube	Monitor and confirm tube placement before feeding.
Nasopharyngeal irritation; mucosal erosion; otitis media	Large bore vinyl or rubber feeding tubes for prolonged time periods	Consider use of soft, small-bore feeding tubes or feeding by tube enterostomy.
	Improper positioning or place-	Position tube properly and tape correctly;

TABLE 8–5. POSSIBLE ADVERSE REACTIONS TO TUBE FEEDINGS *Continued*

PROBLEM	POSSIBLE CAUSES	MANAGEMENT STRATEGY
	ment	choose tube of correct size for patient.
	Decreased salivary secretions due to lack of chewing; mouth breathing	Keep mouth and lips moist. Allow chewing of sugarless gum, gargling, or sucking on anaesthetic lozenges if appropriate.
Gastrointestinal Complications		
Nausea and vomiting; cramping; distention	Improper location of tube	Periodically confirm tube position.
	Rapid increase in rate, volume, or concentration	Return to slower rate, and advance by smaller increments. Advance only when tolerated at current rate.
	High osmolality	Dilute to isotonic strength if gastric residuals are consistently high. Increase concentration over several days. Consider change to isotonic formula.
	Delayed gastric emptying	Check gastric residuals every 4 to 6 hours on continuous feedings or prior to each bolus. Monitor for drugs or disease states that may influence gastric or intestinal motility.
	Lactose intolerance	Change to lactose-free formula
	Cold formula	Warm to room temperature before use.
	Obstruction	Stop formula feeding immediately

Table continued on following page

TABLE 8–5. POSSIBLE ADVERSE REACTIONS TO TUBE FEEDINGS *Continued*

PROBLEM	POSSIBLE CAUSES	MANAGEMENT STRATEGY
	Excessive fat in formula	Switch to lower-fat formula. Reduce fat in modular feedings.
Constipation	Inadequate fiber or fluid intake	Monitor intake and output; add free water if intake is not greater than output by 500 to 1,000 mL/day. Use formula with added fiber.
	Medications	Evaluate medication side effects; suggest stool softener or bulk-forming laxative.
	Inactivity	Increase patient activity if possible.
Diarrhea; defined as passage of more than 200 g of stool per 24 hours or the passage of liquid stools	Protein-energy malnutrition; decreased oncotic pressure due to serum albumin below 3.0 g/dL	Use isotonic or elemental formula at slow rate initially. If severe, suggest antidiarrheal therapy or parenteral nutrition.
	Infectious origin; microbial contamination of formula	Confirm with stool, blood, or formula cultures. Review tube-feeding handling and infection control procedures.
	Malabsorption of fat or other nutrients	Evaluate for pancreatic insufficiency; use pancreatic enzyme replacements if indicated. Change to low-fat or elemental formula.
	Bolus feeding; dumping syndrome	Change to continuous feeding, or decrease bolus volume and increase frequency of feeding.
	Hyperosmolar formula	Reduce rate and increase gradually; dilute formula

TABLE 8–5. POSSIBLE ADVERSE REACTIONS TO TUBE FEEDINGS *Continued*

PROBLEM	POSSIBLE CAUSES	MANAGEMENT STRATEGY
		or change to isotonic product.
	Medications	Consider antidiarrheal agents such as Kaopectate, paregoric, or Lomotil. Change to fiber-containing formula.
Metabolic Complications		
Hyperosmolar dehydration	Administration of hypertonic formula with inadequate water	Initiate hypertonic feedings at reduced rates; dilute; or consider use of isotonic formula.
Fluid overload or overhydration	Refeeding of patients with PEM; common in patients with cardiac, renal, or hepatic disease	Restrict fluids; use concentrated formula.
	Prolonged use of over dilute formula	Advance formula concentration as tolerated.
Hyponatremia	Congestive heart failure, cirrhosis, hypoalbuminemia, edema, ascites	Apply diuretic therapy; restrict fluids. Use concentrated formula.
	Excess gastrointestinal losses	Monitor serum levels and hydration status, and replace sodium as needed.
Hypernatremia	Dehydration	Assure adequate fluid intake.
Hypokalemia	Acidosis, insulin administration, diarrhea, marked malnutrition, diuretic therapy	Monitor electrolytes daily; supplement potassium as needed.
Hyperkalemia	Renal insufficiency	Perform frequent biochemical monitoring.

Table continued on following page

TABLE 8–5. POSSIBLE ADVERSE REACTIONS TO TUBE FEEDINGS *Continued*

PROBLEM	POSSIBLE CAUSES	MANAGEMENT STRATEGY
Other serum electrolyte or mineral abnormalities	Various	Use formula containing low levels of potassium. Monitor serum levels regularly, making individualized adjustments as needed.
Essential fatty acid (EFA) deficiency	Formula with low levels of EFA used over prolonged time periods	Provide a minimum of 4% of the caloric intake from EFAS. Add 5 mL safflower oil daily.
Glucose intolerance; hyperglycemia hyperosmolar nonketotic coma	Diabetes mellitus; or temporary insulin resistance caused by trauma or sepsis	May need to stop feeding and to rehydrate patient. Monitor blood sugar frequently, making adjustments in insulin dose. Avoid formulas high in simple sugars.
Increased respiratory quotient; excess CO_2 production; respiratory insufficiency	Overfeeding of calories, especially in the form of carbohydrates	Reduce the respiratory quotient by balancing the calories provided from fat, protein, and carbohydrate. Increase the percentage of calories provided as fat by using high-fat formula or adding modular fat.

American Dietetic Association. Handbook of clinical dietetics. New Haven: Yale University Press, 1992; 138–139. Reprinted wtih permission.

schedule to avoid metabolic complications that can arise during parenteral nutrition. In many facilities, a consultant health care team will advise the staff and can be called when problems arise (see also Section 6-6).

TABLE 8–6. SUGGESTED MONITORING FOR PARENTERAL NUTRITION

PARAMETER	FREQUENCY
Blood glucose	Every 6 hr
Body weight	Daily
Estimation of nutrient intake	Daily
Fluid intake and output	Daily
Serum electrolytes, BUN, serum creatinine, serum calcium, and phosphorous	Daily
Serum magnesium, liver enzymes and bilirubin	Daily
Serum triglycerides, cholesterol, and albumin; 24-hr urinary urea nitrogen	Once weekly
Vital signs	Every 8 hr

Acute and Chronic Renal Failure

Acute renal failure is a functional disturbance of the kidneys severe enough to cause alteration in plasma biochemistry. Chronic renal failure results from permanent damage to the kidney following progressive decrease in renal function. Whether renal failure is acute or chronic, adjustment in nutrient intake is needed.

- In acute renal failure, nutritional therapy is planned to decrease the protein content of the diet while providing adequate calories to avoid catabolism of body proteins.

- During chronic renal failure, nutritional management must be designed to decrease renal solute load while maintaining nutritional status.

- The client with chronic renal failure will be placed on some type of kidney dialysis in order to maintain life.

- Nutrient guidelines for the client on dialysis must account for protein, sodium, potassium, phosphorus, calcium and fluids.

- Nutrient care plans are designed by the registered dietician for individual client conditions.

Fat-Modified Diets

Medical nutrition therapies that rely on fat restriction are indicated when fat digestion and absorption are impaired due to exocrine pancreatic insufficiency. Restriction of all fats may be required for the nutritional management of the client with small-bowel resection. Pancreatic enzyme replacement accompanies dietary fat restriction in the nutrition therapy of chronic pancreatitis. Fat intake is reduced to approximately 50 grams per day or about 15–20% of calories from fat and gradually increased to tolerance in combination with enzyme replacement. The average dietary fat intake in the U.S. population is about 37% of calories from fat. To achieve a restricted-fat diet the daily meal plan in Table 8-7 can serve as a guide.

Cardiovascular Disease Nutrition

Fat-modified nutritional therapies are also used for treatment and prevention of cardiovascular disease (CVD). For cardiovascular health total fat intake is recommended at no more than 30% of calories. As mentioned above, the average dietary fat intake in the United States is approximately 37% of calories. The report from the National Cholesterol Education Program Expert Panel, recently revised, guides the medical nutrition and drug therapy for adults at risk for CVD. Dietary intervention remains the first line of treatment for elevated plasma total cholesterol. Medical nutrition therapy is designed to reduce plasma cholesterol while maintaining a nutritionally adequate eating pattern. The Food Guide Pyramid discussed in Section 8-1 can be used as a guide with modification of total and kinds of dietary fats.

- The first level of nutritional treatment is a food intake pattern with no more than 30% of calories from total fat and less than 300 mg cholesterol per day and 8–10% of calories from saturated fat.

TABLE 8–7. DAILY MEAL PLAN FOR THE RESTRICTED-FAT (50 g) DIET

FOOD	AMOUNT	FAT
Skim milk	2 or more cups	none
Lean meat, fish, poultry	6 oz	18–30 g
Whole egg	2 per week	2 g
Vegetables	3 or more servings	none
Fruit	2 or more servings	none
Breads, cereals, starch	6 or more servings	trace
Fats	3 servings	15 g
TOTAL FAT		35–47 g

- For an estimate of the fat content of food refer to the exchange lists in Table 8-8. Remember, cholesterol is only found in association with fat from animal sources and that most saturated fat is also from animal fats.

- Further reductions of saturated fat to 7% of calories and total cholesterol to no more than 200 mg per day may be required as a second step if plasma cholesterol levels remain elevated.

- Weight reduction for the overweight client and increased physical activity are important adjunctive therapies for the treatment of high plasma cholesterol.

- Potassium regulation is frequently critical in management of CVD. For foods with high potassium content, refer to Table 8-9.

Diabetes Mellitus and Calorie-Controlled Nutrition Management

Medical nutrition therapy that regulates caloric or macronutrient intake can be used to treat clients with diabetes mellitus or clients who need to gain, lose, or maintain body weight. Diabetes mellitus is a chronic condition characterized primarily by elevation of blood glucose, although

Text continued on page 382

TABLE 8–8. EXCHANGE LISTS FOR DIABETES NUTRITION MANAGEMENT

STARCH/BREAD LIST

Each item in this list contains approximately 15 g carbohydrate, 3 g protein, a trace of fat, and 80 kcal. Whole-grain products average about 2 g fiber per serving. Some foods are higher in fiber. Starch exchanges can be chosen from any of the items on this list. The general rule for starch foods not on this list is that:

½ cup of cereal, grain, or pasta is one serving.

1 oz of a bread product is one serving.

Cereals/Grains/Pasta

*Bran cereals, concentrated	⅓ cup
*Bran cereals, flaked	½ cup
(such as Bran Buds, All Bran)	
Bulgur (cooked)	½ cup
Cooked cereals	½ cup
Cornmeal (dry)	2½ T
Grape-nuts	3 T
Grits (cooked)	½ cup
Other ready-to-eat unsweetened	¾ cup
cereals	
Pasta (cooked)	½ cup
Puffed cereal	1½ cup
Rice, white or brown (cooked)	⅓ cup
Shredded wheat	½ cup
*Wheat germ	3 T

Dried Beans/Peas/Lentils

*Beans and peas (cooked)	⅓ cup
(such as kidney, white, split,	
blackeye)	
*Lentils (cooked)	⅓ cup
*Baked beans	¼ cup

Starchy Vegetables

*Corn	½ cup
*Corn on cob, 6-in long	1
*Lima beans	½ cup
*Peas, green (canned or frozen)	½ cup
*Plantain	½ cup
Potato, baked	1 small (3 oz)
Potato, mashed	½ cup
Squash, winter (acorn, butternut)	¾ cup
Yam, sweet potato, plain	⅓ cup

TABLE 8–8. EXCHANGE LISTS FOR DIABETES NUTRITION MANAGEMENT *Continued*

Bread

Bagel	½ (1 oz)
Bread sticks, crisp, 4-in long × ½ in	2 (⅔ oz)
Croutons, low-fat	1 cup
English muffin	½
Frankfurter or hamburger bun	½ (1 oz)
Pita, 6-in across	½
Plain roll, small	1 (1 oz)
Raisin, unfrosted	1 slice (1 oz)
*Rye, pumpernickel	1 slice (1 oz)
Tortilla, 6-in across	1
White (including French, Italian)	1 slice (1 oz)
Whole wheat	1 slice (1 oz)
Taco shell, 6-in across	2
Waffle, 4½-in square	1
Whole wheat crackers, fat added (such as Triscuits)	4–6 (1 oz)

Crackers/Snacks

Animal crackers	8
Graham crackers, 2½-in square	3
Matzoth	¾ oz
Melba toast	5 slices
Oyster crackers	24
Popcorn (popped, no fat added)	3 cups
Pretzels	¾ oz
Rye crisp, 2-in × 3½-in	4
Saltine-type crackers	6
Whole wheat crackers, no fat added (crisp breads, such as Finn, Kavli, Wasa)	2–4 slices (¾ oz)

Starch Foods Prepared with Fat
(Count as 1 starch/bread serving, plus 1 fat serving)

Biscuit, 2½-in across	1
Chow mein noodles	½ cup
Corn bread, 2-in cube	1 (2 oz)
Cracker, round butter type	6
French fried potatoes, 2-in to 3½-in long	10 (1½ oz)
Muffin, plain, small	1

Table continued on following page

TABLE 8–8. EXCHANGE LISTS FOR DIABETES NUTRITION MANAGEMENT *Continued*

Pancake, 4-in across	2
Stuffing, bread (prepared)	¼ cup

*Foods with 3 or more grams of fiber per serving.

MEAT LIST

Each serving of meat and substitutes on this list contains about 7 g protein. The amounts of fat and number of calories vary, depending on the kind of meat or substitute chosen. The list is divided into three parts based on the amount of fat and calories: lean meat, medium-fat meat, and high-fat meat. One ounce (one meat exchange) of each of these includes:

	Carbohydrate (g)	Protein (g)	Fat (g)	Calories
Lean	0	7	3	55
Medium-fat	0	7	5	75
High-fat	0	7	8	100

Lean Meat and Substitutes
(One exchange is equal to any one of the following items.)

Beef:	USDA Good or Choice grades of lean beef, such as round, sirloin, and flank steak; tenderloin; and chipped beef†	1 oz
Pork:	Lean pork, such as fresh ham; canned, cured or boiled ham;† Canadian bacon,† tenderloin.	1 oz
Veal:	All cuts are lean except for veal cutlets (ground or cubed). Examples of lean veal are chops and roasts.	1 oz
Poultry:	Chicken, turkey, Cornish hen (without skin)	1 oz
Fish:	All fresh and frozen fish	1 oz
	Crab, lobster, scallops, shrimp, clams (fresh or canned in water†)	2 oz
	Oysters	6 medium
	Tuna† (canned in water)	¼ cup
	Herring (uncreamed or smoked)	1 oz
	Sardines (canned)	2 medium

TABLE 8–8. EXCHANGE LISTS FOR DIABETES NUTRITION MANAGEMENT *Continued*

Wild Game:	Venison, rabbit, squirrel	1 oz
	Pheasant, duck, goose (without skin)	1 oz
Cheese:	Any cottage cheese	¼ cup
	Grated Parmesan	2 T
	Diet cheeses† (with less than 55 kcal/oz	1 oz
Other:	95% fat-free luncheon meat	1 oz
	Egg substitutes with less than 55 kcal per ¼ cup	¼ cup

Medium-Fat Meat and Substitutes
(One exchange is equal to any one of the following items.)

Beef:	Most beef products fall into this category. Examples are: all ground beef, roast (rib, chuck, rump), steak (cubed, Porterhouse, T-bone), and meatloaf.	1 oz
Pork:	Most pork products fall into this category. Examples are: chops, loin roast, Boston butt, cutlets.	1 oz
Lamb:	Most lamb products fall into this category. Examples are: chops, leg, and roast.	1 oz
Veal:	Cutlet (ground or cubed, unbreaded)	1 oz
Poultry:	Chicken (with skin), domestic duck or goose (well-drained of fat), ground turkey	1 oz
Fish:	Tuna† (canned in oil and drained)	¼ cup
	Salmon† (canned)	¼ cup
Cheese:	Skim or part-skim milk cheeses, Ricotta	¼ cup
	Mozzarella	1 oz
Other:	Diet cheeses† (with 56–80 kcal/oz)	1 oz
	86% fat-free luncheon meat†	1 oz
	Egg (high in cholesterol, limit to 3 per week)	1

Table continued on following page

TABLE 8–8. EXCHANGE LISTS FOR DIABETES NUTRITION MANAGEMENT *Continued*

	Egg substitutes with 56–80 kcal per ¼ cup	¼ cup
	Tofu (2½ in x 2¾ in x 1 in)	4 oz
	Liver, heart, kidney, sweetbreads (high in cholesterol)	1 oz

High-Fat Meat and Substitutes

Remember, these items are high in saturated fat, cholesterol, and calories, and should be used only three (3) times per week. (One exchange is equal to any one of the following items.)

Beef:	Most USDA Prime cuts of beef, such as ribs, corned beef†	1 oz
Pork:	Spareribs, ground pork, pork sausage† (patty or link)	1 oz
Lamb:	Patties (ground lamb)	1 oz
Fish:	Any fried fish product	1 oz
Cheese:	All regular cheeses,† such as American, Blue, Cheddar, Monterey, Swiss	1 oz
Other:	Luncheon meat,† such as bologna, salami, pimento loaf	1 oz
	Sausage,† such as Polish, Italian	1 oz
	Knockwurst, smoked	1 oz
	Bratwurst†	1 oz
	Frankfurter† (turkey or chicken)	1 frank (10/lb)
	Peanut butter (contains unsaturated fat)	1 T
	Count as one high-fat meat plus one fat exchange:	
	Frankfurter† (beef, pork, or combination)	1 frank (10/lb)

†Foods with 400 mg or more of sodium per exchange.

VEGETABLE LIST

Each vegetable serving on this list contains about 5 g carbohydrate, 2 g protein, and 25 kcal. Vegetables contain 2–3 grams of dietary fiber. Vegetables are a good source of vitamins and minerals. Fresh and frozen vegetables have more vitamins and less added salt. Unless otherwise noted, the serving size for vegetables (one vegetable exchange) is:

½ cup of cooked vegetables or vegetable juice.
1 cup of raw vegetables.

TABLE 8–8. EXCHANGE LISTS FOR DIABETES NUTRITION MANAGEMENT *Continued*

Artichoke (½ medium)	Mushrooms, cooked
Asparagus	Okra
Beans (green, wax, Italian)	Onions
Bean sprouts	Pea pods
Beets	Peppers (green)
Broccoli	Rutabaga
Brussels sprouts	Sauerkraut†
Cabbage, cooked	Spinach, cooked
Carrots	Summer squash (crookneck)
Cauliflower	Tomato (one large)
Eggplant	Tomato/vegetable juice†
Greens (collard, mustard, turnip)	Turnips
	Water chestnuts
Kohlrabi	Zucchini, cooked
Leeks	

Starchy vegetables such as corn, peas, and potatoes are found on the Starch/Bread list.

†400 mg or more sodium per exchange.

FRUIT LIST

Each item on this list contains about 15 g carbohydrate, and 60 kcal. Fresh, frozen, and dry fruits have about 2 g fiber per serving. Fruit juices contain very little dietary fiber. The carbohydrate and calorie content for a fruit serving are based on the usual serving of the most commonly eaten fruits. Use fresh fruits or fruits frozen or canned without sugar added. Whole fruit is more filling than fruit juice and may be a better choice for those who are trying to lose weight. Unless otherwise noted, the serving size for one fruit serving is:

½ cup of fresh fruit or fruit juice.

¼ cup of dried fruit.

Fresh, Frozen, and Unsweetened Canned Fruit

Apple (raw, 2-in across)	1 apple
Applesauce (unsweetened)	½ cup
Apricots (medium, raw) or	4 apricots
Apricots (canned)	½ cup, or 4 halves
Banana (9-in long)	½ banana
*Blackberries (raw)	¾ cup
*Blueberries (raw)	¾ cup
Cantaloupe (5-in across)	⅓ melon
(cubes)	1 cup
Cherries (large, raw)	12 cherries

Table continued on following page

TABLE 8–8. EXCHANGE LISTS FOR DIABETES NUTRITION MANAGEMENT *Continued*

Cherries (canned)	½ cup
Figs (raw, 2-in across)	2 figs
Fruit cocktail (canned)	½ cup
Grapefruit (medium)	½ grapefruit
Grapefruit (segments)	¾ cup
Grapes (small)	15 grapes
Honeydew melon (medium) (cubes)	⅛ melon 1 cup
Kiwi (large)	1 kiwi
Mandarin oranges	¾ cup
Mango (small)	½ mango
*Nectarine (1½-in across)	1 nectarine
Orange (2½-in across)	1 orange
Papaya	1 cup
Peach (2¾-in across)	1 peach, or ¾ cup
Peaches (canned)	½ cup, or 2 halves
Pear	½ large, or 1 small
Pears (canned)	½ cup, or 2 halves
Persimmon (medium, native)	2 persimmons
Pineapple (raw)	¾ cup
Pineapple (canned)	⅓ cup
Plum (raw, 2-in across)	2 plums
*Pomegranate	½ pomegranate
*Raspberries (raw)	1 cup
*Strawberries (raw, whole)	1¼ cup
Tangerine (2½-in across)	2 tangerines
Watermelon (cubes)	1¼ cup

Dried Fruit

*Apples	4 rings
*Apricots	7 halves
Dates	2½ medium
*Figs	1½
*Prunes	3 medium
Raisins	2 T

Fruit Juice

Apple juice/cider	½ cup
Cranberry juice cocktail	⅓ cup
Grapefruit juice	½ cup
Grape juice	⅓ cup

TABLE 8–8. EXCHANGE LISTS FOR DIABETES NUTRITION MANAGEMENT *Continued*

Orange juice	½ cup
Pineapple juice	½ cup
Prune juice	⅓ cup
*3 or more grams of fiber per serving	

MILK LIST

Each serving of milk or milk products on this list contains about 12 g carbohydrate and 8 g protein. The amount of fat in milk is measured in percent (%) of butterfat. The calories vary, depending on the kind of milk chosen. The list is divided into three parts based on the amount of fat and calories: skim/very low fat milk, low-fat milk, and whole milk. One serving (one milk exchange) of each of these includes:

	Carbo-hydrate (g)	Protein (g)	Fat (g)	Calories
Skim/Very low fat	12	8	trace	90
Low fat	12	8	5	120
Whole	12	8	8	150

Skim and Very Low Fat Milk

Skim milk	1 cup
½% milk	1 cup
1% milk	1 cup
Low-fat buttermilk	1 cup
Evaporated skim milk	½ cup
Dry nonfat milk	⅓
Plain nonfat yogurt	8 oz

Low-Fat Milk

2% milk	1 cup fluid
Plain low-fat yogurt (with added nonfat milk solids)	8 oz

Whole Milk

The whole milk group has much more fat per serving than the skim and low-fat groups. Whole milk has more than 3¼% butterfat. Try to limit choices from the whole milk group as much as possible.

Whole milk	1 cup
Evaporated whole milk	½ cup
Whole plain yogurt	8 oz

Table continued on following page

TABLE 8–8. EXCHANGE LISTS FOR DIABETES NUTRITION MANAGEMENT *Continued*

FAT LIST

Each serving on the fat list contains about 5 g fat and 45 kcal. The foods on the fat list contain mostly fat, although some items may also contain a small amount of protein. All fats are high in calories and should be carefully measured. Everyone should modify fat intake by eating unsaturated fats instead of saturated fats. The sodium content of these foods varies widely. Check the label for sodium information.

Unsaturated Fats

Avocado	⅛ medium
Margarine	1 tsp
‡Margarine, diet	1 T
Mayonnaise	1 tsp
‡Mayonnaise, reduced calorie	1 T
Nuts and Seeds:	
Almonds, dry roasted	6 whole
Cashews, dry roasted	1 T
Pecans	2 whole
Peanuts	20 small or 10 large
Walnuts	2 whole
Other nuts	1 T
Seeds, pine nuts, sunflower (without shells)	1 T
Pumpkin seeds	2 tsp
Oil (corn, cottonseed, safflower, soybean, sunflower, olive, peanut)	1 tsp
‡Olives	10 small or 5 large
Salad dressing, mayonnaise-type	2 tsp
Salad dressing, mayonnaise-type, reduced-calorie	1 T
‡Salad dressing (all varieties)	1 T
†Salad dressing, reduced-calorie	2 T
(Two tablespoons of low-calorie salad dressing is a free food.)	

Saturated Fats

Butter	1 tsp
‡Bacon	1 slice
Chitterlings	½ oz
Coconut, shredded	2 T
Coffee whitener, liquid	2 T

TABLE 8–8. EXCHANGE LISTS FOR DIABETES NUTRITION MANAGEMENT *Continued*

Coffee whitener, powder	4 tsp
Cream (light, coffee, table)	2 T
Cream, sour	2 T
Cream (heavy, whipping)	1 T
Cream cheese	1 T
‡Salt pork	¼ oz

‡If more than 2 servings eaten, these foods have 400 mg or more sodium.

FREE FOODS

A free food is any food or drink that contains less than 20 kcal/serving, and can be taken in unlimited amounts. Two or three servings per day of those items that have a specific serving size can be eaten.

Drinks
Bouillon† or broth
without fat
Bouillon, low sodium
Carbonated drinks, sugar-free
Carbonated water
Club soda
Cocoa powder,
unsweetened (1 T)
Coffee/Tea
Drink mixes, sugar free
Tonic water, sugar-free

Nonstick pan spray

Fruit
Cranberries,
unsweetened (½ cup)
Rhubarb, unsweetened
(½ cup)

Vegetables (raw, 1 cup)
Cabbage*
Celery*
Chinese cabbage*
Cucumber
Green onion
Hot peppers
Mushrooms

Salad greens
Endive
Escarole
Lettuce
Romaine*
Spinach*

Sweet substitutes
Candy, hard, sugar-free
Gelatin, sugar-free
Gum, sugar-free
Jam/Jelly, sugar-free
(2 tsp)
Pancake syrup, sugar free
(1–2 T)
Sugar substitutes
(saccharin, aspartame)
Whipped topping (2 T)

Condiments
Catsup (1 T)
Horseradish
Mustard
Pickles†, dill,
unsweetened
Salad dressing, low-calorie
(2 T)
Taco sauce (1 T)
Vinegar

Table continued on following page

TABLE 8–8. EXCHANGE LISTS FOR DIABETES NUTRITION MANAGEMENT *Continued*

Radishes
Zucchini*

Seasonings can be very helpful in making food taste better. Be careful of how much sodium is used. Read the label, and choose those seasonings that do not contain sodium or salt.

Basil (fresh)	Lemon juice
Celery seeds	Lemon pepper
Cinnamon	Lime
Chili powder	Lime juice
Chives	Mint
Curry	Onion powder
Dill	Oregano
Flavoring extracts (vanilla, almond, walnut, peppermint, butter, lemon, etc.)	Paprika
	Pepper
	Pimento
Garlic	Spices
Garlic powder	Soy sauce†
Herbs	Soy sauce, low sodium ("lite")
Hot pepper sauce	
Lemon	Wine, used in cooking (¼ cup)
	Worcestershire sauce

*3 g or more of fiber per serving.
†400 mg or more of sodium per serving.

COMBINATION FOODS

These combination foods do not fit into only one exchange list. It can be quite hard to tell what is in a certain casserole dish or baked food item. This is a list of average values of some typical combination foods.

Food	Amount	Exchanges
Casseroles, homemade	1 cup (8 oz)	2 starch, 2 medium-fat meat, 1 fat
Cheese pizza,† thin crust	¼ of 15 oz or ¼ of 10 in	2 starch, 1 medium-fat meat, 1 fat
Chili with beans*† (commercial)	1 cup (8 oz)	2 starch, 2 medium-fat meat, 2 fat
Chow mein*† (without noodles or rice)	2 cups (16 oz)	1 starch, 2 vegetable, 2 lean meat

TABLE 8–8. EXCHANGE LISTS FOR DIABETES NUTRITION MANAGEMENT *Continued*

Macaroni and cheese†	1 cup (8 oz)	2 starch, 1 medium-fat meat, 2 fat
Soup		
Bean*†	1 cup (8 oz)	1 starch, 1 vegetable, 1 lean meat
Chunky, all varieties†	10¾ oz can	1 starch, 1 vegetable, 1 medium-fat meat
Cream† (made with water)	1 cup (8 oz)	1 starch, 1 fat
Vegetable† or broth†	1 cup (8 oz)	1 starch
Spaghetti and meatballs† (canned)	1 cup (8 oz)	2 starch, 1 medium-fat meat, 1 fat
Sugar-free pudding (made with skim milk)	½ cup	1 starch

If beans are used as a meat substitute:

Dried beans,* peas,* lentils*	1 cup (cooked)	2 starch, 1 lean meat

FOODS FOR OCCASIONAL USE

Moderate amounts of some foods can be used in the meal plan, in spite of their sugar or fat content, as long as blood glucose control is maintained. The following list includes average exchange values for some of these foods. Because they are concentrated sources of carbohydrate, the portion sizes are very small.

Food	Amount	Exchanges
Angel food cake	1/12 cake	2 starch
Cake, no icing	1/12 cake, or a 3-in square	2 starch, 2 fat
Cookies	2 small (1¾-in across)	1 starch, 1 fat
Frozen fruit yogurt	1/3 cup	1 starch
Gingersnaps	3	1 starch
Granola	¼ cup	1 starch, 1 fat
Granola bars	1 small	1 starch, 1 fat
Ice cream, any flavor	½ cup	1 starch, 2 fat

Table continued on following page

TABLE 8–8. EXCHANGE LISTS FOR DIABETES NUTRITION MANAGEMENT *Continued*

Ice milk, any flavor	½ cup	1 starch, 1 fat
Sherbet, any flavor	¼ cup	1 starch
Snack chips,‡ all varieties	1 oz	1 starch, 2 fat
Vanilla wafers	6 small	1 starch, 1 fat

*3 or more g fiber per serving.

†400 mg or more of sodium per exchange

‡If more than one or two servings are eaten, these foods have 400 mg or more of sodium.

Mahan LK and Arline MT. Krausels food, nutrition and diet therapy. 8th ed. Philadelphia: WB Saunders, 1992. Reprinted with permission.

abnormalities of lipid and protein metabolism also occur. Medical nutrition therapy is planned to achieve optimal blood glucose concentration, meet nutrient requirements for growth, development, or maintenance of healthy body weight, and prevent or delay metabolic complications associated with diabetes. Food intake patterns are planned to achieve a goal of carbohydrate, protein, and fat calories based on individual nutritional status and current medical therapy.

DISTRIBUTION OF CALORIES

Most food patterns will provide 45–50% of calories from carbohydrate, 15-20% of calories from protein, and 30–35% of calories from fat. The distribution of calories during the day is just as important as the overall dietary prescription. In order to achieve as smooth a course of blood glucose as possible, caloric intake is distributed throughout the day in a pattern, such as 20% of calories at breakfast, 40% at lunch and 40% at dinner. The prohibition of sucrose or "sugar" is of much less importance than generally appreciated. In fact many studies confirm that the glycemic effect of carbohydrate is identical for sugars and starches. Glycemic differences can only be demonstrated for different amounts of total carbohydrate. In other words, sucrose has no more potent glycemic effect than orange juice or spaghetti noodles at the same level of total carbohydrate.

TABLE 8–9. POTASSIUM-REGULATED DIET

Whenever possible, hypokalemia should be treated by increasing dietary potassium.

FOODS HIGH IN POTASSIUM
(300 to 500 mg or 7.6 to 12.5 mEq per average serving)

Fruits	Meats	Vegetables	Milk
Oranges	Hamburger	Raw toma-	Milk of all
Bananas	Beef chuck	toes	kinds
Grapes	Lamb	Artichokes	Yogurt
Strawber-	Ham	Raw carrots	
ries	Pork	Cooked	
Avocados	Veal	white or red	
Apricots	Fish	beans	
Dates	Turkey	Black-eyed	
Melons		peas	
Canta-		Celery	
loupe		Mushrooms	
Raisins		Cooked	
Prunes		chard	
Peaches		Parsnips	
Persim-		Lima beans	
mons		White pota-	
		toes	
		Cooked spin-	
		ach	
		Radishes	

FOODS LOWER IN POTASSIUM (50 to 150 mg or 1.25 to 3.8 mEq per average serving)

Fruits	Grains	Vegetables	Other
Berries of	Cereals, cooked	Green or wax	Cheeses of all
all kinds	or dry	beans	kinds
	Bread (all	Beets	Eggs
	kinds)	Mixed vege-	Canned soups
		tables	Candies
		Onions	Desserts
		Green pep-	Wine
		pers	
		Raw lettuce	
		Salad greens	

Many clients who require insulin injections to control blood glucose will require 5–10% of lunch and/or dinner calories to be used for food intake between meals or at bedtime.

INDIVIDUALIZED MANAGEMENT

For optimal management of diabetes, the client should follow an individualized meal plan designed in consultation with a registered dietician. Frequently the meal plan will be based on the food groups found in the exchange lists in Table 8-8. Complications of diabetes may require additional medical nutrition therapy such as modification of the type of fat for CVD or reduced sodium intake for hypertension or renal disease. All clients with diabetes would be well advised to reduce the amount of saturated fat to 10% of total calories as a preventive measure.

Recently the Diabetes Complication and Clinical Trial has confirmed that aggressive treatment of insulin-dependent clients decreases the progression of complications. This means that the relationship between insulin therapy and food intake is carefully titrated. In situations where meals are delayed, i.e. extended clinic appointments or delayed diagnostic tests where food has been withheld, unexpected low blood glucose episodes and hypoglycemic reactions may occur. The best treatment of hypoglycemic reactions is prevention through anticipation. Health care professionals should help clients anticipate low blood glucose episodes in hospital and clinic settings and intervene with carbohydrate-containing drinks or snacks.

Body Weight Management

A food intake plan that limits total caloric intake below weight maintenance requirements will result in a decrease in body weight. A decrease in body weight of significantly overweight individuals (body mass index greater than 30 kg/m^2) is indicated for the medical nutrition therapy of such conditions as hyperlipidemia, hypertension, impaired glucose tolerance, diabetes mellitus, osteoarthritis, or problems with lower extremity joints, and sleep apnea. Most commonly the need for calorie-limited nutrition therapy will be identified by the registered dietician or ordered by the physician; however, if you suspect the need for a decrease in body weight to improve the health of the client, call the registered dietician responsible for the nutrition care of the client. When a client needs to follow a specified meal plan to achieve a lower, higher, or sometimes even to maintain current body weight, the exchange list (see Table 8-8) system of developing a calorie-specific meal plan is useful. The guidelines of estimating caloric requirement provided in Section 8-3 can be used to arrive at an appropriate reduced calorie prescription.

- A moderate caloric decrease, 500–1000 calories below caloric requirement for weight maintenance, will result in gradual weight loss.

- Very-low-calorie diets, 400–800 calories, are usually provided in liquid or powder formulations and, like any method of reducing caloric intake, will result in weight loss. However, at the same time they lower basal energy expenditure and have not been shown to have any long-term advantage.

- Ideally, a revised food intake plan designed to help a client achieve a more healthful body weight results in permanent behavior change and long-term maintenance of desired weight.

- Calorie-limited diets are contraindicated for some populations. Despite the added risk of obesity, calorie-reduced regimens are not appropriate during pregnancy.

- When the overweight client is undergoing treatment for malignant conditions that may result in severe anorexia or decreased food intake, reduced calorie diets should not be recommended.

- Also, health risks associated with overweight in the elderly have been found to be less significant than for younger individuals. Calorie-limited food intake plans should be used with caution in individuals over 65 years of age. Body mass index associated with lowest mortality in this age group is about 5 kg/m^2 higher than in younger adults, 27.8 kg/m^2 for men and 27.3 kg/m^2 in women.

Sodium-Restricted Nutrition Therapy

Food intake plans are limited to a prescribed level of sodium. Table salt, which chemically is sodium chloride, is restricted and foods that naturally contain the mineral sodium are limited. The purpose of the diet is to decrease the osmolarity of the extracellular fluid for management of diseases, such as high blood pressure, congestive heart failure, and severe liver disease.

- The physician order for a sodium-restricted diet should be given in milligrams or milliequivalents of sodium.

- Severe sodium-restricted diets have been replaced by drug therapy.

- At a minimum, sodium-restricted diets limit the amount of salt used in food preparation and added at the table. Obviously salty, highly processed, salt-preserved, and salt-pickled foods are omitted.

- The individual food pattern is established by the dietitian to match the client's food preferences.

8-6 CULTURAL DIVERSITY OF FOOD HABITS

The proportion of the United States population from different racial and ethnic groups is steadily increasing. While people from a given culture may have similar health attitudes, beliefs, and practices, there are many variations within each cultural group due to education, age, religion, socioeconomic status, geographic location, and length of time in the United States that make it difficult to summarize food habits by culture, race, or ethnicity. Consequently, factors such as economics, religion, customs, and fads influence eating habits and patterns, as well as individual preferences. Whatever the ethnic or cultural background, culturally sensitive nutrition counseling promotes better communication and positive behavior changes.

Religions and diet are also closely connected. Many religions do not permit followers to eat certain foods. Buddhists are not allowed to eat any meat. Moslems can eat no pork. Hindus consider the cow sacred, and may consume no animal foods except dairy products. Orthodox Jews avoid certain kinds of foods, including pork, nonkosher meats, and shellfish. The Seventh-Day Adventists promote ovolactovegetarianism.

Some people choose their diet on the basis of fads and myths. Eating habits have long been partly controlled by beliefs about what is fit to eat. Today, some people avoid white bread or processed foods, because they fear that substances added during flour milling or processing make these foods impure. Others eat "natural" or organically grown food to ensure a healthy diet, while some groups have encouraged strict vegetarianism for the purpose of achieving a certain "spiritual" level. Brief descriptions of several ethnic and cultural food patterns follows.

African-American

African-American food habits are often referred to as "soul food" or the quality of food that transcends its ability to nourish the body and reaches to nourish the spirit. The diet includes a high intake of vegetables, fruits, legumes, fish, and poultry. However, most of the desired food preparation techniques add relatively large amounts of fat and salt or rely on frying. Foods are boiled for long periods of time, so many nutrients are in the broth. In counseling, acknowledge what is good about food habits and recommend only the changes that are needed based on an assessment and treatment. Questions which need to be answered include: Can I still eat fried foods? How can I give food flavor or taste without adding fat, meat and/or salt?

Hispanic

Hispanic food habits include three cultures: Mexican-American, Puerto Rican, and Cuban-American. Their foods have origin in three major cultural groups, American Indian, Spanish, and African. The Mexican-American traditional soups, stews, and dishes that incorporate vegetables, meat, and bean-based dishes and puddings are nutrient-dense. Encourage the use of corn-based tortillas, fresh fruits or drinks, milk-based hot beverages, tortillas made without fat, and lower-calorie puddings. The Puerto Rican diet is an amalgam of traditional and popular foods in the United States. Traditional diet patterns of rice, beans, mixed dishes and thick stews or soups made with roots and tubers or tropical items have expanded to include hamburgers, pizza, and ready-to-eat cereals. Data on the Cuban-American diet are sparse. Most persons eat black beans and rice, starchy vegetables, and corn-based dishes such as the Cuban tamale. This cultural preference toward highly seasoned or hot dishes encourages the use of high amounts of sodium. Emphasize the use of spices which do not contain sodium. Some Hispanics erroneously equate "low sodium" with "bland," and that all seasonings are omitted. When advising a Hispanic client, identify the individual's place of origin, primary language, and education level. Linguistic diversity among Hispanic subgroups complicate the direct translation of printed materials and oral instructions.

Chinese

The Chinese have been in the United States since the mid-1800s. Today there are more than 800,000 Chinese in the United States, half of whom were born here. Whether native-born Chinese or second- or third-generation Chinese-American, food maintains a central role in their lives. Four major regions, each with its own distinctive taste, exists in China. Traditionally, food plays a vital role in the prevention and treatment of various diseases and physical conditions. Eating styles include a morning meal of thick rice soup flavored with pork or fish, noodles, or vegetables. The afternoon and evening meals generally begin with soup followed by a vegetable dish, mixed dishes with meat, or seafood. Dairy foods are not a major part of the traditional diet. Many Chinese adults have lactose intolerance. Salted, dried, and pickled foods and marinade and dipping sauces raise the sodium content of meals. Recommend more ginger, scallions, garlic, vinegar, pepper, and coriander. If lower fat is required, recommend reducing the amount of oil used in cooking.

Asian Indian

Food practices of Asian Indians are shaped by geographical region and religious traditions. In India 80% of the population follows vegetarian food habits. Cows are considered sacred, thus beef is taboo. Muslims do not eat pork, so non-vegetarians choose between chicken, lamb, goat, and seafood. Everyday meals consist of grains, mainly rice and wheat, legumes, fruits, and vegetables. While many Asian Indians cling to their ethnic food habits, their diets have been influenced by high-calorie, high-fat foods in the United States, especially among the children. In India transportation is frequently on foot or bicycle. Here in the United States, travel is by car and the busy lifestyle leaves little time for exercise. Coupled with the change in dietary patterns, many Asian Indians living in the United States develop obesity, hypertension, and signs and symptoms of insulin resistance.

REFERENCES

Bantle JP, Laine CW, Thomas JW. Metabolic effects of dietary fructose and sucrose in type I and II diabetic subjects. J Am Med Assoc 1986; 256:3241–3246.

Bronner Y, Burke C, Joubert BJ. African-American/soul foodways and nutrition counseling. Top Clin Nutr 1994; 9:20–27.

Committee on Diet and Health, Food and Nutrition Board, National Research Council. Diet and health: implications for reducing chronic disease risk. Washington, DC: National Academy Press, 1989.

Coulston AM, Hollenbeck CB, Swislocki ALM, Reaven GM. Persistence of hypertriglyceridemic effect of low fat, high carbohydrate diets in NIDDM patients. Diabetes Care 1989; 12:94–101.

Ensminger AH, Ensminger ME, Konlande JE, Robson JRK. Foods and nutrition encyclopedia. Ann Arbor: CRC Press, 1994:576–583, 1913–1920.

Goodrick GK, Foreyt JP. Why treatments for obesity don't last. J Am Diet Assoc 1991; 91:1243–1247.

Harris JA, Benedict FG. A biometric study of basal metabolism in man. Pub. No. 279. Washington, DC: Carnegie Institution, 1991.

Institute of Medicine. Nutrition during pregnancy. Washington, DC: National Academy Press, 1990.

Kozier B et al. *Techniques in clinical nursing,* Menlo Park, CA: Addison Wesley, 1993.

Mahan LK, Arline MT. Krause's food, nutrition and diet therapy. 8th ed. Philadelphia: WB Saunders, 1992.

Phillips PA, Rolls BJ, Ledingham JGG, Forsling ML, Morton JJ, Crowe MJ, Wollner L. Reduced thirst after water deprivation in healthy elderly men. New Engl J Med 1984; 311:753–759.

Public Health Service. Surgeon general's report on nutrition and health. Pub. No. DHHS 88-50210. Rockville, MD: US Department of Health and Human Services, 1988.

Rodriguez JC. Diet, nutrition, and the Hispanic client. Top Clin Nutr 1994; 9:28–39.

Sridaran G, Kolhatkar RR. Ethnic food practices of Asian Indians. Top Clin Nutr 1994; 9:45–48.

Summary of the second report of the national cholesterol education program (NCEP) expert panel on detection, evaluation, and treatment of high blood cholesterol in adults (Adult Treatment Panel II). J Am Med Assoc 1993; 269:3015–3023.

Tayback M, Kumanyika S, Chee E. Body weight as a risk factor in the elderly. Arch Intern Med 1990; 150:1065–1072.

The American Dietetic Association. Handbook of clinical dietetics. 2nd ed. New Haven: Yale University Press, 1992:119–147.

The Diabetes Control and Complications Trial Research Group. The effect of intensive treatment of diabetes on the development and progression of long-term complications in insulin-dependent diabetes mellitus. N Engl J Med 1993; 329:977–986.

Thomas AE, McKay DA, Cutlip MB. A nomograph method for assessing body weight. Am J Clin Nutr 1976; 29:302–304.

US Department of Agriculture. The food guide pyramid. Home and Garden Bulletin No. 252. Washington, DC: Government Printing Office, 1992.

US Department of Agriculture and US Department of Health and Human Services. Nutrition and your health: dietary guidelines for Americans. Home and Garden Bulletin, No. 232. Washington, DC: Government Printing Office,1990.

US Senate Select Committee on Nutrition and Human Needs. Dietary goals for the United States. 2nd ed. Washington DC: Government Printing Office, 1977.

Wu-Jung CJ. Understanding food habits of Chinese Americans. Top Clin Nutr 1994; 9:40–44.

CHAPTER 9

INFECTIOUS DISEASES AND INFECTION PREVENTION

9-1 **Basic Epidemiology**

9-2 **Infection Prevention Measures**

9-3 **Disease-Causing Microorganisms**

9-4 **Communicable and Infectious Diseases**

A primary goal of nursing is to be aware of infection-causing conditions and to take actions to both prevent and cure infections.

9-1 BASIC EPIDEMIOLOGY

Epidemiology is the study of the distribution and causes of disease within a population. A clear understanding of the epidemiology of infections is very important in carrying out the nurse's role in planning and delivering health care.

A basic fact about all infections is that six components or links must be present for any infection to occur. In Figure 9-1, a chain is used to illustrate the six factors necessary for infection. If an infectious agent enters a susceptible host and begins to multiply, varying responses may occur within the host. Figure 9-2 describes the spectrum of host responses to an infection by an infectious agent.

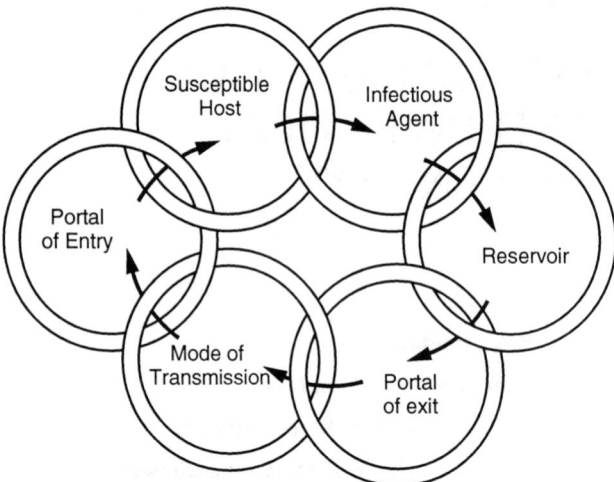

Figure 9–1. The six components of the infectious disease process. From Soule B. The APIC curriculum for infection control practice Vol. I. Kendall/Hunt Publishing Co, 1987. Used with permission.

COMMUNICABLE DISEASE DEFINITIONS AND VOCABULARY

Causative Agent   A biological, physical, or chemical entity capable of causing disease

Carrier   A person with a subclinical infection who may transmit illness to others

Reservoir (of Infectious Agents)   A person, animal, arthropod, plant soil, or substance in which an infectious agent normally lives and multiplies, on which it depends primarily for survival, and where it produces itself in such a manner that it can be transmitted to a susceptible host

Portal of Entry   The path by which an infectious agent enters the susceptible host

Mode of Transmission   The mechanism for transfer of an infectious agent from a reservoir to a susceptible host

Susceptible Host   A person lacking resistance to a particular pathogenic agent

Portal of Exit   Path by which an infectious agent leaves the reservoir

Endemic   The usual presence of disease within a geographic area

COMMUNICABLE DISEASE
DEFINITIONS AND VOCABULARY *Continued*

Epidemic   An excess over the expected occurrence of disease within a geographic area

Pandemic   An epidemic that affects several countries or continents

Outbreak   Synonymous with epidemic, but a term often preferred when dealing with the public; does not evoke the same fear response as the term "epidemic"

Unrecognized (Asymptomatic, Subclinical) Infection   An infectious process running a course similar to that of clinical disease but below the threshold of clinical symptoms

Recognized (Symptomatic, Clinical) Infection   An infection resulting in clinical signs and symptoms (disease)

Colonization   Presence of microorganisms in or on a host with growth and multiplication but without tissue invasion or damage

Contamination   The presence of microorganisms on inanimate objects, in substances, or in the environment

Cross-infection   Infection caused when pathogenic microorganisms are transmitted between individuals

Endogenous Infection   The host's normal flora becomes displaced (e.g., *Escherichia coli* from the colon enters the urinary tract and causes a urinary tract infection)

Exogenous Infection   An infection caused by environmental pathogens

Latent Infection   A phase in an established infection during which the causative organism is dormant in the host, sometimes for years, e.g., latent syphilis

Nosocomial Infection   An infection that was not present or incubating in a client on admission to a health care facility and is temporarily associated with that admission. A nosocomial infection may be present at the time of admission and the infection is related to previous hospitalization at the same facility. Nosocomial infections also include infections acquired in the hospital but appearing after discharge. This term also applies to infections acquired by health care providers if exposure to the infection is related to their work in the health care facility.

Subclinical, Silent, Inapparent, or Asymptomatic Infection   A laboratory-verified infection that shows no symptoms.

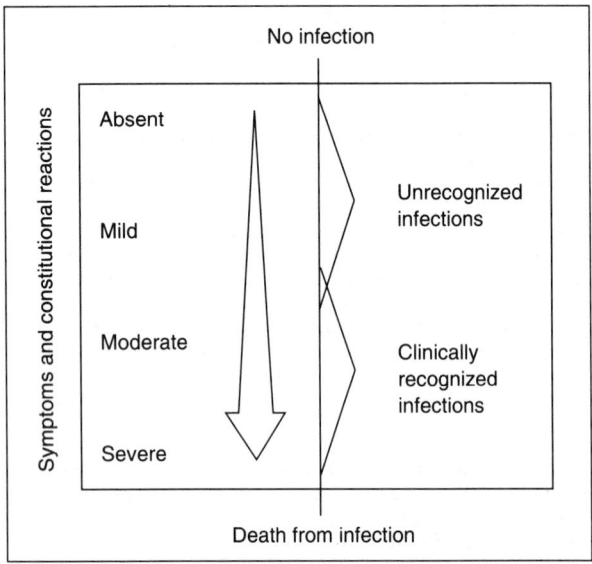

Figure 9–2. Various host responses to infection by an infectious agent. From Soule B. The APIC curriculum for infection control practice Vol. I. Kendall/Hunt Publishing Co, 1987. Used with permission.

Although effective vaccines, improved general hygiene, sanitary conditions and antibiotic therapy have made many infectious diseases among the most easily preventable and treatable illnesses, new organisms continue to arise as causes of disease. In addition, as longevity increases and improvements in medical technology continue, the use of invasive procedures and immunosuppressive therapies continue to rise as well. Thus, organisms that previously caused no harm can gain entrance to the body and cause infection.

Prevention of disease depends on breaking the chain of infection. Primary strategies are eliminating the pathogen, strengthening host immunity, and interrupting the mode of transmission. In the clinical setting, key infection control actions include handwashing, using anti-microbial agents, wearing gloves when in contact with body fluids and implementing isolation barriers when appropriate.

9-2   INFECTION PREVENTION MEASURES

Infection prevention activities focus on breaking the infection chain. Breaking the chain requires interrupting one or more of the components of the infectious disease process. By following the basic principles of hand washing, Universal Precautions and Body Substance Isolation, OSHA Bloodborne Pathogen Standard compliance, appropriate isolation techniques, and immunization recommendations, nurses can play a vital role in breaking the chain of infection.

Hand Washing and Skin Protection

- Hand washing is the most effective means of preventing the spread of pathogens. Wash hands for 10–15 seconds with soap and running water:
  - Before and after each client contact
  - After contact with client's body fluids
  - Before and after performing an invasive procedure
  - After removing gloves
  - Before and after contact with eyes, nose, or mouth
  - Before contact with food
  - After using rest room
- Examine hands for any cuts, abrasions, or breaks in skin and cover with waterproof dressing or bandage.
- Health care providers who have exudative lesions or weeping dermatitis should refrain from all direct client care and from handling client care equipment until the condition resolves.

Universal Precautions and Body Substance Isolation

Universal Precautions is a system of barrier protection and is intended to prevent parenteral, mucous membrane, and non-intact skin exposure to bloodborne pathogens in clients and personnel in the health care setting. Body Substance Isolation (BSI) is another system of barrier protection. Universal Precautions focuses primarily on blood and certain body fluids that may contain blood, and have been implicated in the transmission of bloodborne pathogens. Body Substance Isolation includes the isolation of *all* moist body substances from *all* clients.

Body Substance Isolation is composed of two parts. The primary focus of BSI is on the isolation of moist body substances through the use of barrier protection during care of *all* clients regardless of their diagnosis. The secondary focus is the disease-driven component that is used for the client with confirmed or suspected highly communicable infectious disease transmitted by the airborne/respiratory route. Respiratory isolation is usually required.

OSHA Bloodborne Pathogen Standard

The Federal Occupational Health and Safety Administration (OSHA) Bloodborne Pathogen Standard mandates that the administration of health care facilities take an active role in protecting employees from occupational exposure to bloodborne pathogens. The standard includes the fundamental concept of Universal Precautions and requires the caregiver to assess the likelihood of exposure to blood and body fluids prior to each procedure or client contact.

The standard includes the following requirements:

- Specific identification of all employees who are occupationally exposed to blood or body fluids

- Development of a written exposure control plan that requires specified work practices, engineering controls, and personal protective equipment to be used

- Offering hepatitis B vaccinations to any employees considered to be occupationally exposed to blood or body fluids

- Development of post-exposure follow-up procedures and documentation

- Mandatory training programs
- Record keeping to document compliance with the regulation

TERMS DESCRIBING THE COMPONENTS OF THE OSHA BLOODBORNE PATHOGEN STANDARD

Engineering controls Measures and devices that localize or remove hazards from personnel or the work site. Examples: "sharps" disposal containers, splash guards, needle-free devices.

Personal protective equipment Specialized clothing or equipment worn for protection from exposure to blood or body fluids. Examples: gloves, masks, goggles, aprons.

Post-exposure follow-up Confidential medical consultation and treatment provided immediately after an exposure. Post-exposure management includes counseling, hepatitis B vaccine if not previously given, HIV testing of blood from employee and source client, if available, and post-exposure prophylaxis, if indicated. All records and documents are confidential.

Work practice controls Habits and practices that reduce the risk of exposure to blood or body fluids. Examples are hand washing, *not* recapping needles, and refraining from eating and drinking in work areas where there is high risk of occupational exposure to blood or body fluids. See Table 9-1 for more specific guidelines.

Infectious substance The following materials are defined by the CDC as infectious, requiring observance of Universal Precautions: blood, semen, vaginal secretions, cerebrospinal fluid, synovial fluid, pericardial fluid, pleural fluid, peritoneal fluid, amniotic fluid, saliva (in dental procedures), any body fluid visibly contaminated with blood, any unidentified body fluid, any unfixed tissue or organ other than intact skin, any cell, tissue or organ culture containing human immunodeficiency virus (HIV), or any culture medium or other solution containing hepatitis B virus (HBV). Universal Precautions do not apply to feces, saliva, nasal secretions, sputum, sweat,

---

TABLE 9–1. UNIVERSAL PRECAUTIONS—WORK PRACTICE CONTROLS

Hand Washing

A vital part of disease prevention—see Sec. 9-2 to review.

Gloves

Wear gloves when touching blood and body fluids containing blood, or surfaces or items soiled with blood or body fluids, or when contamination with blood may occur. Change gloves between client contacts. Wear gloves if you have any cuts, scratches, or breaks in the skin.

Masks, Goggles, Glasses, Face Shields

Wear protective eyewear and other barriers to protect the mucous membranes of your mouth, nose, and eyes during procedures that are likely to generate droplets of blood or other body fluids to which Universal Precautions apply.

Disposal of Needles and Sharps

Place used disposable needle units (*uncapped and unbroken*), scalpel blades, and other sharp objects in puncture resistant containers, kept near place of use.

Laundry

Handle soiled linen as little as possible and with minimal agitation. Place linen soiled with blood or body fluids in leakage-resistant bags at the site where used.

Specimens

Use well-constructed containers with secure lids to transport all specimens. Do not contaminate outside of container when collecting specimens.

Blood Spills

Use a chemical germicide approved for use in your facility to decontaminate work surfaces after a spill of blood or body fluids.

Infective Wastes

Follow agency policies for disposal of infective wastes, both when disposing of and decontaminating contaminated materials.

---

tears, vomitus, or urine unless traces of blood are present.

Isolation Systems

Isolation systems are designed to break the chain of infection by:

- Controlling or eliminating the infective agent
- Controlling or eliminating the reservoir
- Interrupting transmission

Many health care facilities have replaced disease-specific and category isolation with Universal Precautions and Body Substance Isolation. Disease-specific and category isolation require a specific or confirmed diagnosis prior to initiating isolation procedures. Many infections go unnoticed since the client may not be exhibiting infection symptoms or the confirming laboratory results have not been received. In most cases, when the infectious disease is known or suspected, the client does not require a private room nor isolation precautions because the infection is not highly communicable, and secretions/excretions can be contained with Universal Precautions. Table 9-2, Precautions for the Client with Infectious Diseases, lists selected infectious diseases and the role of the nurse in preventing transmission within the health care facility. When Universal Precautions/ Body Substance Isolation measures are followed for all clients and when Respiratory Isolation is used for the client with highly communicable infections, maximum protection for both client and health care personnel is achieved.

RESPIRATORY ISOLATION

Respiratory isolation procedures are initiated for the client confirmed of suspected highly communicable diseases transmitted by the airborne route. Table 9-3, Precautions for the Client with Airborne Communicable Infectious Diseases, lists diseases requiring respiratory isolation. Specific requirements for respiratory isolation:

- Private room
- Keep door closed
- Signs designating respiratory isolation
- Mask for susceptible persons who come in contact with the client
- Hand washing before and after caring for the client
- Use of body substance isolation principles

TABLE 9–2. PRECAUTIONS FOR THE CLIENT WITH INFECTIOUS DISEASES

The client with the following infectious diseases requires Universal Precautions, but usually does not require a private room. Regardless of the client's infection status, the nurse must assess the client's condition to determine if the client's secretions/excretions can be contained within his or her immediate environment. If so, the client may be placed in a room with other clients and Universal Precautions are to be observed. If not, then a private room is recommended.

Acquired Immunodeficiency Syndrome (AIDS)
Amebiasis
Aspergillosis
Campylobacteriosis
Cat Scratch Fever
Cholera
Clostridium difficile Entero-colitis
Coccidioidomycosis
Creutzfeld-Jakob Disease
Cryptococcosis
Cryptosporidiosis
Cytomegalovirus (CMV) Infection
Diarrhea
Encephalitis
Gas Gangrene
Gastroenteritis
Giardiasis
Gonorrhea
Hansen's Disease (Leprosy)
Hepatitis A, B, C, or D
Herpes Simplex Infection
Human Immunodeficiency Virus (HIV) Infection
Impetigo
Influenza
Kawasaki Syndrome
Legionellosis
Listeriosis
Malaria
Meningitis (not Meningococcal)
Methicillin-Resistant *Staphylococcus aureus* (MRSA) Infection
Mycoplasma Pneumonia
Pediculosis (Lice)
Pneumococcal Pneumonia
Pneumocystis Carinii Pneumonia (PCP)
Poliomyelitis
Pseudomonas Infection
Q Fever
Rabies
Respiratory Syncytial Virus (RSV) Infection
Rotavirus Infection
Salmonellosis
Scabies
Shigellosis
Staphylococcus aureus Infection
Streptococcal Disease
Syphilis
Toxic Shock Syndrome
Toxoplasmosis
Tuberculosis (Extra-Pulmonary)
Tularemia
Typhoid Fever
Wound Infection/Abscess
Yersiniosis

**TABLE 9–3. PRECAUTIONS FOR THE CLIENT
WITH AIRBORNE COMMUNICABLE
INFECTIOUS DISEASES**

The client with the following airborne communicable
infectious diseases requires respiratory isolation as well as
body substance/isolation.

Anthrax
Chickenpox
Diphtheria
Ebola-Marburg virus
Hemorrhagic fever
Lassa fever
Measles
Meningococcal infections (for 24 hr after effective therapy
　started)
Mumps
Pertussis
Rubella
Tuberculosis, Pulmonary
Varicella zoster

It is recommended by the Center for Disease Control
that the client with suspected or confirmed active tuberculosis be placed in a private room with negative air flow
ventilation, and that caregivers wear particulate respirator
masks when in contact with such clients.

Immunity and Immunization

When considering immunization and immunity, the
needs of the health care provider are as important as the
community at large in order to prevent transmission of
communicable disease. The risk to the health care worker
is high due to the multiple exposures he/she faces daily.

HEALTH CARE PROVIDERS

It is important for each health care provider to know their
own immune status. Table 9-4 describes recommended

TABLE 9–4. RECOMMENDED IMMUNIZATIONS FOR HOSPITAL AND OUTPATIENT FACILITY PERSONNEL

VACCINES	PRIMARY SCHEDULE AND BOOSTER(S)	INDICATIONS	MAJOR PRECAUTIONS OR SPECIAL CONSIDERATIONS
Hepatitis B Inactived virus vaccine (plasma-derived or yeast-derived vaccine)	3 doses, with 2nd and 3rd given 1 and 6 mo after first. Need for boosters unknown. Alternative schedule: 4 doses at 0, 1, 2, and 12 mo. Dose: 1.0 mg (IM)	Personnel who have regular or potential contact with client's blood or tissue fluids and are not known to be previously infected or immune should be immunized. If 2nd dose not given until ≥ 4 mo after first, give 3rd dose 3–5 mo after 2nd. Do not start over if schedule is interrupted. Can start series with one manufacturer's vaccine and finish with another.	Serologic screening for susceptibility before immunization need not be done unless the hospital considers it cost-effective or a potential vaccinee requests it.
Influenza Inactivated whole virus and split virus vaccine	Annual fall immunization with current vaccine. Either whole or	Personnel and volunteers who have extensive contact with client	History of anaphylactic hypersensitivity to eggs.

**TABLE 9–4. RECOMMENDED IMMUNIZATIONS
FOR HOSPITAL AND OUTPATIENT
FACILITY PERSONNEL** *Continued*

VACCINES	PRIMARY SCHEDULE AND BOOSTER(S)	INDICA-TIONS	MAJOR PRECAUTIONS OR SPECIAL CONSIDER-ATIONS
	split virus vaccine may be used. Dose: 0.5 ml (IM)	should be immunized.	
Measles Live virus vaccine	2 doses, at least 1 mo apart. No booster. Dose: 0.5 ml (SC)	Personnel born in 1957 or later should be considered immune only if they have documented measles sero-positivity or documented receipt of two doses of measles vac-cine on or af-ter the first birthday. Those born in 1956 or earlier should be considered susceptible unless they have docu-mentation of seropositivity or receipt of one dose of measles vac-	Pregnancy: immu-nocompromised persons; history of anaphylactic hy-persensitivity to egg or neomycin; receipt of immune globulin or blood/blood product in preceding 3 months. Previous immuni-zation is *not* a con-traindication. MMR is vaccine of choice if recipi-ents possibly are susceptible to measles or mumps as well as to ru-bella.

Table continued on following page

TABLE 9–4. RECOMMENDED IMMUNIZATIONS FOR HOSPITAL AND OUTPATIENT FACILITY PERSONNEL *Continued*

VACCINES	PRIMARY SCHEDULE AND BOOS-TER(S)	INDICA-TIONS	MAJOR PRECAUTIONS OR SPECIAL CONSIDER-ATIONS
		cine on or after the first birthday.	
Rubella Live virus vaccine	1 dose No booster Dose: 0.5 ml (SC)	All personnel should be immune to rubella. Persons lacking documentation of vaccine on or after 1st birthday or laboratory evidence of immunity should be considered susceptible.	Pregnancy; immunocompromised persons; history of anaphylactic hypersensitivity to neomycin. Previous immunization is *not* a contraindication. MMR is vaccine of choice if recipients possibly are susceptible to measles or mumps as well as to rubella.
Polio Inactivated virus vaccine (IPV) or live virus Vaccine (OPV) or any combination of IPV and OPV.	IPV: 2 doses 4–8 weeks apart; 3rd dose 6–12 mo after 2nd. Dose: 0.5 ml (SC). OPV: 2 doses 6–8 weeks apart with a 3rd dose of 6–12 mo after the 2nd.	Personnel who may have direct contact with acute polio clients should complete a primary series.	a) It is prudent on theoretical grounds to avoid immunizing pregnant women. b) OPV should not be given to immunocompromised individuals or to persons with known immunocompromised family members. Use IPV in such situations. c) Anaphylactic hypersensitivity to neomycin.

TABLE 9–4. RECOMMENDED IMMUNIZATIONS FOR HOSPITAL AND OUTPATIENT FACILITY PERSONNEL *Continued*

VACCINES	PRIMARY SCHEDULE AND BOOSTER(S)	INDICA-TIONS	MAJOR PRECAUTIONS OR SPECIAL CONSIDER-ATIONS
Tetanus/ Diphtheria	All adults, hospital personnel included, should receive Td (tetanus-diphtheria) toxoid boosters every 10 years. For those who have never received these toxoids, the primary immunization series with Td is 2 doses 4–8 weeks apart with a 3rd dose 6–12 months after the 2nd.		

immunizations for hospital and medical outpatient facility personnel. The provider who is nonimmune to any of the common childhood communicable diseases is susceptible to that disease, and may acquire the disease in the community or hospital, putting the nonimmune client at risk. Health care providers must document that they are immune to measles, mumps, and rubella. A vaccine is not yet available for varicella. Nurses with uncertain varicella history must confirm their immune status by serologic testing. Hepatitis B vaccination is recommended for all health care workers who have contact with blood and body fluids.

Influenza immunization is recommended for health care providers and high risk persons, and should be administered in the fall season from mid-October to mid-November.

COMMUNITY

Comprehensive immunization is one of the most important means of controlling disease. Table 9-5 lists the immunization schedule for children. It is also recommended that the elderly and persons who are chronically ill receive influenza and pneumococcal vaccines. Travelers

TABLE 9–5. IMMUNIZATION SCHEDULE FOR CHILDREN

AGE	IMMUNIZATION*
2 mo	Diphtheria/pertussis/tetanus; polio; Haemophilus influenzae b (Hib); Hepatitis B
4 mo	Diphtheria/pertussis/tetanus; polio; Hib; Hepatitis B
6 mo	Diphtheria/pertussis/tetanus; polio (optional); Hib; Hepatitis B
15 mo	Measles/mumps/rubella
15–18 mo	Diphtheria/pertussis/tetanus; polio; Hib; TB tine test
4–5 yr	Diphtheria/pertussis/tetanus; polio booster; TB tine test; measles/mumps/rubella
15 yr and every 10 yr thereafter	Diphtheria/tetanus booster

*Before immunization, obtain from the child's parents a history of allergy and past reaction to immunization. Ascertain if the child receives corticosteroid or any other drugs that suppress the immune response. After immunization, instruct parents to report a severe reaction. Give them a record of immunization.

to or immigrants from endemic areas are required to have appropriate immunizations.

9-3 DISEASE-CAUSING MICROORGANISMS

Bacteria

Many bacteria have adapted in a harmless way to life within the human body. Other bacterial are harmful and may cause human disease. Harmful bacteria are termed pathogens, and their infection of body tissue results in a characteristic illness. The identification of a bacterium suspected of being the cause of an infection is one of the major tools for the objective diagnosis of infectious diseases.

EXAMPLES OF COMMON BACTERIAL INFECTIONS

GRAM-POSITIVE COCCI

Staphylococcal Infections
Abscesses
Bacteremia, septicemia
Bloodstream infections
Carbuncles
Cellulitis
Empyema
Endocarditis
Enterocolitis
Food poisoning
Furuncles (boils)
Hepatic abscess
Impetigo
Osteomyelitis
Perinephric abscess
Pneumonitis
Skin and soft tissue infection
Splenic abscess

Streptococcal Infections
Arthritis
Empyema
Impetigo
Mastoiditis
Meningitis
Necrotizing fasciitis
Otitis media
Pericarditis
Peritonsillar abscess
Peritonitis
Pneumonitis
Scarlet fever
Sinusitis
Streptococcal sore throat

GRAM-NEGATIVE COCCI

Meningococcal Infections
Endocarditis
Gonorrhea
Meningitis
Meningococcemia (simple, fulminant, chronic)

Others
Pneumonia
Purulent conjunctivitis
Sinusitis

GRAM-POSITIVE BACILLI

Actinomycosis
Anthrax
Botulism
Diphtheria
Erysipeloid
Gas gangrene
Listeriosis
Nocardiosis
Tetanus

GRAM-NEGATIVE BACILLI

Brucellosis
Chancroid
Cholera
Haemophilus influenzae infection
Nosocomial infections (e.g., *Escherichia coli*)
Plague (black death)
Pseudomonas infections
Rat-bite fever
Salmonellosis
Shigellosis
Tularemia
Whooping cough (pertussis)

EXAMPLES OF COMMON BACTERIAL INFECTIONS *Continued*

MYCOBACTERIUM	SPIROCHETES
Leprosy	Leptospirosis
Tuberbulosis	Relapsing fever (tick, fowl-nest, cabin, or vagabond fever)
	Syphilis

Viruses

The estimated 400 viruses that infect humans are classified according to their size and shape (spherical, rod-shaped, or cubic), or means of transmission (respiratory, fecal-oral, or sexual). Protection by means of immunization (e.g., against influenza virus) is difficult because of the many different strains that cause illness. Most viruses resist available antiviral drugs.

EXAMPLES OF VIRAL INFECTIONS

RESPIRATORY VIRAL INFECTIONS	RASH-PRODUCING VIRAL INFECTIONS	ENTERIC VIRAL INFECTIONS
Adenovirus infection	Herpes simplex infection	Echovirus infection
Common cold	Herpes zoster (shingles)	Herpangina
Influenza (grippe, flu)	Measles (rubeola)	Poliomyelitis
Parainfluenza	Roseola infantum (exanthem subitem)	Rotavirus infection
Respiratory syncytial virus infection	Rubella (German measles)	
	Varicella (chicken pox)	

ARBOVIRUS INFECTIONS	MISCELLANEOUS VIRUS INFECTIONS
Colorado tick fever	AIDS (human immuno-deficiency virus [HIV])
Dengue	

EXAMPLES OF VIRAL INFECTIONS
Continued

ARBOVIRUS INFECTIONS	MISCELLANEOUS VIRUS INFECTIONS
Yellow fever	Cytomegalovirus (CMV) infection
	Infectious mononucleosis
	Lassa fever
	Mumps
	Rabies
	Warts (verrucae)

Chlamydiae

Once thought to be large viruses, chlamydiae now constitute a separate order, family, and genus. Although they are intracellular pathogens, they resemble bacteria in that they possess both RNA and DNA, divide by binary fission, have bacterial ribosomes, and have a cell wall. Chlamydial infections often produce nonspecific symptoms or no symptoms at all, which makes diagnosis difficult. Sexually transmitted chlamydia can go undetected for years, and can cause sterility.

EXAMPLES OF CHLAMYDIAL INFECTIONS

Neonatal inclusion conjunctivitis
Pelvic inflammatory disease
Salpingitis
Trachoma

Fungi (Mycoses)

Fungi are single-celled organisms that may infect the skin and superficial tissues, subcutaneous tissues and bone, or the internal organs, bloodstream, or lungs.

EXAMPLES OF FUNGAL INFECTIONS

Aspergillosis
Blastomycosis
Candidiasis
Chromomycosis

EXAMPLES OF FUNGAL INFECTIONS
Continued

Coccidioidomycosis
Cryptococcosis
Histoplasmosis
Sporotrichosis
Tinea-Ringworm
Zygomycosis

Rickettsia

Rickettsia are small, gram-negative, bacteria-like organisms that can induce life-threatening infections. Most often these microbes are carried by fleas, ticks, or mites, which then infect the host by biting. These infections are relatively uncommon in the United States, but are on the rise with the increase of outdoor activities such as backpacking and camping.

EXAMPLES OF RICKETTSIAL INFECTIONS

Epidemic typhus
Q Fever
Rickettsial pox
Rocky Mountain spotted fever
Scrub typhus
Trench fever

Protozoa

These are one-celled organisms that belong to the animal kingdom. Along with helminths, protozoa account for a major proportion of the diseases caused by infectious agents worldwide. Although most prevalent in the developing countries, some of these infections are becoming clinically recognized pathogens in the developed countries.

EXAMPLES OF PROTOZOAN INFECTIONS

African trypanosomiasis (sleeping sickness)
Amebiasis (amebic dysentery)

EXAMPLES OF PROTOZOAN INFECTIONS *Continued*

Amebic meningoencephalitis
Giardiasis (giardiasis enteris, lambliasis)
Leishmaniasis
Malaria
South African trypanosomiasis (Chagas' disease)
Toxoplasmosis

Helminths (Worms)

Helminthiasis is prevalent is many parts of developing and developed countries. Fortunately, there are effective, safe, orally administered chemotherapeutic agents for most worm infections.

EXAMPLES OF HELMINTHIC INFECTIONS

Ascariasis (roundworm infections)
Enterobiasis (pinworm disease, oxyuriasis, seatworm or threadworm infection)
Hookworm disease (uncinariasis)
Schistosomiasis (bilharziasis)
Strongyloidiasis (threadworm infection)
Taeniasis (tapeworm disease)
Toxocariosis (visceral larva migrans [VLM])
Trichinosis (trichiniasis, trichinellosis, found in inadequately cooked pork)
Trichuriasis (whipworm disease)

9-4 COMMUNICABLE AND INFECTIOUS DISEASES

Predisposing factors to the acquisition of communicable and infectious diseases are advanced age or disability, malnutrition, poor hygiene, alcoholism, neoplastic disease, diabetes, or other chronic disease, drug abuse, trauma, childbirth, invasive procedures, multiple sexual partners, or any other condition that compromises immunity and exposes the individual to pathogens. Table 9-6 lists incubation

Text continued on page 426

TABLE 9–6. SELECTED COMMUNICABLE INFECTIOUS DISEASES

NAME	AGENT	INCUBATION PERIOD	INFECTIOUS PERIOD	MODE OF TRANSMISSION	SYMPTOMS	TREATMENT
AIDS (acquired immuno-deficiency syndrome)	Human immuno-deficiency virus (HIV)	1–3 mo from infection to development of HIV antibodies; 2 mo–10 yr from infection to diagnosis of AIDS	Unknown; presumed to extend throughout life	Direct contact through body opening (mouth, vagina, rectum, skin lesion, or by intravenous route) with body fluids, primarily blood or semen, of infected person	Initially, fever, fatigue, anorexia, unexplained extreme weight loss, lymphadenopathy, skin rashes, chronic diarrhea, and lack of resistance to infection	Treatment of secondary opportunistic infections with antibiotics, also drugs such as zidovudine (AZT)
Amebiasis (Amebic dysentery)	*Entamoeba histolytica*	3 days to several mo	During period of passing of feces contaminated with cysts; may last for years	Fecal-oral route, contaminated food or water	Vary with severity-diarrhea (sometimes intermittent), blood and mucus in feces, abdominal discomfort	Chemotherapeutics or antibiotics
Botulism (*Clostridium botulinum*)	Refer to Table 9-8, Foodborne Illnesses Caused by Toxin-Producing Bacteria					
Campylobacter	Refer to Table 9-7, Foodborne Illnesses Caused by Bacteria					

Clostridium Perfringens - Food poisoning (*Clostridium welchii*)	Refer to Table 9-8, Foodborne Illnesses Caused by Toxin-Producing Bacteria					
Chickenpox (varicella)	Refer to Table 9-12, Differential Diagnosis of Common Exanthems					
Common cold	Rhinoviruses	12–72 hr	24 hr before onset to 5 days after onset	Direct oral contact or spread by droplets or fomites	Pharyngitis, nasal congestion, headache, fever, chills, myalgia, arthralgia, malaise, cough	Symptomatic
Diphtheria	*Corynebacterium diphtheriae*	2–5 days	Several hr before onset, usually 2 weeks during infection	Contact with droplets from mouth, nose, or throat of infected person or carrier	Sore throat, fever, coryza, malaise, grayish patches (pseudomembranes) on tonsils and mucosa of throat and nose	Antitoxin, antibiotics
Gastroenteritis due to enteroviruses, rotaviruses, paroviruses	Refer to Table 9-11, Foodborne Illnesses Caused by Viruses					
Giardiasis	Refer to Table 9-10, Foodborne Illnesses Caused by Parasites					

Table continued on following page

TABLE 9–6. SELECTED COMMUNICABLE INFECTIOUS DISEASES *Continued*

NAME	AGENT	INCUBATION PERIOD	INFECTIOUS PERIOD	MODE OF TRANSMISSION	SYMPTOMS	TREATMENT
Gonococcal Infection	*Neisseria gonorrhoeae*	2–9 days or longer	During infection	Sexual contact with exudates from mucous membranes of infected persons	In the male, acute anterior urethritis with burning on urination; serous discharge, becoming profuse, greenish yellow and often blood tinged. In the female, often asymptomatic	Ceftriaxone and doxycycline
Hepatitis A	Hepatitis A virus (HAV)	15–45 days	From latter half of incubation period to a few days after onset of jaundice	Person-to-person transmission via fecal-oral route; ingestion or parenteral inoculation with infected blood or blood products; sexual contact	Acute infection, fever, anorexia, nausea, vomiting, fatigue, lassitude, headache, abdominal discomfort, sometimes followed by jaundice (which may last 1–2 weeks)	Symptomatic

Hepatitis B	Hepatitis B virus (HBV)	45–180 days	From several weeks before onset of symptoms through clinical course of disease	Parenteral exposure to infected blood and blood products; contaminated needles, syringes, and IV equipment; sexual contact	Insidious onset; symptoms similar to those in infectious hepatitis. Severity ranges from inapparent cases to fulminating, fatal cases of acute hepatic necrosis	Symptomatic
Hepatitis C	Hepatitis C virus (HCV)	2–6 weeks	From 1 or more weeks before onset of symptoms through clinical course of disease	Parenteral exposure to infected blood and blood products; contaminated needles, syringes, and IV equipent. The importance of person-to-person contact and sexual activity in the transmission is not well defined.	Slow onset, anorexia, abdominal discomfort, nausea, vomiting, progressing to jaundice less frequently than hepatitis B	Symptomatic

Table continued on following page

TABLE 9–6. SELECTED COMMUNICABLE INFECTIOUS DISEASES *Continued*

NAME	AGENT	INCUBATION PERIOD	INFECTIOUS PERIOD	MODE OF TRANSMISSION	SYMPTOMS	TREATMENT
Hepatitis Delta	Hepatitis D virus (HDV)	Not firmly established	From several weeks before onset of symptoms through clinical course of disease	Parenteral exposure to blood and blood products, contaminated needles, syringes, and IV equipment; sexual contact.	Abrupt onset with symptoms resembling Hepatitis B infection. Seen in conjunction with Hepatitis B infection.	Symptomatic
Herpes simplex	Herpes simplex virus (HSV 1 & 2)	2–12 days	While lesions are present; before crusting	Direct contact	Fever, pharyngitis, erythema, edema, then primary typical lesions erupting, rupturing and leaving painful ulcers and yellow crusts. Fever, genital lesions occur with HSV2. Lesions on hands are called herpetic whitlow. Healing begins 7–10	Symptomatic. Acyclovir for treatment of primary infection.

Refer to Table 9-12, Differential Diagnosis of Common Exanthems

Disease	Causative agent	Incubation	Transmission	Symptoms	Treatment
Infectious mononucleosis				days after initial onset and is complete within 3 weeks.	
Influenza	Influeza virus (types A and B)	24–72 hr	Direct contact, droplet infection, hand transmission to eyes or nose from articles freshly contaminated with respiratory secretions of infected persons	Sudden onset, chills and fever, prostration, aches and pains in back and limbs, coryza, sore throat, bronchitis	Symptomatic; antibiotics for secondary infection.
Legionellosis "Legionnaire's Disease," "Pontiac Fever"	Legionella pneumophila, other legionellae	Legionnaire's disease 2–10 days; Pontiac fever 5–66 hr	Person-to-person transmission has not been documented; Airborne transmission via aerosol-producing devices; transmission into post-operative	Fever (39°–40.5°), chills, non-productive cough (if respiratory infection), abdominal pain, diarrhea	Erythromycin

Table continued on following page

TABLE 9–6. SELECTED COMMUNICABLE INFECTIOUS DISEASES *Continued*

NAME	AGENT	INCUBATION PERIOD	INFECTIOUS PERIOD	MODE OF TRANSMISSION	SYMPTOMS	TREATMENT
				cardiac surgery wound during bathing of client with contaminated tap water		
Malaria	*Plasmodium vivax, Falciparum malariae*	12–30 days	1–3 yr for vivax malaria; as long as plasmodia gametocytes are present in blood	Bite of female anopheline mosquito; transfusion of blood of infected persons	Chills, fever, headache, and myalgia interspersed with periods of well-being. Acute attacks (paroxysms) occur when erythrocytes rupture lasting 1–4 hr	Antimalarial drugs; chloroquine by mouth.
Measles (rubeola)	Refer to Table 9-12, Differential Diagnosis of Common Exanthems					
Meningococcal meningitis	*Neisseria meningitidis*	2–10 days	Until organisms are no longer present in upper respiratory	Droplet spread and direct contact with discharges from nose and throat	Sudden onset, fever, intense headache, stiff neck, nausea, vomiting; frequently, petechial rash;	Antibiotics, sulfonamides

Disease	Causative agent	Incubation period	Period of communicability	Method of transmission	Signs and symptoms	Treatment
			secretions (usually 24 hr after initiation of appropriate therapy)	of infected persons and carriers.	delirium and coma.	
Mumps	Mumps virus	12–26 days	From about 6 days before appearance of symptoms until swelling subsides (about 9 days)	Droplet spread and direct contact with saliva of infected persons	Slight fever, malaise, nausea, irritability, swelling, inflammation and tenderness of salivary glands.	Symptomatic
Pediculosis	Various species of lice	Eggs of lice hatch in 1 week	While lice remain alive on infested person or in clothing	Direct contact with an infested person or with clothing, linen, or headgear on which lice or eggs exist.	Itching; skin excoriation; matted, foul-smelling, lusterless hair (in severe cases)	Antiparasitic shampoo (gamma benzene hexachloride)
Pertussis (whooping cough)	Bordetella pertussis	7 days, not longer than 21 days	7 days after exposure to 3 weeks after onset of paroxysmal cough	Direct contact with respiratory secretions of infected persons, indirect contact with freshly	Catarrhal stage; hacking nocturnal cough, anorexia, sneezing, listlessness, low-grade fever, injected conjunctiva. Paroxysmal stage	Antibiotics, ampicillin, erythromycin

Table continued on following page

TABLE 9–6. SELECTED COMMUNICABLE INFECTIOUS DISEASES *Continued*

NAME	AGENT	INCUBATION PERIOD	INFECTIOUS PERIOD	MODE OF TRANSMISSION	SYMPTOMS	TREATMENT
				contaminated fomites.	(after 7–14 days); spasmodic recurrent characteristic paroxysmal coughing that may expel tenacious mucus and cause complications.	
Plague, pneumonia	*Yersinia pestis*	1–6 days	Duration of illness	Aerosolized droplets of sputum	Fever, swollen, inflamed lymph nodes	Antibiotics
Pneumonia, pneumococcal	*Pneumococci*	1–3 days	While infectious agent is present in oral and nasal discharges.	Spread by droplet or direct oral contact; indirect contact with fomites freshly contaminated with respiratory discharges.	Acute infection, sudden onset with chills and fever, often pain in the chest, usually cough and dyspnea.	Antibiotics

Disease	Causative Agent	Incubation Period	Period of Communicability	Mode of Transmission	Symptoms	Treatment
Poliomyelitis	Poliovirus (types I, II and III)	7–12 days	7–10 days before and after onset	Direct contact with feces or secretions from pharynx	Acute illness; fever, malaise; variable, but usually include headache and stiffness of neck and spine.	Symptomatic
Rabies	Rabies virus	From 10 days to 2 years, average 50–60 days	In biting animals 3–5 days before onset of symptoms and throughout course of disease.	Virus transmitted in the saliva of an infected animal; rarely, person to person.	Fulminating encephalitis, almost inevitably fatal; depression, fever, headache, anorexia, nausea, sore throat, malaise, restlessness, hyperesthesia of skin, hypersensitivity to light and sound, convulsions, paralysis.	Rabies vaccine and/or rabies immune globulin when bitten by rabid animal; symptomatic once symptoms occur.
Ringworm	Several species of fungi	Unknown for tinea pedis (athlete's foot) 10–14 days for tinea corpis	While lesions present on body and viable spores exist on fomites	Contact with skin lesions of infected persons and animals and with contaminated shower stalls or other articles.	Ring-shaped scaly or dry lesions on the skin or scalp; itching; inflammation and pain in severe cases.	Antifungals, e.g., griseofulvin, by mouth, clotrimazole, miconazole

Table continued on following page

TABLE 9–6. SELECTED COMMUNICABLE INFECTIOUS DISEASES *Continued*

NAME	AGENT	INCUBATION PERIOD	INFECTIOUS PERIOD	MODE OF TRANSMISSION	SYMPTOMS	TREATMENT
Rubella (German measles)	Refer to Table 9-12, Differential Diagnosis of Common Exanthems					
Salmonellosis	Refer to Table 9-7, Foodborne Illnesses Caused by Bacteria					
Scabies	*Sarcopetes scabiei*	Several days to weeks	Until mites and eggs are destroyed	Direct contact with skin, clothing or bedding of an infected person.	Characteristic burrow of itch mite, not inflammatory unless scratched; severe itching, especially when warm	Micticides
Scarlet fever	Refer to Table 9-12, Differential Diagnosis of Common Exanthems					
Shigellosis	Refer to Table 9-7, Foodborne Illnesses Caused by Bacteria					
Staphylococcal food poisoning	Refer to Table 9-8, Foodborne Illnesses Caused by Toxin-Producing Bacteria					
Streptococcal foodborne illness	Refer to Table 9-8, Foodborne Illnesses Caused by Toxin-Producing Bacteria					
Streptococcal sore throat	*Streptococcus pyogenes*	1–3 days	10–21 days if untreated; or 24 hr after penicillin therapy started	Direct contact with respiratory secretions of infected	Fever of 101°–104°F; sore throat with severe pain on swallowing, red pharynx, tonsilar	Antibiotics; penicillin or erythromycin

				persons, or contaminated food.	exudate, edematous tonsils and uvula, swollen glands, malaise and weakness, nasal discharge, anorexia.	
Syphilis	*Treponema pallidum*	10–90 days	During primary and secondary stages and mucocutaneous recurrences, infectiveness ends within 24 hr of adequate penicillin treatment	Sexual contact, saliva, semen, vaginal discharges, blood or exudates from moist skin lesions of infected persons; during birth.	Ulcer appears at site of inoculation (usually the genitals); constitutional symptoms and generalized lesions of skin and mucous membranes follow; may recur over several years. Late (tertiary stage) manifestations involve circulatory and central nervous systems.	Antibiotics; penicillin, erythromycin, tetracycline
Trichinosis	*Trichinella spiralis*	1–28 days	Not transmitted person to person	Ingestion of undercooked, infected pork	Variable with stage and degree of infection; sometimes asymptomatic. Stage 1: anorexia, nausea, vomiting, diarrhea, abdominal pain, fever.	Thiabendazole, supportive therapy

Table continued on following page

TABLE 9–6. SELECTED COMMUNICABLE INFECTIOUS DISEASES *Continued*

NAME	AGENT	INCUBATION PERIOD	INFECTIOUS PERIOD	MODE OF TRANSMISSION	SYMPTOMS	TREATMENT
					Stage 2: edema, facial and muscle pain, itching burning skin, high fever, sometimes cardiac and respiratory difficulty.	
Tuberculosis	*Mycobacterium tuberculosis*	4–12 weeks from infection to primary lesion	As long as infectious tubercle bacilli are discharged in sputum	Airborne and droplet spread from sputum of infected persons	Any symptomatic or nonspecific symptoms such as fatigue, weakness, anorexia, weight loss, night sweats, low-grade fever, cough.	Daily doses of isoniazid, ethambutol, or rifampin for 8–9 mo.

| Typhoid Fever | *Salmonella typhi* | 7–21 days | Until typhoid bacilli no longer appear in excreta; can be as long as 3 mo after onset of symptoms | Ingestion of food or water contaminated by feces or urine of patient or carrier. | Chills, fever, headache, backache, anorexia, diarrhea, or constipation, epistaxis, generalized aching, frequently bronchitis. Rose-colored raised rash that appears in crops on about the 7th day on the abdomen, chest and back. | Antibiotics |

period, modes of transfer, symptoms, and treatment for selected communicable and infectious diseases.

Foodborne Illnesses

Foodborne illnesses, food poisoning, foodborne intoxication, and foodborne infections are common terms applied to illnesses acquired through consumption of contaminated food or water. Tables 9-7 through 9-11 describe foodborne illnesses caused by bacteria, toxin-producing bacteria, parasites, viruses, and toxins from shellfish and fish. These tables include the mode of action, incubation period, symptoms, transmission, and the communicability of these foodborne illnesses.

Common Exanthems

Exanthems are skin eruptions or rashes that occur as a symptom of acute viral or coccal disease, or sensitivities related to some medications. Table 9-12 describes common exanthems and includes causative agent, incubation period, period of communicability, signs/symptoms, site, character, and onset/duration.

Reportable Communicable Diseases

The first step in the control of communicable disease is its rapid identification, followed by notification to the local health authority that the disease exists within a specific jurisdiction. State and county administrative practices on diseases to be reported may vary because of different conditions and disease frequencies. Health department personnel are also available to conduct epidemiologic investigations. Reportable disease information contributes to county, state, and national analysis of epidemiologic trends.

- Diseases are to be reported to local health authorities by mail, telephone, or telegraph. Along with the disease or suspected disease and the means of exposure if known, such reports should include the client's name, address, age, race, and sex. The list of reportable diseases varies from state to state, but usually includes those listed in Table 9-13.

Text continued on page 441

TABLE 9-7. FOODBORNE ILLNESSES CAUSED BY BACTERIA

DISEASE	MODE OF ACTION	INCUBATION PERIOD	SYMPTOMS	SOURCE	TRANSMISSION	COMMUNICABILITY
Campylobacter	Bacterial infection	3–5 days range of 1–10 days	Diarrhea, abdominal pain, fever, nausea, vomiting, malaise, may last 1–10 days	Animals (cattle, dogs, sheep, rodents, birds, poultry)	Contaminated food, ingestion, cross contamination of uncooked foods, unpasteurized milk, water, contact with infected animals, people.	Person-to-person
Salmonellosis	Bacterial infection and/or enterotoxin	6–72 hr, usually 12–35 hr	Sudden onset of abdominal pain, diarrhea is more frequent than vomiting, fever, lasts longer than 24 hr.	Humans, domestic and wild animals, raw meat and poultry products, eggs. Animal feeds and fertilizers prepared from meat, meal, bones.	Meat, poultry, eggs, pies, lightly cooked food, unpasteurized milk, surfaces contaminated by raw foods, rodents, man.	Communicable from person-to-person by fecal-oral route.

Table continued on following page

TABLE 9–7. FOODBORNE ILLNESSES CAUSED BY BACTERIA *Continued*

DISEASE	MODE OF ACTION	INCUBATION PERIOD	SYMPTOMS	SOURCE	TRANSMISSION	COMMUNICABILITY
Shigellosis	Bacterial infection	1–7 days, median 1–3 days	Abdominal cramps, diarrhea, fever, vomiting; blood, pus, or mucus in stools.	Infected food handlers especially handling liquids or moist foods that require no further cooking. Found in milk, dairy products.	Direct or indirect fecal-oral transmission.	Person-to-person.
Vibrio parahaemolyticus	Bacterial infection	15–24 hours	Abdominal pain, nausea, vomiting, diarrhea.	Shellfish, saltwater fish.	Inadequately cooked fish, shellfish, especially shrimp.	Not communicable from person-to-person

Yersinia enterocolitica	Bacterial infection	3–7 days, generally under 10 days	Acute watery diarrhea, fever, headache, nausea, malaise, mimics flu. Sometimes fever, headache, chills and blood mucous diarrhea lasts 1–2 days.	Raw vegetables, meats, water, and unpasteurized milk.	Fecal-oral transmission and drinking/eating fecally contaminated foods and water. Isolated from raw milk, ice cream, mussels, oyster. Person-to-person as well as contaminated food.

From Communicable Diseases Control Manual, San Mateo County Department of Health Service. San Mateo, CA, 1991. Reprinted with permission.

TABLE 9–8. FOODBORNE ILLNESSES CAUSED BY TOXIN-PRODUCING BACTERIA

DISEASE	MODE OF ACTION	INCUBATION PERIOD	SYMPTOMS	SOURCE	TRANSMISSION	COMMUNICABILITY
Staphylococcal poisoning (*S. aureus*)	Heat stable enterotoxin	1–6 hr, usually 2–4 hr	Violent, abrupt onset of nausea, vomiting, cramps, prostration and sometimes diarrhea. Subnormal temperature and blood pressure. Duration of illness is 12–72 hr.	Human skin and nasal carriers. Bovine origin in milk outbreaks.	Pastries, custards, salads, sliced meats, improperly stored foods.	Person-to-food-to-person. Not person-to-person.
Bacillus cereus	Bacterial infection, heat labile or heat stable enterotoxin.	1–6 hr vomiting, 6–16 hr diarrhea.	Nausea and vomiting or abdominal pain and diarrhea. Duration 24 hr.	Organism found in soil, raw, dried and processed foods.	Food kept at room temperature. Rice, vegetables, meat dishes.	Not communicable person-to-person.
Clostridium perfringens (*C. welchii*)	Bacterial infection and/or heat	6–24 hr, usually 10–12	Sudden onset of abdominal colic followed by	Human, cattle, pigs, vermin, soil.	Stews, meat pies, reheated meats and gravies.	Not communicable person-to-person.

	labile enterotoxin.	hr.	diarrhea. Nausea occurs but vomiting is rare. Duration is less than 24 hr.		Occasionally fresh meat.	Not communicable person-to-person.
Streptococcus	Heat stable toxin	2–18 hr	Nausea, sometimes vomiting, colic and diarrhea. Rapid recovery.	Food products contaminated by insects, animal, or human excreta. Nasal carriers.	Improperly cooked or stored foods, salads, sliced meats.	Not communicable person-to-person.
Botulism (*Clostridium botulinum*)	Heat labile toxin	12–36 hr, up to several days.	Weakness, dizziness, headache, constipation, double vision, cranial and motor nerve paralysis. Respiratory failure.	Soil, intestinal tract of animals and fish.	Ingestion of food containing performed toxin due to improperly home-canned foods, or improperly processed commercial foods.	Not communicable from person-to-person.

From Communicable Diseases Control Manual, San Mateo County Department of Health Service. San Mateo, CA, 1991. Reprinted with permission.

TABLE 9–9. FOODBORNE ILLNESSES CAUSED BY TOXINS FROM SHELLFISH AND FISH

DISEASE	MODE OF ACTION	INCUBATION PERIOD	SYMPTOMS	SOURCE	TRANSMISSION	COMMUNICABILITY
Shellfish intoxication (paralytic shellfish poisoning)	Heat stable toxin (generally).	Minutes to hours.	Prickly feeling in lips, tongue, finger tips immediately after eating, followed by ataxia, paralysis.	Gonyaulax catanella, a plankton abundant between May through October (mussel quarantine period.)	Mussels and possibly other shellfish that are plankton feeders.	Not communicable from person-to-person.
Ciguatera poisoning	Heat stable toxin.	3–5 hr	Tingling, numbness of mouth; abdominal cramps; nausea, vomiting, diarrhea (6–8 hr).	Numerous varieties of tropical fish. Example: Barracuda.	Ingestion of tropical reef fishes especially gonads, intestines, roe. Older fish are more toxic.	Not communicable from person-to-person.

			headache, myalgia, dizziness, blurred vision, paralysis. Sensitory phenomenon may persist for months.		
Scromboid poisoning (histamine like)	Bacterial decomposition after fish is caught will release toxin.	Few minutes to 1 hr.	Headache, dizziness, nausea, vomiting, peppery taste, burning throat, facial swelling, flushing, urticaria, epigastric pain.	Mackerel, tuna, mahimahi, Pacific dolphin, bonito, albacore.	Consumption of mackerel, tuna, etc. that are not promptly refrigerated.	Not communicable from person-to-person.

From Communicable Diseases Control Manual, San Mateo County Department of Health Service. San Mateo, CA, 1991. Reprinted with permission.

TABLE 9–10. FOODBORNE ILLNESSES CAUSED BY PARASITES

DISEASE	MODE OF ACTION	INCUBA-TION PERIOD	SYMPTOMS	SOURCE	TRANS-MISSION	COMMUNI-CABILITY
Anisakiasis (larval nematodes)	After fish are caught, larvae move out of internal organs into fish muscles.	Few hours (stomach involvement) few days to weeks (intestinal involvement).	Abdominal cramps, vomiting. Epigastric pain, sometimes hematemesis. Occasional migration of worm upward to be coughed up.	Uncooked salt-water fish or squid (sushi).	Consumption of fish infected with larvae especially uncooked, cooked less than 140° or stored at −4°F for less than 60 hr.	Not communicable from person-to-person
Giardiasis	Protozoan infection	5–25 days (or longer) median 7–10 days.	May be asymptomatic, diarrhea, steatorrhea, abdominal cramps, bloating, fatigue, weight loss, anemia.	Infected individuals, contaminated water.	Fecal-oral ingestion of cysts in fecally contaminated water.	Communicable from person-to-person.

From Communicable Diseases Control Manual, San Mateo County Department of Health Service. San Mateo CA, 1991. Reprinted with permission.

TABLE 9–11. FOODBORNE ILLNESSES CAUSED BY VIRUSES

DISEASE	MODE OF ACTION	INCUBATION PERIOD	SYMPTOMS	SOURCE	TRANSMISSION	COMMUNICABILITY
Gastroenteritis due to enteroviruses, rotaviruses, paroviruses	Viral infection	24–48 hr	Severe diarrhea, nausea, vomiting, malaise, may last 1–10 days.	Viral shedding from individuals.	Fecal-oral, fecal-respiratory.	Communicable from person-to-person.

From Communicable Diseases Control Manual, San Mateo County Department of Health Service. San Mateo CA, 1991. Reprinted with permission.

TABLE 9-12. DIFFERENTIAL DIAGNOSIS OF COMMON EXANTHEMS (Skin rashes)

CONDITION/ AGENT	INCUBA-TION PERIOD	PERIOD OF COMMUNI-CABILITY	SIGNS/ SYMPTOMS	SITE	ERUPTION/ CHARACTER	ONSET/ DURATION
Chicken pox (varicella) Varicella zoster virus	14–21 days	One day before onset of symptoms until all crops of vesicles have crusted over.	Moderate fever, chills, headache, malaise, occasional sore throat	Usually first on trunk, later on face, neck, extremities; infrequently on palms and soles	Lesions discrete; progress from macule-papule to vesicle to crusting; appear in crops; so various stages develop simultaneously	Shortly after onset of symptoms; last a few days to 2 weeks.
Drug rash	History of drug use.	None	Variable, including fever, generalized; sometimes restrictive to exposed surface	Generalized; sometimes restrictive to exposed surface	May be morbilliform, scarlatiniform, erythematous, acneform, vesicular, bullous, purpuric or exfoliating.	Variable

	Incubation	Communicability	Symptoms	Rash location	Rash description	Rash timing
Erythema Infectiosum (Fifth disease) (Slapped Cheek) Parvovirus B19	5–10 days	Greatest before onset of rash. Not communicable after rash appears.	Low grade fever, occasional arthralgias	Starts on cheeks, spreads to arms, legs, trunk.	Maculopapular; often blotchy or reticular.	Shortly after onset of symptoms; lasts 5–10 days; may recur for several weeks.
Infectious mono-nucleosis Epstein-Barr virus	10–50 days	Undetermined.	Malaise, headache, fatigue, sore throat, splenomegaly, temperature fluctuations lymphadenopathy.	Most prominent over trunk.	Occurs in about 15% of cases as a morbilliform, scarlatiniform or vesicular rash.	Appears 5–14 days after onset of illness; lasts about 3 days.
Measles (rubeola) Measles virus	7–14 days	From 2–4 days before appearance of rash until 2–5 days after onset.	Fever, coryza, cough conjunctivitis, malaise photophobia, Koplik's spots, mild pruritus.	Starts around ears, on face, neck spreading over trunk, limbs; limbs escape in mild cases.	Maculopapular; brownish pink in color and irregularly confluent in severe cases, or petechial. Discrete in mild cases.	3–5 days after onset of symptoms; last 4–7 days.

Table continued on following page

TABLE 9–12. DIFFERENTIAL DIAGNOSIS OF COMMON EXANTHEMS (Skin rashes) *(Continued)*

CONDITION/ AGENT	INCUBATION PERIOD	PERIOD OF COMMUNICABILITY	SIGNS/ SYMPTOMS	SITE	ERUPTION/ CHARACTER	ONSET/ DURATION
Rosela infantum (Exanthem subitum) (Sixth disease) Human Herpes virus-6	5–15 days	Unknown.	Infants and preschool children affected. Characteristic disappearance of high fever upon appearance of rash.	Chest and abdomen with moderate involvement of face and extremities.	Either diffuse macular or maculopapular.	On about 4th day rash appears as temperature drops suddenly to normal; lasts 1–2 days.
Rubella (German measles) Rubella virus	14–21 days	Shortly before onset of symptoms until rash disappears; infected newborns are usually infective for many months.	Malaise, fever, headache, rhinitis, postauricular and suboccipital lymphadnopathy with tender nodes.	Face, neck and spreading to trunk and limbs.	Fine pinkish macules which become confluent and often scarlatiniform or pin point in third day.	1–2 days after onset of symptoms; lasts about 1–3 days.

Disease					
Scarlet fever Group A hemolytic streptococci	3–5 days. Occasionally slightly shorter or longer.	Usually 24 hr before onset of symptoms, until 2–3 weeks thereafter, or even longer if complicated by sinusitis, otitis media.	Sore throat, chills, fever, headache, vomiting, strawberry tongue; cervical lymphadenopathy; circumoral pallor, rapid pulse.	Face, neck, chest, abdomen, spreading to extremities. Entire body surface may be involved.	Diffuse pinkish-red flush of skin, blanching on pressure.	On 2nd day; lasts 4–10 days.

From Communicable Diseases Control Manual, San Mateo County Department of Health Service. San Mateo CA, 1991. Reprinted with permission.

TABLE 9–13. REPORTABLE COMMUNICABLE DISEASES

Acquired Immune Deficiency Syndrome (AIDS)
Amebiasis
Anthrax
Botulism (infant, foodborne, wound)
Brucellosis
Campylobacteriosis
Chancroid
Chlamydial infection (*C. trachomatis*)
Cholera
Coccidioidomycosis
Conjunctivitis (acute infection of the newborn, specify etiology)
Cryptosporidiosis
Cysticercosis
Dengue
Diarrhea of the newborn, outbreaks
Diphtheria
Encephalitis: viral, bacterial, fungal, parasitic (specify etiology)
Foodborne illness (food poisoning)
Giardiasis
Gonococcal infections
Granuloma inguinale
Hemophilus influenzae, invasive disease
Hepatitis A
Hepatitis B, cases and carriers (specify)
Hepatitis C
Hepatitis Delta (D)
Hepatitis, unspecified
Kawasaki syndrome (mucocutaneous lymph node syndrome)
Legionellosis
Leprosy (Hansen's disease)
Leptospirosis
Listeriosis
Lyme Disease
Lymphogranuloma venereum
Malaria
Measles (rubeola)
Meningitis: viral, bacterial, fungal, parasitic (specify etiology)
Meningococcal infections
Mumps
Non-gonococcal urethritis (excluding laboratory confirmed chlamydial infections)
Pelvic Inflammatory Disease (PID)
Pertussis (whooping cough)
Plague
Poliomyelitis, paralytic
Psittacosis
Q Fever
Rabies, human and animal
Relapsing fever
Reye syndrome
Rheumatic fever, acute
Rocky Mountain spotted fever
Rubella (German measles)
Salmonellosis (other than typhoid fever)
Shigellosis
Streptococcal infections (outbreaks and cases in food handlers and dairy workers only)
Syphilis
Tetanus
Toxic shock syndrome
Trichinosis
Tuberculosis
Tularemia
Typhoid fever, cases and carriers
Typhus fever
Yellow fever

- For more information or help with infectious diseases, contact your state or local health department. If in a health care facility, contact the infection control practitioner.

- The Center for Disease Control (CDC) recommends that every health care institution subscribe to or have access to *Morbidity and Mortality Weekly Report* (MMWR), a publication that reports on current trends in communicable diseases. Subscriptions are available through the National Technical Information Service, 5285 Port Royal Road, Springfield, VA 22161 (702) 487-4650.

Acquired Immunodeficiency Syndrome

Although more is known about AIDS than when it was first discovered in the mid 1980s, a cure is not available at this time. Worldwide, scientists are diligently working toward this goal.

In January 1993, the Centers for Disease Control (CDC) published the expanded AIDS case definition. This means that individuals who are *HIV infected* are counted as persons with AIDS if they have one of the opportunistic infections or cancers listed in Table 9-14, or if they have any of the following:

- T4 cell count of less than 200

- The percent T4 is less than 14

- More than one bout of pneumonia in a 12-mo period (not PCP)

- Cervical cancer

- Pulmonary tuberculosis

The reason for this new definition is to have a better idea of the number of HIV-infected persons in the United States. It is not meant to have any clinical or prognostic implications. One major benefit to a community in having a more accurate account of HIV-infected persons would be for planning for service needs. In addition, state and federal funding levels are often based on actual case numbers.

TABLE 9–14. LIST OF CONDITIONS IN THE 1993 AIDS SURVEILLANCE CASE DEFINITION

More than a dozen opportunistic infections and several cancers are considered to be sufficiently specific indicators of the underlying immunodeficiency to be included in the case definition of AIDS.

Candidiasis of bronchi, trachea, or lungs
Candidiasis, esophageal
Cervical cancer, invasive*
Coccidioidomycosis, disseminated or extrapulmonary
Cryptococcosis, extrapulmonary
Cryptosporidiosis, chronic intestinal (> 1 mo duration)
Cytomegalovirus disease (other than liver, spleen, or nodes)
Cytomegalovirus retinitis (with loss of vision)
HIV encephalopathy
Herpes simplex: chronic ulcer(s) (> 1 mo duration); or bronchitis, pneumonitis, or esophagitis
Histoplasmosis, disseminated or extrapulmonary
Isosporiasis, chronic intestinal (> 1 mo duration)
Kaposi's sarcoma
Lymphoma, Burkitt's (or equivalent term)
Lymphoma, immunoblastic (or equivalent term)
Lymphoma, primary in brain
Mycobacterium avium complex or *M. kansasii,* disseminated or extrapulmonary
Mycobacterium tuberculosis, any site (pulmonary* or extrapulmonary)
Mycobacterium, other species or unidentified species, disseminated or extrapulmonary
Pneumocystis carinii pneumonia
Progressive multifocal leukoencephalopathy
Salmonella septicemia, recurrent
Toxoplasmosis of brain
Wasting syndrome due to HIV

*Added in 1993 expansion of the AIDS surveillance case definition.

- See also Table 9-15 for other prevalent sexually transmitted diseases and the National Association hotline telephone numbers.

- Table 9-6 lists clinical information about AIDS.

- Public education is critically important in abating fears associated with AIDS. Nurses should be actively

TABLE 9–15. SEXUALLY TRANSMITTED DISEASES

Acquired Immunodeficiency Syndrome (AIDS)	Herpes
Amebiasis	Lambliasis
Balantis	Lymphogranuloma venereum
Candidiasis	Molloscum contagiosum
Chancroid	Nongonoccal urethritis
Chlamydia trachomatis infection	Pediculosis
Condyloma acuminatum (genital warts)	Proctitis (multiple causes)
Corynebacterium vaginale	Reiter's syndrome
Cytomegalovirus	Salmonellosis
Donovanosis	Scabies
Gardnerella vaginalis vaginitis	Shigellosis
Giardiasis	Syphilis
Gonorrhea	Trichomoniasis
Granuloma inguinale	
Hemophilus vaginitis	
Hepatitis	

engaged in helping to educate the public. The following organizations can offer information and referral services on AIDS and related issues:

- Public Health Service AIDS Hotline 800-342-2437

- San Francisco AIDS Foundation Hotline 800-367-2437

Sexually Transmitted Diseases

Sexually transmitted diseases are among the most prevalent infections worldwide. Gonorrhea is now reaching epidemic proportions in the United States, as is Acquired Immune Deficiency Syndrome (AIDS).

The following organizations offer information and referral services on sexually transmitted diseases:

- National AIDS Hotline, 800-342-2437

- National Herpes Hotline, 919-361-8488

- National Sexually Transmitted Diseases Hotline/American Social Health Association, 800-227-8922

Tuberculosis

Tuberculosis was thought to be nearly eradicated in the United States. Recently the disease has become more prevalent in the United States for a variety of reasons, including changing demographics, decreased access to medical and public health care systems, and an increase of people with weakened immune systems. The usual infectious agent of tuberculosis is *Mycobacterium tuberculosis*. Tuberculosis is a curable disease in the vast majority of cases, if symptoms are recognized and medical treatment is instituted in a timely manner.

Tuberculosis is transmitted via airborne droplets containing the tubercle bacilli when a contagious person coughs and a susceptible person inhales the droplets. The likelihood of inhaling these infectious droplets increases in enclosed, crowded, or poorly ventilated living areas. Once inhaled, the bacilli travel to the air sacs of the lungs and multiply, causing infection to begin. Tuberculosis infections involving the lungs are the most common and the most communicable. Laryngeal tuberculosis is also communicable. Extrapulmonary tuberculosis, that is, tuberculosis involving other organs, is generally not communicable.

Most people with latent tuberculosis infection remain entirely well, have no manifestations of active tuberculosis disease during their life span, and are not infectious to other people. The tuberculosis infection can usually be recognized in such people by a positive (redness and induration >10 mm) reaction to the tuberculin skin test, an intradermal injection of mycobacterial protein.

Symptoms of active pulmonary tuberculosis disease include fatigue, fever, night sweats, weight loss, cough, chest pain, hemoptysis, and hoarseness. Antituberculosis therapy can be used to eradicate active disease.

Risk Reductions for Community and Health Care Settings

Specific actions to reduce the risk of tuberculosis transmission in the community and health care setting should include:

- Screen clients for active tuberculosis and tuberculous infection

- Provide rapid diagnostic services

- Prescribe appropriate curative and preventive therapy
- Maintain physical measures to reduce microbial contamination of the air
- Screen healthcare facility personnel for tuberculosis infection and tuberculosis
- Prompt investigation and control of outbreaks

  Additional recommendations applicable to all healthcare settings:

- Early identification and preventive treatment of the client with tuberculous infection at high risk for active tuberculosis
- Early identification and treatment of the client with active tuberculosis
- Potential supplemental environmental approaches
  - High-efficiency filtration
  - Germicidal UV irradiation
  - Disposable particulate respirator masks for filtration of exhaled air
- Procedure-specific precautions
  - Diagnostic sputum induction
  - Bronchoscopy
- Decontamination: cleaning, disinfecting, and sterilization
- Documentation of surveillance of tuberculosis transmission
  - Routine skin testing
  - Evaluation of health care personnel after unprotected exposure or with positive PPD test
  - Work restrictions

TERMS ASSOCIATED WITH TUBERCULOSIS

Acid-fast Bacilli (AFB)   Bacteria that retain certain dyes even when washed with an acid solution.

TERMS ASSOCIATED WITH TUBERCULOSIS *Continued*

	Usually AFB are mycobacteria. A presumptive diagnosis of TB is often made on the basis of a positive "AFB smear"; the diagnosis is not confirmed until a culture is grown and identified as *M. tuberculosis.*
Anergic	The state of being immunologically suppressed and therefore unable to produce a tuberculin skin test reaction, even though infected with tubercle bacilli.
Disseminated (miliary) TB	When large numbers of tubercle bacilli have been spread through the bloodstream to many parts of the body. Miliary refers also to the appearance of the chest film in disseminated tuberculosis (looks like scattered millet seeds).
Extrapulmonary	Tuberculosis outside the lungs. In the U.S. about 15% of reported cases involve extrapulmonary sites, such as kidney, pleura, lymph nodes, etc.
High-risk Medical Procedures	Procedures that induce cough or sputum production and cause a potential to spread droplet nuclei, e.g., bronchoscopy, sputum induction.
Lymph Nodes	Small nodules of specialized immune cells located throughout the body (also called lymph glands or glands).
Mantoux Tubercullin Skin Test	The most reliable and best standardized technique for tuberculin testing, given by injecting 0.1 ml of PPD-tuberculin into the superficial layers of the skin (usually the forearm) with a needle and syringe.
Mycobacterial	The genus to which *Mycobacterium tuberculosis* and all other mycobacteria (e.g., *M. avium* complex, *M. kansasii*) belong.
Mycobacterium Tuberculosis	The bacterium that causes TB—often abbreviated *M. tuberculosis.*
Particulate Respirator Device	A particulate respirator face mask that is designed to filter out particles 1–4 microns in diameter.

TERMS ASSOCIATED WITH TUBERCULOSIS *Continued*

Pulmonary	Referring to the lungs. Most tuberculosis cases in the United States (approximately 85%) are pulmonary.
Tubercle Bacilli	Often used to refer to *Mycobacterium tuberculosis* (and to *Mycobacterium bovis*).
Ultraviolet Light	A form of radiation between visible light and x-ray that is effective in killing many bacteria including tubercle bacilli.

REFERENCES

Benenson A. Control of communicable diseases in man. American Public Health Association, 1990.

Castle M. Hospital infection control: principles and practice. New York: John Wiley & Sons, 1980.

Centers for Disease Control and Prevention. Guidelines for preventing the transmission of tuberculosis in health care settings, with special focus on HIV-related issues. MMWR December 7, 1990; 39:RR17.

Centers for Disease Control and Prevention. Draft guidelines for preventing the transmission of tuberculosis in health care facilities, second edition. *Federal Register* 1993; 58[195]: 52810–52854.

Centers for Disease Control and Prevention. Revised classification system for HIV infection and expanded surveillance case definition for AIDS among adolescents and adults. MMWR December 18, 1992; 41:RR-17.

Department of Labor, Occupational Safety and Health Administration. OSHA bloodborne pathogen standard code of federal regulations, Title 29. CFR Part 1910. December 6, 1991.

Hoeprich PD, Jordan MC (eds). Infectious diseases, 4th ed. Philadelphia: JB Lippincott, 1989.

Hopkins C. AIDS-implementation of universal precautions and body fluid precautions. Infectious diseases clinics of North America Vol. 3, No. 4. December 1989; pp. 747–762.

Immunizations required for child care center entry. California Administrative Code, Title 17, Sections 6000–6075.

Jackson M, Lynch P. An attempt to make an issue less murky: a comparison of four systems for infection prevention. Infection Control and Hospital Epidemiology Vol. 12, No. 7. July 1991; pp. 448–450.

San Mateo County Department of Health Service, Communicable Diseases Control Manual. San Mateo, CA, 1991.

State of California Department of Health Services, Infectious Diseases Branch, Immunization Unit, Berkeley, CA, December 1990.

Williams W et al. Vaccines of importance in the hospital setting: problems and developments. Infectious disease clinics of North America, Vol. 3, No. 4. December 1989; pp. 701–722.

THE CLIENT UNDERGOING SURGERY

The concept of the client having surgery in the hospital has changed. The trend in health care continues to be away from inpatient and toward more outpatient surgery. More outpatient surgery places additional responsibility on the nurse. The nurse must be able to quickly assess the client for complications and client teaching must be of the highest caliber. Additionally, inpatient postoperative stays have been shortened to the point that many clients remain in the hospital for 24–72 hours.

Surgery may be done for diagnostic, curative, palliative, or cosmetic reasons. The role of the nurse is all-encompassing. Nursing is responsible for the client preoperatively, maintaining surveillance of the client during surgery, and monitoring and preventing complications postoperatively. In many settings, postoperative care is being provided by specially trained home care nurses.

10-1 PREOPERATIVE PREPARATION

The role of the nurse in preoperative preparation is key. Many times the nurse is the first person to identify client issues and concerns. With the advent of outpatient surgery, the nurse may be implementing preoperative teaching several days prior to surgery. It is not uncommon to find the nurse performing a preoperative assessment and client teaching on the telephone the night prior to surgery. Key areas to focus on for preoperative preparation:

- Assess the client for the following:

    - Understanding of the surgical procedure, anesthesia, and hospitalization (if hospitalization is anticipated)

    - The client's responsibilities preoperatively

    - Client's response to stress

    - Knowledge of postoperative status

    - Areas of concern

- Perform a baseline nursing assessment to evaluate client risk factors and notify the physician if appropriate. Assess for:

  - A history of chronic illness (e.g., diabetes, COPD, cardiac disease)

  - Presence of cold, sore throat, or an acute illness in the last 7 days

  - Review of client medications, especially steroids, insulin, oral hypoglycemics, aspirin, and anti-inflammatories (Table 10-1).

- If preoperative labwork, EKG or chest x-rays are ordered, review the results and notify the physician if abnormalities exist. If ordered tests are not available on the chart, obtain a telephone report or request a fax. Notify the surgical team of missing lab results prior to surgery.

- Review the chart for the presence of a correctly completed consent form(s). Many states have regulatory requirements concerning the nature of the consent and the type of consents required for surgery. The nurse may be requested to obtain the signed consent. It is the responsibility of the physician to explain the risks and benefits of surgery. The nurse may be responsible for obtaining the actual signature of the client or legally responsible person.

- The following criteria should be met prior to a client or designee signing the consent form:

  - The client/designee is mentally competent and unaffected by drugs that could alter thinking.

  - The client/designee understands the nature of the surgery and inherent benefits/risks.

  - The client/designee does not feel pressured into consenting to surgery but does so willingly.

- If there are questions the nurse does not feel comfortable clarifying or the nurse questions the client's understanding of the procedure or risks involved, the client/designee should delay signing the consent form and the nurse must notify the physician and operating room (OR) immediately.

TABLE 10–1. SURGICAL RISK FACTORS AND POTENTIAL COMPLICATION

Nurse and physician should identify the following risk factors and anticipate potential complications.

	INCREASED LIKELIHOOD OF
Advancing Age	Multiple organ degenerative diseases
	Dehydration
	Sensitivity to central nervous system, depressants, analgesics, anesthetics (reduced dosages and careful monitoring are required)
Obesity	Prolonged surgery due to inaccessibility of surgical site
	Wound infection, dehiscence, and/or incisional herniation
	Delayed recovery from anesthesia due to increased absorption by adipose tissue
Nutritional Deficiencies	Delayed healing (especially if proteins and vitamins C and B complex are low).
Impaired Respiratory Status	Pulmonary obstruction
	Pneumonia (surgery should be delayed if client has an upper respiratory tract infection)
Impaired Cardiovascular Status	Myocardial infarction
	Thromboembolism
	Hemorrhage
	Fluid and electrolyte imbalances
Renal Impairment	Urinary infection
	Fluid and electrolyte imbalances
	Toxicity
Liver Damage	Bleeding tendencies
	Poor wound healing
	Infection
Diabetes	Infection
	Hypoglycemia or hyperglycemia (insulin-dependent clients are usually placed on sliding scale)
	Thromboembolism
Medication Use	Incompatibility of medications with anesthetic agents (steroids, tranquilizers, antibiotics)
	Increased bleeding (anticoagulants)
	Potassium deficiency (diuretics)
	Hypotension, shock (antihypertensives)

- Prior to surgery, discuss the client's NPO status, the need to discuss with the MD which daily medications should be discontinued, and any preoperative preps. On the day of surgery, review or initiate preoperative teaching as shown in Table 10-2. Answer any questions that the client or family/significant others may have. Review the preoperative teaching outline and provide written/audio visual material as available. Document content of preoperative teaching and the client's/significant others' understanding of the material presented.

- Complete the necessary preoperative checklists and forms as shown in Table 10-3. Do not leave areas blank. If information is unavailable, state this. If the client is unable to provide information, identify who is providing the client's medical history.

- Review discharge planning and special client needs, especially if the client will be released the same day or within 24 hr.

- On the day of surgery, administer ordered preoperative medications and perform required surgical preps.

10-2 POSTOPERATIVE CARE

Routinely, the postoperative client is observed in a post-anesthesia care unit (PACU) until vital signs are stable and the client is responsive. With local anesthesia or some minor procedures, the client may be recovered by the OR nurse or preoperative nurse in a special discharge unit.

After leaving the PACU, the client will either be released to home or transferred to a nursing unit. The emphasis of this section is on nursing unit-based care though several frequently occurring outpatient surgeries will be discussed.

The focus of postoperative surgical nursing is *monitoring and anticipation/prevention* of complications. Sound nursing judgment is based on knowledge of the symptoms of complications commonly associated with surgery in general as well as the particular type of surgery the client has undergone.

TABLE 10–2. OUTLINE FOR PREOPERATIVE TEACHING

1. **About surgery and anesthesia**
   - ☐ Nature and duration of surgery
   - ☐ Type of anesthesia
   - ☐ Time surgery scheduled

2. **What to expect the day before surgery**
   - ☐ Skin prep
   - ☐ Enemas
   - ☐ NPO after midnight
   - ☐ Bedtime sedation
   - ☐ Diagnostic measures (e.g., blood drawn, ECG)

3. **What to expect the day of surgery**
   - ☐ Hygienic measures
   - ☐ Removal of dentures, cosmetics, etc.
   - ☐ Hospital attire
   - ☐ Care of possessions
   - ☐ Insertion of tubes (e.g., nasogastric, urinary)
   - ☐ Preoperative medications
   - ☐ Time to go to surgery
   - ☐ When family can visit
   - ☐ Where family can wait during surgery

4. **What to expect after surgery**
   - ☐ PACU stay (and intensive care unit if necessary)
   - ☐ Availability of analgesic
   - ☐ Equipment in use postoperatively (e.g., IV, oxygen, tubes and catheters, elastic stockings)

5. **Postoperative preventive techniques** (see Table 10-6)
   - ☐ Deep breathing and coughing techniques
   - ☐ Incisional splinting
   - ☐ Leg exercises
   - ☐ Turning in bed, getting out of bed, ambulating

TABLE 10–3. PREOPERATIVE CHECKLIST: THE DAY OF SURGERY

Client Preparation

☐ Morning care completed

☐ All nail polish, cosmetics, hairpins removed

☐ Dentures, prostheses, wigs, contact lenses removed

☐ Hospital gown in place (caps and boots required in some hospitals)

☐ All valuables taken by the family or locked in hospital safe. If client wishes to wear a wedding ring, it is secure with gauze or tape around the finger.

☐ Preoperative teaching reinforced. All client's questions answered.

The Client's Chart

☐ All orders and procedures have been completed and recorded in the client's chart.

☐ The consent form is signed and on the chart.

☐ Baseline assessment information including vitals and peripheral pulses is documented and on the chart.

☐ Pertinent laboratory data is current and on the chart.

On Call to Surgery

☐ Client is assisted in voiding (or catheterized if undergoing gynecologic procedure).

☐ Preoperative medications are given as ordered, either 30 to 60 min before prescribed time of surgery or "on call" when notified by the operating room.

☐ Client is instructed not to smoke or get out of bed.

☐ Side rails are raised.

I. Postoperative Assessment and Care
A. Assessment

- All institutions have standards for postoperative monitoring. Traditionally the client is monitored and vital signs are taken according to a predetermined schedule (e.g. q 15 min × 4, q 30 × 4, q 1 × 2, then every 4 hr). Frequency of vital signs is determined by the status of the client post PACU and the client's condition.

- **Respirations.** Notify the physician immediately if respiratory distress or abnormal breathing patterns exist. Signs of abnormal breathing patterns include: shallow, rapid breathing, snoring, stridor, wheezing, apprehension, restlessness or confusion. Listen for bilateral breath sounds and observe for tracheal deviation. Observe the chest for asymmetry, use of accessory muscles or unequal lung expansion. If a client is on a pulse oximeter and is unable to maintain his baseline oxygen level, administer oxygen and call the physician. In the event that a client experiences respiratory distress, prepare to institute emergency measures (oxygen, intubation, mechanical ventilation, medication).

- **Pulse.** Compare the preoperative and postoperative pulse values. Assess for the rate and quality of the pulse. The pulse may be slightly elevated, but should be within 10% of the client's preoperative values. Changes in the numerical value, or irregularities in the "quality" of the pulse should be reported. Correlate pulse rate and quality with the overall client picture (output, blood pressure, mentation).

- **Blood Pressure.** Blood pressure is an indirect measure of cardiac output. Compare the postoperative values with the preoperative values. Fluid volume deficit/overload, anesthesia, hypothermia and pain can have an impact on the blood pressure. Watch for a postoperative drop of more than 15–20 mm Hg.

- **Temperature.** A client may return from the PACU slightly hypothermic. This is due to the cold OR environment and anesthesia. During the first 48 hr the client may experience a slight elevation in temperature (38°C/100.4°F) that usually reflects the surgical stress response. A temperature ele-

vation may also be caused by respiratory congestion, atelectasis, or less frequently by dehydration. After the first 48 hr, a moderate to marked
elevation in temperature (above 37.5–38°C) is
usually caused by an infection. Unless a client is
awake and alert, temperatures should be taken
using the axillary or tympanic route.

- Initiate a quick physical assessment. Notify the
physician if the client has not voided, experiences increased pain, abnormal respiration or
mental status changes. See Table 10-4 for other
areas to be reviewed.

- Monitor the client for postoperative complications. Notify the physician immediately if you
suspect a complication. Be prepared with observable data and current vital signs. See Table 10-5.

B. Early ambulation along with coughing and deep
breathing is the most significant nursing measure to
prevent postoperative complications. It is usually
ordered within hours of surgery but may be delayed one to two days with certain orthopedic
surgeries.

- To prevent syncope when the client ambulates,
raise the head of the bed and allow the client to
adjust to the increased head elevation. Take the
client's blood pressure. Then have the client dangle the legs. Orthostatic blood pressures should
be taken. If the blood pressure does not adjust to
the resting pressure, wait until it does. Question
the client for dizziness or lightheadedness.

- Once the blood pressure has equalized and the
client states he or she is comfortable, assist the
client to slowly stand by the bedside. This may
take two staff members depending on the client's
size, surgical procedure, ability to ambulate, and
hospital equipment.

- The client should be assisted to the chair or bathroom for the first 24 hr postoperatively (or
longer depending on the client's condition). If
the client feels faint, assist back to the chair or

Text continued on page 464

TABLE 10–4. NURSING ASSESSMENT AND CARE OF CLIENT ON POSTOPERATIVE ADMISSION TO THE CLINICAL UNIT

☐ Record time of client's return to the unit

☐ Take baseline vitals, compare with preoperative values

☐ Assess neurologic status
Level of consciousness
Orientation
Movement of extremities

☐ Assess wound, dressing, and drainage tubing
Type and amount of drainage
Connect tubing to gravity or suction drainage

☐ Assess color and appearance of skin

☐ Assess urinary status
Time of voiding
Presence or absence of urge to void
Bladder distention
Urinary output (report if <30 ml/hr)
Presence and patency of catheter

☐ Assess pain and discomfort

☐ Position for safety and comfort (usually on side with rails up with head of bed elevated 30–45 degrees)

☐ Intravenous infusion
Type of solution
Amount remaining
Flow rate
Appearance and location of IV site

☐ Attach call light within reach

☐ Place emesis basin and tissues within reach

☐ Check and carry out postoperative orders

☐ Determine emotional condition and support

TABLE 10–5. POSTOPERATIVE COMPLICATIONS

PROBLEM, SIGNS AND SYMPTOMS	PREVENTION	INTERVENTIONS
Shock Tachycardia, hypotension, thready pulse, diaphoresis, restlessness, anxiety, fever, cold, clammy skin, lip cyanosis *Hypovolemic:* visible bleeding, low hemoglobin and hematocrit, ringing in ears, seeing spots *Septic:* warm, flushed diaphoretic skin *Cardiogenic:* distended neck veins, chest pains *Neurogenic:* hypotension with slow pulse, warm extremities	Mentally and physically prepare the client. Have blood available. Measure any blood loss accurately. Minimize operative trauma. Monitor vital signs and assess client frequently. Prevent infection. Identify high-risk individuals.	• Keep airway open • Arrest hemorrhage using pressure control. Elevate legs. • Restore circulating blood volume—peripheral IVs, central venous pressure line, plasma expanders. • Begin blood transfusion when blood is available. • Obtain blood for lab—pH, PO_2, PCO_2, and hematocrit. • Insert urinary catheter to monitor hourly output. • Reassure the client even if you think you cannot be heard. • Keep client warm. • Administer ordered drugs—ionotropics, vasodilators, antimicrobials, corticosteroids. • Continue flow sheet, monitoring of vital signs, observations,

Table continued on following page

TABLE 10–5. POSTOPERATIVE COMPLICATIONS
Continued

PROBLEM, SIGNS AND SYMPTOMS	PREVENTION	INTERVENTIONS
		and interventions throughout impending shock.
Hemorrhage See "shock" above. Arterial bleeding— bright red and comes out in spurts. Venous bleeding—dark in color and bubbles out. Bleeding may also be internal.	See "shock" above.	• Treat the client for shock. • Inspect wound as possible site for bleeding— apply gauze pad pressure dressing. • Ice lavage for internal bleeding.
Pulmonary Complications Dyspnea, hyperpnea, rales, shallow, decreased, or noisy respirations, knifelike pain in the chest, unexplained rise in temperature	Report evidence of upper respiratory infection to surgeon. Position client on side or turn head to prevent aspiration of vomitus. Reinforce preoperative teaching about breathing exercises. Assist with early ambulation. Carefully monitor client's status and progress.	• Promote full aeration of lungs— turning, coughing, deep breathing, incentive spirometer. • Ambulate when possible. • Hydrate the client. • Initiate specific measures for particular pulmonary problems (e.g., cool mist for bronchitis, antibiotics for infections, etc.)
Pulmonary Embolism Symptoms vary according to size and location of embolism: sharp, stabbing pains in the	Prevent stasis of blood in the extremities due to dependent position of the legs, prolonged sitting, immobility,	• Restore cardiopulmonary function—oxygen by face mask with client in upright position, cardiac monitoring,

TABLE 10–5. POSTOPERATIVE COMPLICATIONS
Continued

PROBLEM, SIGNS AND SYMPTOMS	PREVENTION	INTERVENTIONS
chest, anxiety, cyanosis, dyspnea, rapid pulse, pallor, clinical shock. In some cases it may be manifested by a subtle deterioration in the client's condition with no explainable cause.	or restrictive clothing. Encourage high fluid intake. Insist on leg exercises and antiembolism stockings. Avoid leaving catheters (e.g., central venous pressure) in veins for long periods.	drugs to maintain blood pressure, treat for heart failure if present. • Anticoagulant therapy. • Reassure and quiet the client, administer morphine to control panic. • Surgical intervention may be necessary.
Deep-vein Thrombosis Pain or cramp in the calf, progressing to painful swelling of the whole leg. Slight fever, chills, perspiration. Marked tenderness over anteromedial surface of the thigh.	Hydrate the client. Insist on leg exercises and ambulation as soon as allowed by physician. Avoid any restrictive devices i.e., tight straps that would impair circulation. Low-dose heparin (5000 U SQ q 8–12 hr 2 hr preoperatively and 7 days postoperatively or until fully ambulatory, SCDs)	• Anticoagulant therapy, IV, IM or po. • Control pain, swelling, and venous stagnation by wrapping the legs from toes to groin with elastic bandage.
Intestinal Obstruction Sharp, colicky, abdominal pains with pain-free intervals.	Assess carefully for bowel sounds and passage of flatus. Identify high-	• Relieve abdominal distention by passing an NG suction tube. • Replace electro-

Table continued on following page

TABLE 10–5. POSTOPERATIVE COMPLICATIONS
Continued

PROBLEM, SIGNS AND SYMPTOMS	PREVENTION	INTERVENTIONS
As obstruction becomes complete, pain-free intervals become shorter, and there may be vomiting. No bowel movements unless obstruction is partial, then there may be diarrhea. Most commonly occurs on third to fifth postoperative day.	risk individuals: those with surgery on lower abdomen and pelvis. Inflammatory adhesions may cause intestines to kink.	lytes by IV tube. • Surgical intervention may be necessary.
Paralytic Ileus No bowel sounds. No passage of flatus or feces from the rectum. X-rays reveal a dilated bowel, with gas distributed throughout the digestive tract.	Assess carefully for bowel sounds and passage of flatus. Do not give fluids too soon.	• Nasogastric suction • IV fluids • Rectal tube to relieve flatus.
Wound Infection Local: induration (hardening of the area), redness, pain, drainage, foul smell. Systemic: elevated temp., pulse.	Strict asepsis in all aspects of care. Encourage optimal nutritional level. Prophylactic antibiotics if risk is high.	• Obtain cultures and send to laboratory. • Assist surgeon with stitch removal, wound irrigation, drain insertion. • Administer antibiotics as prescribed. • Warm, moist dressing may be prescribed.
Wound Dehiscence Client states something gave way in his wound. In an in-	Identify clients at risk: the elderly, those with weak or pendulous abdominal	• Stay with the client and have someone notify the surgeon immediately.

TABLE 10–5. POSTOPERATIVE COMPLICATIONS
Continued

PROBLEM, SIGNS AND SYMPTOMS	PREVENTION	INTERVENTIONS
testinal wound the edges of the wound part, and intestines push out.	walls, those with pulmonary or cardiac problems. Apply abdominal binder for clients at risk.	• If intestines are exposed, cover with sterile moist dressings. • Keep client on absolute bed rest. Instruct client to bend knees to relieve pressure on abdomen. • Reassure client, keep quiet and relaxed. • Prepare for surgical repair of wound.
Emotional/ Psychological Disturbances Insomnia, restlessness, agitation, delusions, hallucinations, bright and roving eyes, suicidal thoughts	Physically and emotionally prepare the client. Identify clients at risk: those with disturbances of body image, alcoholism, prior emotional disturbances, exhaustion.	• Carefully describe client behavior to physician. • Spend time with and support the client. • Administer tranquilizing medications as ordered. • Prevent harm to client or others—monitor frequently, restrain as last resort.

ease client to the floor. Assist the client back to bed with assistance once recovered.

C. **Monitor and assist in maintaining fluid and electrolyte balance.** Adequate fluid and electrolytes are essential to prevent cardiac irregularities and facilitate healing. See Chapter 5 for further information.

- Intake and output measurements are essential in the first 24–48 hr. Clients with foley catheters, IVs, feeding or gastric tubes require intake and output until the tubes are removed.

- During the first 24–48 hr the client may be third-spacing fluid. Careful observation of the difference between intake and output is important. After 48 hr the client usually begins to diurese and may experience a greater output than intake.

- Thirst is a sign of dehydration and may be annoying to the client. Good oral hygiene and adequate fluid replacement should assist in relieving the problem. Provide ice chips if ordered. Avoid lemon swabs since they may irritate the oral mucosa.

- The client with excess fluid loss may experience hypokalemia. Potassium should be monitored and replaced as needed. The dosage of potassium replacement is dependent on the client's medications, dietary intake, renal function, and serum potassium levels.

D. **Resuming oral intake**

- Generally the client may resume oral intake as soon as the gag reflex returns, although this depends on the nature of the surgery. Check the physician's orders for resumption of oral intake. With bowel surgery the client is usually kept NPO until bowel sounds are heard. Bowel sounds should be checked every shift and usually return within 24–48 hr.

- Intravenous fluids are usually discontinued when the client can tolerate and maintain an adequate intake.

- The client's diet is advanced from clear liquids to solids according to tolerance. See Section 8-5.

E. Elimination

- Fluids, bowel movements, and flatus should be recorded.

- If the client has resumed a full diet and a bowel movement has not occurred in 2–3 days, the physician may order a stool softener, suppository or an enema. Immobility, diet, and the administration of narcotics all may contribute to postoperative constipation.

F. Wound care

- The client's wound dressing should be assessed upon arrival from the PACU and frequently for the first few days postoperatively.

- The initial dressing should be reinforced and the physician notified if excessive drainage is occurring.

- Check the surgical record to see if a drain is present.

- Wounds with drains are expected to drain more than closed wounds.

- Document the type of wound dressing, the presence or absence of drainage, tubes, and drains and the color and consistency of drainage.

- Note the odor of the wound and the amount of drainage. See Section 10-4 for dressing change procedure, wound irrigation, and suture removal.

II. Postoperative discomforts

A. Nausea and vomiting are experienced by approximately 10–30% of the surgical population. Factors that contribute to nausea and vomiting include: anesthetic, age, sex, weight, type of surgical procedure, postoperative pain, and a history of motion sickness.

- Administer antiemetic as ordered.

- Administer pain medication as ordered.

- Position client on side or elevate the head of the bed 30–45 degrees as medically indicated. If the client begins to vomit, turn the client on side to prevent aspiration.

- Begin oral intake when nausea subsides. Early oral intake in the absence of bowel sounds may cause vomiting.

- Have suction equipment available for the client unable to expel vomitus.

B. Pain control. Pain is one of the greatest fears a client verbalizes.

- During the first 24–48 hr postoperatively, the client should be medicated according to a pain scale. See Section 2-3.

- Pain medication should be given prior to the onset of severe pain.

- The use of epidurals and PCA pumps assist in this effort. The nurse can also use alternative methods to assist the client in minimizing pain.

C. Urinary retention

- Most clients void within 6–8 hr of surgery.

- If the client has not voided within this time frame (or one specified by the physician), palpate and percuss the bladder for distention. Request an order to straight catheterize the client.

- The client must have a minimum of 30 ml/hr of urine to facilitate kidney function.

- Assess the urine for concentration, specific gravity and smell. Urine should be pale yellow in color and odorless. Certain surgeries or drugs may alter the color of urine.

D. Restlessness. May be caused by pain, bladder distension, abdominal distension, fear, anxiety, lack of oxygen, hemorrhage, or shock.

- The client may need pain medication or emergency interventions (in the case of shock, sepsis, emboli).

- Evaluate the client, their vital signs and observe for urinary output, bleeding, or mentation changes. If all the critical factors appear normal, pain medication, changing the bed linen, talking with the client, or giving a back massage may reduce restlessness.

III. Postoperative complications. The key to excellent surgical nursing is the detection and management of potential life-threatening complications. While the list below is not all-inclusive, it reviews several key life-threatening disorders that may affect any surgical client. (See Table 10-5 for a detailed list.)

 A. Atelectasis and pneumonia. To detect atelectasis or pneumonia, a comprehensive respiratory assessment must be done a minimum of once a shift. Thoracic surgical procedures require more frequent respiratory assessments since the risk of lung compromise is greater. Excellent pulmonary toilet (coughing and deep breathing, incentive spirometry and adequate fluid intake) can assist in preventing these disorders.

- Encourage coughing and deep breathing and incentive spirometry during waking hours (except in certain neurosurgical and ophthalmic surgery cases when it is contraindicated).

- Administer antibiotics and bronchodilators as ordered.

- Elevate the head of the bed if not medically contraindicated.

- Assist the client in turning at least every 2 hr. For the client who is unable to turn, special rotating beds may be helpful.

- Review laboratory data and x-rays.

- Notify physician of changes in the client's respiratory status.

- Administer oxygen as ordered.

- Suction the client as needed.

- Document findings reviewing breath sounds, respiratory rates, presence or absence of sputum, the use of accessory muscles, and skin color.

B. Pulmonary embolism and thrombophlebitis. Immobility and client positioning in surgery may predispose an individual to venous stasis. If a clot is formed in the vein it may break away and lodge in the lung tissue obstructing the flow of blood and decreasing oxygenation. Prevention is the key to decreasing the risk of thrombophlebitis and pulmonary embolism.

- Client at risk for phlebitis (previous history, selected surgical interventions, or a long time on the surgical table) should be preoperatively fitted with antiembolism hose and sequential compression devices (SCDs).

- Early ambulation and preventive administration of anticoagulants can decrease clot formation.

- Careful observation for the signs of embolism or thrombi formation are important.

    - The client with emboli may exhibit the following: chest pain, shortness of breath, rapid, shallow respirations, cyanosis, restlessness, rales over affected area, pink frothy sputum.

    - The client with phlebitis may exhibit leg pain, increase in temperature in the calf, reddened area of the leg. Homan's sign may be present.

- If the client experiences an emboli, it is an emergency. Notify the physician immediately. The following interventions are used to treat the client experiencing an emboli: oxygen therapy, analgesics, Heparin, elevation of the head of the bed, frequent blood gas analysis, radiographic analysis and emotional support. Continuous assessment of the client's clotting time is done to titrate the appropriate amount of Heparin.

- If the client experiences thrombophlebitis, careful assessment of his or her PT and PTT is done.

IV Heparin may be ordered to prevent clot formation. Warm compresses and elevation of the leg are usually ordered. Antiembolic hose or SCD machines should not be used on the affected leg, since they may assist in releasing a clot.

C. **Sepsis and septic shock.** A potentially life-threatening condition, sepsis and septic shock occur when there is an infection in the blood. Sepsis may be due to the type of surgical procedure, break in asepsis, client history of chronic illness, use of steroids or multiple antibiotics. Numerous lines, tubes and drains have also been implicated in sepsis.

- Monitoring changes in vital signs, urine output and mentation are key. Observe for a widening pulse pressure and client restlessness.

- Notify physician if sepsis is suspected. Usually wound and blood cultures will be ordered.

- Large amounts of fluids, antibiotics and oxygen will be ordered to maintain vital organs and fight infection.

- In the case of septic shock, the client is usually transferred to an intensive care unit where continuous monitoring can be provided.

D. **Wound infection and dehiscence and evisceration.** Wound infections are the most common surgical complication. Dehiscence occurs when the wound edges come apart. Evisceration is the complete opening of the wound with spillage of the abdominal contents. A history of taking steroids, obesity, break in asepsis and smoking predispose a client to dehiscence and evisceration.

- Observe the wound for its integrity and drainage. Document the amount, color, consistency and odor of drainage.

- Monitor vital signs, especially temperature. Since many wound infections occur 5–7 days post-surgery, the client may develop an infection after discharge. Excellent client education is required.

- Listen for client complaints of increasing pain, pulling, or bulging.

- Request an order to culture wound drainage if an infection is suspected.

- In the event of an evisceration, cover the abdominal contents with sterile soaked gauze pads, place the client in low Fowler's position and call the physician. Monitor vital signs and prepare the client for emergency surgery.

- Wound infections are typically treated with antibiotics, irrigations and frequent dressing changes.

- Document changes in wound status.

  E. **Hemorrhage.** Hemorrhage and loss of fluid volume usually occur with a break in suture or a missed unsutured blood vessel. The client will experience changes in vital signs, mental status, and/or decreased urine output. With internal bleeding observable blood may not be present on the dressing since the abdomen can hold a significant quantity of blood. Usually internal bleeding is signified by increasing pain, abdominal tenseness and changing vital signs.

- Monitor vital signs. Check for a rapid, weak pulse. The skin may be cool and clammy. Respirations will be rapid, shallow and weak. The urine output will have decreased or not be present.

- Typical interventions include: IV crystalloids to increase blood pressure and restore urine output, assessment of volume deficit and return to surgery for exploration. Supplemental oxygen is usually provided.

10-3 NURSING CARE IN SELECTED TYPES OF SURGERY

The field of invasive surgery has changed drastically in the last five years. Lasers and endoscopes have replaced many surgeries that required large incisions and prolonged recovery time. While the client may no longer require extensive hospitalization or wound management, monitoring for complications is still crucial. Excellent preoperative assessments and postoperative teaching is required since the client may no longer be hospitalized or spend a significant amount of time in the hospital.

Abdominal Surgery

The client having abdominal surgery is at risk for fluid and electrolyte imbalances. Careful monitoring of intake and output is important. Observe for signs of complications including: peritonitis, sepsis, paralytic ileus, and hemorrhage. If the client has an NG tube, careful oral hygiene is important. See Section 10-4 for procedure for nasogastric insertion, gastric decompression and irrigation. Bowel sounds and the presence of flatus should be assessed every shift. Diet is usually advanced when nausea and vomiting have decreased, bowel sounds are heard and the GI tract can tolerate fluids.

CHOLECYSTECTOMY

Cholecystectomy is the removal of the gallbladder. It is performed when stones impede bile flow and cause pain. It may be incisional or laparoscopic with laser.

Incisional Cholecystectomy

- If the client has a T-tube, facilitate drainage by making sure the drainage bag is flowing to gravity and the tube is patent. The tube may be clamped several days postoperatively to allow bile to travel to the intestine to assist with digestion. Asepsis is important when handling the bag or tube.

- Many times a penrose drain is inserted. Check the operative record for its presence.

- Assess the amount, color, and consistency of drainage.

- Careful skin care must be maintained around the tube site, since bile is highly caustic and will irritate the skin.

- If an NG tube is present, maintain NG to low suction.

- Monitor vital signs and watch for signs of abdominal pain, fever, or jaundice (indicating blockage).

- Encourage coughing and deep breathing (Table 10-6) since the incision is high and hypoventilation and atelectasis may occur.

- Discharge instructions may include T-tube management, avoidance of heavy lifting, signs and symptoms of biliary obstruction and infection, use of pain medication and follow up physician visits.

Laparoscopic Laser Cholecystectomy

- Usually 3–4 small stab wounds are present and may be sutured or closed with steri strips. The stab wounds are usually covered with bandages.

- Since carbon dioxide is used to inflate the abdomen for visualization, the client typically experiences shoulder pain that can be severe. Assist the client in repositioning (the semi-Fowler's position may help), and encourage ambulation.

- The client is usually discharged 1–2 days postoperatively and can return to work within 1 week.

- Discharge instructions may include care and management of stab wounds, avoidance of heavy lifting, signs and symptoms of infection, use of pain medication, and return physician appointment.

BOWEL SURGERY WITH AN OSTOMY

Ostomies may be permanent or temporary. Permanent colostomies or ileostomies usually follow surgery for a chronic illness such as Crohn's disease or when a malignancy is present. Temporary colostomies such as the loop or double barrel colostomy may be created to temporarily rest the intestines after trauma or diverticulitis. With temporary colostomies, after healing occurs, the bowel is reanastomosed and bowel function resumes. Common complications of ostomies include: fluid and electrolyte imbalance, sepsis, hemorrhage, and skin excoriation around the stoma site.

- Maintain accurate intake and output. Supplement fluid and electrolytes to maintain balance. Assess lab work on a daily or shift basis.

TABLE 10–6. POSTOPERATIVE PREVENTIVE TECHNIQUES

Teach these and have clients practice these preoperatively. Assist clients in performing these postoperatively.

DEEP BREATHING AND COUGHING

- Place client in a position similar to the one to be assumed after surgery (semi-Fowler's or on side, with head of bed elevated 30 to 40 degrees).
- The client inhales slowly and deeply through the nose, holding the breath for a couple of seconds, and then exhales slowly but completely through the mouth.
- The client's hands are placed lightly over the lower ribs and upper abdomen so the abdomen is felt rising during inspiration and falling during expiration.
- After four to six deep breaths, the client coughs deeply from the lungs rather than the throat.
- Deep breathing often stimulates the cough reflex. If there are secretions they are then moved up out of the respiratory passages and expectorated.
- The client with a thoracic or abdominal incision should splint it while deep breathing and coughing. This is done by holding the two sides of the incision with the hands to relieve the pressure on the wound, or by holding a pillow tightly over the incision to support it.
- Have clients do this exercise several times each hour during the immediate postoperative period.

LEG EXERCISES

- Any leg movements may be helpful but most important is that the client rhythmically contract and relax the calf (gastrocnemius) and thigh (quadriceps) muscles.
  - Have the client alternately flex and extend the ankle by pressing the feet against a footboard or the nurse's hands to accomplish gastrocnemius pumping.
  - For quadriceps setting, the client presses the back of the knee against the bed and then relaxes it. These should be done approximately 10 to 12 times each hour.
- Also desirable are foot circles and knee movements.
  - Have the client draw circles with his or her toes several times an hour.

Table continued on following page

TABLE 10–6. POSTOPERATIVE PREVENTIVE TECHNIQUES *Continued*

- Raising the legs by bending at the knees may be too painful for the client with an abdominal incision.

TURNING IN BED AND AMBULATION (see also Mobility, Impaired Physical, Section 2-11)

- Have clients turn in bed every hour postoperatively to prevent respiratory and circulatory complications.
- The usual sequence is from side to back to side. Show clients how to use the side rails for assistance in turning.
- Most often, clients are ambulated the evening of the day of surgery or on the first postoperative day.
- A helpful technique for minimizing strain on the incision and discomfort when getting up is to turn on the side and then push up to a sitting position. Another one is to raise the head of the bed until sitting erect and then pivot the legs over the side of the bed.

- Observe stoma for color and size. Stoma should be pink to bright red. Report changes in stoma color immediately.

- Assess quality and quantity of stools. Report diarrhea to surgeon. Stools from an ileostomy will be watery at first and later become semisolid or paste-like at approximately 500 ml/day. Stools from a colostomy will be watery in the ascending colon, pasty in the transverse colon and increasingly solid down the descending colon.

- Irrigate stoma only as ordered.

- Refer client to enterostomal therapist for advice on managing the stoma, appliances, and dietary considerations.

- Observe for signs of peritonitis or sepsis due to leaking of stool into the abdominal cavity.

- Provide pain medication as needed.

- Provide emotional support for the client. Refer client to ostomy support groups.

- Discharge instructions should include: managing the stoma, skin care, use of appliances, dietary restrictions or recommendations, body image, support groups, and follow up visits. Encourage the client to drink plenty of fluids and avoid alcohol and diuretics that may increase fluid loss and create a fluid imbalance.

Thoracic Surgery

Surgery to the thoracic cavity is performed for respiratory or cardiac purposes. In this section, respiratory surgeries will be discussed. Surgery on the respiratory tract is performed when the client no longer has the ability to freely clear his or her airway or maintain appropriate gas exchange. This may be due to a congenital deformity, tumor, infection, trauma, or chronic illness. Potential complications with respiratory surgery include: tension pneumothorax, respiratory insufficiency, circulatory insufficiency, and pulmonary embolism (See Table 10-5).

- **Chest tube insertion** is performed to drain the chest of fluid, air or pus and therefore allow the lung to reinflate. With a pneumothorax, the chest tube will restore negative pressure to the pleural space. Chest tube placement can be done at the bedside or in the OR.

  - Review chest tube management as outlined in Section 10-4.

  - Once the chest tube is inserted, monitor vital signs, especially respirations every 15 min and then as ordered. Note respiratory rate, respiratory quality and breath sounds.

  - A chest x-ray will ascertain placement.

  - The closed chest drainage system should be checked for functioning every shift and the amount of drainage documented.

- **Thoracotomy** is the removal of all or part of a lung. It can be performed for tumors, disease, infections or lesions. Types of thoracotomies include: segmental resection, lobectomy, wedge resection and pneumonectomy. Common complications include: hemorrhage, tension pneumothorax, empyema, infection, and dead space in the pleural cavity.

- Positioning of the client is important. The client with a pneumonectomy must be placed on operative side to prevent fluid from affecting the healthy lung. Elevation of the head of the bed can assist lung expansion.

- Coughing and deep breathing as well as incentive spirometry should begin as soon as the client is responsive.

- Breath sounds and vital signs should be done a minimum of once a shift or more often as the client's condition warrants.

- Medicate the client for pain. This will assist the client with moving in bed, range of motion exercises, coughing and deep breathing (see Table 10-6).

- Suction client as required.

- Monitor chest tubes and drainage system.

- Support client emotionally so that anxiety is reduced and breathing is facilitated.

Neurological Surgery

Neurosurgery is performed when medical management has not helped the client or the client is in a life threatening situation. Many neurosurgical procedures involve a craniotomy, which involves opening the skull to expose brain tissue. Potential complications from neurosurgery include: increased intracranial pressure, hemorrhage, CSF leak, meningitis, seizures, infection, and neurological deficits not present before surgery (see Table 10-5).

A. General recommendations for management of the client having cranial surgery

- Observe for signs of increased intracranial pressure including decreased level of consciousness, bradycardia, increase in blood pressure, widening pulse pressure, respiratory pattern changes, increased or decreased respiratory rate, headache, nausea, vomiting, pupillary changes, and seizures.

- Prevent increased intracranial pressure by elevating the head of the bed 20–40 degrees and making sure the client avoids the Valsalva maneuver, rectal stimulation, coughing, straining, sneezing, vomiting and rapid infusion of IV fluids.

- Maintain seizure precautions (see Section 2-13).

- Observe for signs and symptoms of a stress ulcer, abdominal pain, occult blood in the stools, vomitus, or nasogastric aspirate.

- Avoid flexion of the head. Position the client in the lateral or semiprone position. Prevent aspiration of fluids. Observe for partial airway obstruction: noisy respirations, stridor, decreased inspiratory and expiratory volume, restlessness, and cyanosis. *Note:* hypoxia causes increased intracranial pressure.

- Orient the client to person, place, and time.

- Neuro signs should be done a minimum of once a shift.

B. Craniotomy is performed by creating a surgical incision in the skull, allowing the surgeon to visualize the brain tissue. Complications from a craniotomy include increased intracranial pressure, respiratory distress, infection, and hemorrhage. Clients typically are treated with steroids.

- Discuss with the client that a portion of the head will be shaved in the OR. Hair can be saved at client's request.

- Antiembolism hose and SCD machines may be applied in the OR to prevent deep vein thrombosis.

- The client will return from surgery with a large bulky head dressing. Ascertain if a drain is present and its location.

- The client may experience facial swelling and a headache. Medicate for pain as ordered.

- Frequent vital signs and neuro checks will be performed for the first 48–72 hr depending on the client's condition. Many clients go to ICU post-craniotomy but in many hospitals they are sent back to a specialized neurosurgical unit.

- Always compare the client's preoperative and postoperative neurological baseline for changes in status. Notify the physician immediately if a change in the level of consciousness or an increase in the ICP is noted.

- Check for physician orders for client's ability to cough and deep breathe. If ordered, do hourly.

- Monitor client for changes in respiratory status and suction prn. Breath sounds should be done a minimum of once a shift.

- Monitor fluid and electrolytes, assessing laboratory data and intake and output. Supplement the client as ordered.

- Monitor the wound for infection, leakage of CSF, and bloody drainage. Notify the physician if purulent or yellow drainage is noted. Special filter paper is available to test for CSF.

- Provide emotional support to the client who may be self-conscious about hair loss. Help with securing a wig.

- Discharge instructions should include: signs and symptoms of infection, management of the suture line, medication management, changes in mentation, and follow up visits.

C. **Ventricular shunts** are inserted in adults and children who exhibit signs of hydrocephalus. A catheter is inserted into the ventricular system of the brain and tunneled under the skin to another site in the chest or abdomen. In preparation for this surgery, the client should be constantly assessed for signs of increased ICP, seizures, or a change in the client's level of consciousness.

- Review the craniotomy procedure.

- Monitor the client for signs of infection. Use aseptic technique to provide wound care.

- Observe for shunt failure and an increase in ICP. Test the shunt as ordered.

- Slowly elevate the head of the bed according to physician orders. This will allow the client to adjust to the decrease in ICP.

- Unless ordered otherwise, the client should be placed on the nonoperative side. This will prevent pressure on the suture lines and shunt.

- Discharge instructions should include: signs of infection and increased intracranial pressure, management of suture lines, techniques in pumping shunt, medications, signs of shunt failure, and follow up appointments.

Urological Surgery

Urological surgery is fairly commonplace. It is performed for congenital disorders, to correct a medical problem when conservative therapy has failed, or to remove a tumor that may be malignant or impeding urine flow.

A. General recommendations for management of the client having urological surgery

- Observe for and prevent postoperative complications (See Table 10-5.) Key complications include: hemorrhage and shock, pulmonary complications, paralytic ileus, and fluid electrolyte imbalance. Severe pain in the bladder region or abdominal rigidity may indicate bladder obstruction or perforation.

- Maintain patency of drainage tubes, e.g., nephrotomy tube, ureteral catheters. Prevent tubes from kinking or pulling. Irrigate tubes only as ordered using strict aseptic technique.

- Record accurate intake and output as well as characteristic of urine. With urological surgery, urine may be bright red at first but the color should decrease in intensity. Notify the physician of large clots or frank bleeding.

- Encourage at least 2000 cc/day of fluid if not medically contraindicated.

B. Transurethral Resection of the Bladder (TURB) is done to remove small benign or cancerous tumors of the bladder. It is not uncommon for this procedure to be performed numerous times. The TURB can be done with or without the use of a YAG laser. Complications associated with this type of surgery include: hematuria, urinary tract infections, bladder perforations and urinary retention.

- Follow general recommendations in Section A above.

- Encourage fluid intake to assist in flushing the bladder.

- Continuous bladder irrigation may be present. Irrigate the bladder according to the physician instructions. Document intake/outake.

- Assess for signs of a perforated bladder: abdominal rigidity, fever, increasing pain and decreased urine output. Notify physician immediately.

- Medicate for pain and spasms.

- Discharge instructions should include: signs and symptoms of a urinary infection, notification of physician if there is an increase in blood in the urine, importance of fluid intake, restrictions concerning heavy lifting, and sexual intercourse until permitted by physician, review of medications and follow-up visits.

C. Prostatectomy is removal or resection of the prostate gland. It is performed when the prostate enlarges and impedes the flow of urine. The four types of prostate surgery are: transurethral resection, suprapubic, retropubic, and radical perineal prostatectomy. Lasers are presently being introduced into this surgical procedure. One specific complication in this type of surgery is dilutional hyponatremia caused by the frequent irrigation of the bladder in surgery.

- Follow general recommendations in Section A above.

- Since loss of sexual function may be a side effect of the surgery, discuss this with the client and allow the client to discuss issues and concerns.

- Monitor carefully for hemorrhage, infection, and urinary retention.

- Observe for signs and symptoms of dilutional hyponatremia that include: low serum sodium, changes in mentation, seizures, and muscle twitching.

- Continuous or intermittent bladder irrigation may be ordered. Use strict aseptic technique and assess for color of urine and presence of clots.

- Medicate with pain medication and antispasmodics as ordered.

- Discharge instructions should include: the importance of maintaining fluid status, frequently voiding, informing physician of inability to void, observation of urine for increase in bleeding, instruction for no heavy lifting or sexual activity until permitted by MD and use of medications. If client is experiencing incontinence, teach exercises to decrease this, catheter care if client goes home with a catheter and also the importance of follow up appointments.

Endocrine Surgery

Endocrine surgery is performed when medical management or hormonal supplementation is ineffective in controlling the client's endocrinological balance. Endocrine surgery is also performed in the case of benign tumors that may stimulate hormone production or malignancy. Complications in endocrine surgery include: fluid and electrolyte imbalance, cardiac and respiratory issues and mentation changes. Endocrine surgeries may involve the thyroid gland, parathyroid gland, pituitary gland, adrenal glands, pancreas, thymus, and pineal gland.

A. Thyroidectomy is performed when a malignant or benign tumor affects the thyroid, producing a state of hyper or hypo activity. It may also be done for cosmetic reasons (goiter) or when a tumor affects the client's ability to breathe. A thyroidectomy may be partial or complete.

- Observe closely for fluid and electrolyte imbalances and complications of surgery.

- Observe carefully respiratory status and be alert for signs of laryngospasm.

- Position client in semi-Fowler's position to decrease swelling and check to make sure neck bandages are not constricting the trachea.

- A tracheostomy set should be with the client at all times.

- Assess for laryngeal nerve damage by asking client to speak. The client may be hoarse initially.

- Observe for signs of the accidental removal of the parathyroid glands. Signs of hypocalcemia include: muscle spasms, twitching, tingling of lips, fingers and toes, tetany, anxiety, seizures and laryngospasm. Be prepared to administer calcium gluconate as ordered.

- Observe for signs of thyroid storm: elevated temperature (up to 106° F/41.4° C), tachycardia, dehydration, diarrhea, tachypnea, atrial arrhythmias, excessive irritability, delirium, confusion, psychotic behavior, Chvostek's and Trousseau's signs, pulmonary edema and shock.

- Encourage client to place hands behind neck when moving. This will prevent hyperextension and decrease pain.

- Observe for signs and symptoms of infection.

- Observe for signs of hemorrhage. Remember to check behind the neck since blood may flow down the back.

- Discharge instructions should include: medication especially if the entire thyroid was removed, signs and symptoms of hyper/hypothyroidism, suture management and follow-up appointments.

B. Adrenalectomy is performed if the adrenal gland is hyperfunctioning, benign or malignant tumors are present, for hyperaldosteronism and sometimes to treat cancer of the breast and prostate.

- Observe blood pressure closely the first 24–48 hr. Be prepared to administer intravenous fluids, vasopressor and steroids for control of hypotension.

- Observe for signs and symptoms of adrenal crisis: hypotension, weak thready pulse, tachycardia, diaphoresis, nausea, vomiting, muscle cramps, headache, altered mental status, elevation, and then a drop in body temperature and shock.

- Prevent infections and situations that might bring on an adrenal crisis. Place the client in a private room and limit visitors, particularly those with respiratory symptoms. Avoid overexertion, emotional upsets, vomiting, and diarrhea.

- Observe carefully for cardiac insufficiency since the heart has been taxed for a period of time.

- Observe lab data and monitor for hemorrhage as well as potassium levels.

- Supplement with medications as ordered, which may include steroids, insulin, and analgesics.

- Discharge instructions include: medications that will be lifelong if both glands are removed, signs and symptoms of infection, signs of adrenal insufficiency, suture care, and continuous medical follow up, especially when ill.

Breast Surgery

Breast surgery is performed for cosmetic and medical reasons. Benign or malignant tumors can be removed. Breast surgeries performed for malignancies include: lumpectomy, simple mastectomy, radical mastectomy, modified radical mastectomy. Complications include: lymphedema, infection, and decreased muscle strength.

General recommendations for the client having breast surgery

- Observe for and prevent postoperative complications, especially hemorrhage.

- Maintain Hemovac or other suction to drain tubes. Document drainage at least every 8 hr. Teach client how to manage the drainage systems since the client will go home with the drain.

- Check arm and hand of affected side for adequate circulation, sensitivity and motion. Do not take blood pressures, draw blood, or otherwise puncture the affected arm. Elevate the affected arm above the level of the heart while maintaining a position of comfort (for radical mastectomies).

- Do not turn client on affected side.

- Observe surgical site for signs of infection.

- Initiate range of motion exercises for the client with radical mastectomy according to physician order. (See Tables 2-7, 2-8.)

- Provide emotional support for body image and diagnose related issues. Involve significant other(s) as appropriate.

- Discharge instructions should include: signs and symptoms of infection, prevention of lymphedema, strengthening exercises, referral to local and national support groups and prosthesis companies, drainage tube management and follow-up appointments. Many clients will return at a later date for reconstructive surgery.

Ophthalmic Surgery

Ophthalmic surgery is performed for eye disorders that do not respond to medical management, malignancies, and congenital problems. With the advent of lasers, most surgical procedures use lasers that minimize pain, lessen the recovery period and decrease the common surgical complications of hemorrhage and infection.

A. General recommendations for management of the client having opthalmic surgery

- Observe for signs and symptoms of post-operative complications: excessive bleeding or drainage, sudden onset of eye pain, infection, and disorientation.

- Elevate head of bed or position client as ordered by physician. Many clients are released the day of surgery, so emphasize the importance of proper positioning at home.

- Encourage deep breathing. Coughing should not be done postoperatively as it will increase intraocular pressure.

- Maintain the appropriate eye patch or shield as ordered.

- Medicate the client as ordered with eye drops according to schedule.

- If the client is hospitalized, request that the client call the staff for ambulation. Keep the call bell within reach.

- Teach the client to refrain from rubbing the eye, straining with bowel movements, vomiting, bending over, lifting heavy objects, and making sudden head movements. Give an antiemetic if nauseous.

B. Cataract removal repairs an opaque lens caused by age, congenital deformity, or trauma. Surgical procedures include: intracapsular, extracapsular (with or without irrigation and phacoemulsification), and implantation of an intraocular lens. Complications include: hemorrhage, edema, retinal detachment, pupillary block, and corneal breakdown.

- Cataract surgery is usually a same-day procedure so comprehensive teaching must be done.

- Review general instructions especially the wearing of an eye patch and observation of infection.

- Review medications and schedule.

- Client should sleep on unaffected side to decrease ocular pressure.

- Assist with ambulation since clients have decreased visibility.

- Discharge instructions should include: medication administration, signs and symptoms of infection, notifying the physician of pain in eye, safety factors, the wearing of an eye patch, the need to avoid lifting, bending and straining at stools, that the wearing of sunglasses can assist with glare problems and follow up appointments.

C. **Radial keratotomy** is the surgical treatment for myopia. Since the surgery is barely 20 years old, the long-term effects of the surgery are unknown. Complications from this surgery include: infection, over/undercorrecting the myopia, corneal perforation and photophobia.

- The procedure is done on an outpatient basis and uses local anesthetics and sometimes conscious sedation.

- Medicate the client for pain as ordered.

- If an eye patch is not ordered remind the client not to rub the eye.

- Discharge instructions include: administration of eye drops as ordered, use of sunglasses for photophobia (usually goes away in a few months), avoidance of activities that require clear vision till visual disturbances subside, avoidance of contact sports and water until permitted by physician. Makeup should also be avoided until permitted by the physician.

Ear Surgery

Surgery is performed when medical management has failed to cure the disease process. Complications from ear surgery include: bleeding, vertigo, tinnitus, hearing loss, infection, gait disturbance, increased pain, and facial nerve injury.

A. Myringotomy with or without pressure equalization (PE) tube insertion is commonly performed when antibiotic administration is ineffective in controlling fluid in the ear or the client suffers chronic ear infections with or without hearing loss.

- The procedure is done on an outpatient basis using either local or general anesthetics.

- Assess for fluid drainage from ears. If fluid is present, document color, consistency and amount. If the drainage is bright red, report immediately to the physician.

- Discharge instructions: if client has had PE tube placements, water must not enter the ear. Show the client how to make ear plugs with cotton and petrolatum or refer client to stores where ear plugs can be purchased. Inform the client of the signs and symptoms of infection, and the fact that a small amount of drainage from the ear is normal. Have client notify MD of ear pain or excessive drainage. Emphasize that follow up appointments must be kept.

B. Stapedectomy is performed to remove all or part of the stapes due to otosclerosis that inhibits the conduction of sound. The surgery can partially or totally remove the stapes. Some physicians use a laser to perform the surgery. Complications include: infection, facial paralysis, graft dislodgement, headache, and ear pain.

- Position the client according to physician orders.

- Medicate client for nausea and pain.

- Since many clients experience vertigo, have a staff member stay with the client while ambulating. The side rails should be placed in the upright position.

- Use aseptic technique when changing dressings. Document amount, color and consistency of drainage.

- Tell the client to avoid coughing, sneezing, or blowing the nose to prevent dislodging of graft.

- Discharge instructions should include: signs and symptoms of infection, pain or the feeling of movement in the ear, continuous vertigo, proper use of medication, avoidance of water in the ear and a restriction on flying and blowing the nose until the MD permits.

Orthopedic Surgery

Orthopedic surgery is performed to correct congenital abnormalities, repair injury and trauma and to correct diseased bones and joints.

Arthroscopic surgery is performed so that the surgeon can visually inspect the internal joint structures through a scope. The procedure is usually done on an outpatient surgery basis and is done when conservative treatment is not effective.

- The surgery may be done under a local or general anesthetic. If the client had a general anesthetic, encourage coughing, and deep breathing.

- The client will return from surgery with 3–4 stab wounds that are closed with a suture or steri strips covered by a bandage. Observe the dressings for drainage and note the amount, color, and consistency.

- Elevate the extremity and place ice as ordered.

- Discharge instructions are important. Instructions should include signs and symptoms of infection, pain medications ordered, the use of ice to decrease swelling and the use of a cane or crutches if prescribed. Many clients will begin physical therapy after their first postoperative visit.

10-4 SELECTED THERAPEUTIC NURSING PROCEDURES

Before performing any of the therapeutic procedures reviewed in this section, be sure you complete the Checklist of Guidelines for Therapeutic Nursing Procedures (Table 10-7). Specific procedures vary from institution to institution and change as new information is identified. *Always review your own institution's procedure manual to ensure that you are adhering to the standards of your particular facility.* You may wish to modify our selected procedures in pencil.

Sterile Dressing Change

PURPOSE

Maintain cleanliness of an open wound or drain while facilitating healing.

EQUIPMENT

Sterile dressings, clean and sterile gloves, antiseptic solution or swabs, normal saline, tape, waste receptacle.

PROCEDURE

- Verify physician order. Usually the physician will remove the first dressing after surgery.

- Complete the Checklist in Table 10-7.

- Gather all required equipment and wash hands.

- Close windows or turn off fans to prevent drafts and contamination of wound surface.

- Elevate the bed to prevent back strain and turn on lights to increase visibility.

- Open sterile supplies, tear tape and place receptacle in an easily accessible place.

- Don clean gloves and remove old dressing slowly; take care not to dislodge any tubes or drains. Avoid contaminating the wound with the edges of the dressing, the tape or your nonsterile gloves. Touch only the outer surfaces of the dressing.

- If the dressing has dried to the skin or wound, soak with normal saline prior to removing.

**TABLE 10–7. CHECKLIST OF GUIDELINES FOR
THERAPEUTIC NURSING PROCEDURES**

Assessment

- ☐ Review the overall condition of the client: diagnosis, medications, recently performed tests, surgeries and therapies, laboratory data, age, physical and emotional stability.

- ☐ Know the reason the procedure is being performed.

- ☐ Assess the effect the procedure may have on the client.

- ☐ Review the physician's specific instructions (question the physician if a procedure appears to be potentially unnecessary or harmful).

- ☐ Assess the client's ability to tolerate the procedure.

Nursing Interventions

- ☐ Explain the procedure to the client, including purpose and the length of time the procedure will take.

- ☐ Answer any questions the client may have.

- ☐ Gather all equipment at the bedside before you begin.

- ☐ Wash your hands before and after procedures.

- ☐ Provide privacy.

- ☐ Make sure there is adequate lighting.

- ☐ Maintain a matter-of-fact attitude and move swifly and deftly.

- ☐ Encourage the client's participation whenever possible.

- ☐ Instruct client to inhale and exhale slowly before and during particularly tense moments of procedures.

- ☐ Support the client emotionally and promote comfort.

- ☐ Evaluate and document the client's tolerance of the procedure, the efficacy of the procedure and/or any untoward effects.

- Assess the dressing for the amount, color, consistency and odor of drainage. Discard dressing in waste receptacle. Remove gloves and discard.

- Don sterile gloves.

- Cleanse wound with antiseptic solution, normal saline or antiseptic swabs.

- Hold each swab with the tip down and cleanse in the following sequence:

  - Down the incision line from the proximal to distal end by rolling the swab or wiping the gauze over the center of the incision. Discard swab or gauze.

  - Obtain new swab or gauze and wipe down one side of the incision covering approximately 1 in of adjacent tissue. Discard swab/gauze and repeat on other side.

  - If a drain is present, wipe around the drain from the inside out in a circular pattern. Do not wipe over a cleaned area.

- If a drain is present, place a 4-by-4 dressing around the drain and then place another dressing over the entire incision. Use heavier dressings over the drain site areas.

- Remove gloves and secure dressings with tape.

- Lower bed and document findings.

GUIDELINES

- A dressing may be reinforced if unexpected excessive wound drainage occurs and the physician has not ordered a dressing change. The physician should be notified since wet dressings are an open medium for bacteria to infiltrate the wound.

- Wounds should be inspected carefully for redness, edema, skin irritation, type of drainage, and stage of healing. Surgical or traumatic wounds must be observed closely for hemorrhage during the first 24 hr. All wound assessments must be documented.

- Always use Universal Precautions when changing dressings.

Wound Irrigation

PURPOSE

To cleanse the wound of debris, drainage, and old tissue. It also stimulates tissue growth and may assist in the distribution of medication.

EQUIPMENT

Sterile irrigation set including aseptic syringe, solution container, solution receptacle and sterile barrier, sterile gauze, sterile dressing supplies, clean and sterile gloves, ordered irrigation solution, bed protector, sterile red rubber catheter, and waste receptacle.

PROCEDURE

- Complete checklist in Table 10-7.
- See Sterile Dressing Change above.
- Elevate bed to prevent back strain and turn on lights for increased visibility.
- Check physician order.
- Gather equipment and wash hands.
- Open sterile supplies and place bed protector under area to be irrigated.
- Position solution collection receptacle in the proper position for the return flow of the solution. Proper client positioning can assist the flow of the solution into the receptacle.
- Don clean gloves remove and discard old dressing.
- Remove gloves and discard. Pour irrigation solution into sterile solution container.
- Apply sterile gloves.
- Fill the aseptic syringe with irrigating solution and instill directly into the wound or through a catheter that has been placed gently in the wound. Direct the solution over the entire wound, using your nondominant hand to manipulate the solution collection container. Continue irrigating until the prescribed amount of solution has been used.

- Dry wound with a sterile gauze pad and redress using sterile dressing change procedure.

- Document procedure in the chart.

Suture Removal

PURPOSE

To promote continuation of the healing process by discontinuing support no longer needed that may act as a foreign body in the tissue.

EQUIPMENT

Sterile suture removal set including: scissors, forceps and hemostat or staple remover, skin antiseptic, clean and sterile gloves and sterile dressings as indicated.

PROCEDURE

- Check physician's orders, as this is a delegated medical function.

- Complete checklist in Table 10-7.

- Position the client so there is minimal tension on the suture line. A reclining position is best in case there is any nausea or dizziness during the procedure.

- Wash hands and don clean gloves.

- Remove dressing and discard in bag.

- Don sterile gloves.

- Cleanse the site with disinfectant, beginning with the suture line and extending outward for an area of 2 inches. Use sterile swabs or cotton balls and the forceps, with a new cotton ball for each stroke.

- Grasp the first suture with a sterile hemostat or forceps and elevate it so that the portion below the knot is clearly visible.

- With the sterile scissors cut one side of the suture below the knot, close to the skin. Avoid cutting the knot. The key point is to avoid drawing the exposed contaminated portion of the suture through the tissues.

- Remove each suture smoothly and in one continuous motion to minimize pain. The suture should be grabbed by the knot and disposed of in a receptacle. Check to see that the entire suture is removed.

- Sutures may be continuous (formed by one continuous thread) or interrupted (formed by single stitches and inserted separately) or staples may have been used.

- For continuous sutures, grasp each portion to be cut by the suture itself as there is not a knot for each stitch.

- Skin staples are removed in one motion with the staple remover.

- Cleanse area again with disinfectant and cover with a sterile dressing or steri-strips.

- Remove gloves and discard. Wash hands

GUIDELINES

Check with the physician to determine if the client has interrupted sutures or staples as these are often removed in two sequences (every other one at first, with the remainder removed in 24–48 hr).

Nasogastric Tube Insertion, Gastric Decompression, Irrigation, and Gavage

PURPOSE

The introduction of an NG tube into the stomach may be done for the following reasons:

- To prevent or relieve abdominal distension.

- To establish a route for the administration of medications, fluids, or nutrients into the gastric system (gavage).

- To prepare the client for gastric surgery or diagnostic tests.

- To provide a route for solution to be introduced and quickly removed in order to remove irritating substances from the stomach or to decrease bleeding (lavage).

EQUIPMENT

NG tube as ordered, disposable irrigation set, water soluble lubricant, clamp, 1/2 inch adhesive tape, safety pin, rubber band, glass of water with a straw, stethoscope, emesis basin, gloves, and towel. Also suction if ordered, irrigation or feeding solution, 50 cc aseptic syringe, and formula and water if a feeding is ordered.

PROCEDURE

Insertion

- Complete checklist in Table 10-7.
- Wash hands.
- Ask if client has had a history of nasal polyps, injury to the nares or nasal surgery.
- Assess client's vital signs and respiratory status.
- Select the most patent nostril by having the client alternately block one side and breathe through the other. Avoid nares that have had surgery.
- Place towel across the client's chest.
- Don clean gloves.
- Estimate the length of tubing necessary to enter the client's stomach by measuring the distance from the client's earlobe to the tip of the nose and from the nose to the xiphoid process. Mark with tape.
- Lubricate 6–8 in. of the tip of the tubing with the water soluble lubricant.
- Allow client to hold the emesis basin or place it close to the client.
- Insert the tube gently through the selected nostril, aiming back and down. If an obstruction is met, do not force the tube but withdraw it slightly and advance again. If an obstruction is met, try a smaller size tube or try the other nostril.
- Instruct the client to swallow as the tube reaches the pharynx. Sipping water through the straw will help

the swallowing reflex. Continue to advance the tube each time the client swallows, until the tape mark on the tube is at the client's nostril. Immediately withdraw the tube if there are signs of distress such as gasping, coughing, or cyanosis, as this can indicate placement in the trachea.

- Assess for tube patency and correct placement by aspirating stomach contents with a barrel syringe and testing on gastric paper, injecting 10–30 cc of air into the tube and auscultating over the epigastrium with the stethoscope and hearing a whooshing sound. Also check the back of the throat to see if the NG tube is coiled in the pharynx. An x-ray can be used to confirm placement and must be used when feeding tubes are placed.

- Tape the tubing securely to the nose or apply a tube holder, making sure the nares are not obstructed. Weighted intestinal tubes should not be taped.

Decompression (suction)
- Check physician's order for type of suction (continuous or intermittent) and amount of pressure to be used (low is usually 80–100 mm Hg, high is 100–120 mm Hg).

- Assist client to semi-Fowler's position.

- Check for correct placement of the NG tube. When placement is verified, connect the NG tube to the suction correction tubing, using a barrel connector.

- Turn machine on, set the suction at the desired pressure. Make sure the suction is working.

- Coil any extra tubing on the bed, as tubing in a dependent position will make suctioning less effective.

- Keep the air vent open and clear at all times and not in a dependent position.

- Irrigate the NG tube as necessary to maintain patency of the system.

- Assess the system for functioning and the client at least every hour at first then every 2–3 hr thereafter.

- Empty the suction drainage container every shift or when it is two-thirds full. Record output.

- In some situations, such as postoperative gastric resections, bleeding from the stomach is expected. If the blood in the gastric drainage increases in intensity or amount from the base line, notify the physician immediately.

NG Tube Irrigation

Irrigation of a NG tube is indicated to prevent blockages. (Check hospital policy.) It may also be indicated when the NG tube is connected to suction and the suctioned material is not returning as it should, or when a drip tube feeding will not infuse.

- Wash hands and don clean gloves.

- Place client in semi-Fowler's position.

- Turn off the suction or tube feeding and disconnect. Always check for correct placement of the NG tube before instilling fluid to make sure fluid will not enter the lungs.

- Using a 50 cc syringe, instill 20 ml of sterile normal saline into the NG tube. Do not force the solution. Withdraw the 20 ml of solution and discard. Repeat.

- Reconnect the tube to suction or tube feeding and assess for patency and function.

- Record on Intake and Output sheet.

- Disposable irrigation kits should be rinsed well between irrigations and replaced daily.

- If the NG tubes remains blocked, notify the physician or follow hospital protocol.

Gavage (Enteral Feeding) (See also Sec 8-5, in Nutrition chapter)

- Check for physician order.

- Assess for correct placement of the NG tube.

- The head of the bed must be elevated 30–45 degrees before feeding and must remain elevated for at least 30 min to 1 hr afterward to prevent aspiration.

- Assess for bowel sounds and abdominal distension.

- Aspirate residual stomach contents with an aseptic syringe, measure the total amount, and return the residual to the client's stomach.

- Calculate any changes in the volume or the impending tube feeding: as a general rule, subtract aspirated amount from prescribed feeding amount if it is between 50 and 100 cc, and hold feeding if it is more than 100 cc, and check with MD.

- For the syringe method: Remove bulb from aseptic syringe and attach to feeding tube. Hold 6 in above the client's head. Clear the tube with 30–50 cc of water. Pour part of the feeding into the syringe and allow to flow by gravity. Repeat until feeding is completed. Do not allow air to enter the feeding tube. Flush with 30 cc of water.

- Always give medications by the aseptic syringe method. Watch for the following complications in a client receiving tube feedings: nausea, vomiting, gastric distention, diarrhea, aspiration of formula, dehydration, and electrolyte imbalance.

GUIDELINES

- The choice among the variety of gastrointestinal tubes available will be made by the physician based on the purpose of the tube, the size of the client, and availability of the tube. Generally, tubes that are for suctioning purposes are larger in diameter and have an air vent; whereas tubes for the administration of nutrients, fluids or medication are smaller in diameter and have no air vent. Tubes with a weighted tip allow passage through the stomach into the small intestine and are usually used for administering nutrients. Intestinal tubes with a mercury-weighted balloon on the tip are used for relieving bowel obstructions and should be inserted and removed by the physician.

- Prior to intubation, make tubes more or less pliable as needed:

  - place a soft rubber tube in a container of ice

- place a hard plastic tube under warm running water or in a container of warm water

- The client with gastrointestinal tubes needs frequent oral hygiene.

- Never cap or clamp the air vent of a client on gastric suctioning as the air vent helps to decrease the possibility of damage to the intestinal mucosa.

- To ambulate a client on gastric suctioning: turn off suctioning, disconnect NG tube from connecting tubing, insert a catheter plug into lumen of NG tube, and reverse this sequence when ambulation is finished. Newer catheters have anti-reflux valves.

- Frequently assess fluid and electrolyte status of client on gastric intubation because of higher risk for imbalance.

Chest Tube Drainage

PURPOSE

To provide nursing care for the client with chest tubes attached to a closed water-seal drainage system. The most important objectives are to maintain sterility, airtightness, and patency of the system in order to prevent complications.

EQUIPMENT

Two straight 6- to 7-in. hemostats, sterile water-pour bottle, petroleum gauze.

PROCEDURE

- In the immediate postoperative period, check the collection chamber every 30 min, noting volume, color, and consistency of the drainage.

- Mark the level of the fluid, the time, and your initials when you take the measurement on the side of the chamber.

- Tape all connection sites.

- Place the client in low- to semi-Fowler's position. Turn client to affected side, keeping a folded bath blanket under the client to protect the tubes from the client's body weight and prevent obstruction. Change client position frequently.

- *Keep the drainage system below the level of the chest at all times.*

- Assess constantly for signs and symptoms of tension pneumothorax (chest pain, tachypnea, dyspnea, neck vein distention, tracheal deviation, absent lung sounds, increased cardiovascular pressure, decreased BP, cardiopulmonary arrest) and notify physician immediately as this is a life-threatening situation.

- Observe for fluctuations in the fluid column of the water-seal chamber as a sign of proper functioning. Normally fluctuations will stop when there is reexpansion of the lung (usually within 48 to 72 hr of chest-tube insertion). If fluctuations stop or there is continuous bubbling in the water-seal chamber and your client's lungs are not fully expanded, it may be due to one of the following problems: obstructed tubing from clot formation, kinking, patient's position, or suction malfunction. A great deal of bubbling on expiration, or bubbling that continues throughout the respiratory cycle, signals a leak in the system (a small amount may be normal after some thoracic procedures).

- To locate the leak, pinch the tubing near the insertion site for 1 or 2 sec. If the bubbling stops, the leak is proximal to the site you have clamped. After removing the clamp, try to seal the skin around the insertion site with your hands or petroleum gauze. If the bubbling stops now, air has been entering the pleural space at the insertion site. If the bubbling still does not stop, air is entering the thorax from the client's lung and the physician must be notified immediately. If clamping the chest tube near the insertion site does not stop the excessive bubbling, the leak is probably in the tubing and the setup should be changed.

- Continuous bubbling in the suction control section of the drainage system or pleurevac is normal and if it stops, it means there is no suction being applied to the client's pleural space. Rule out air leak by examining all connecting sites, rubber stoppers, and the system. Check for a leak in the suction apparatus, a blocked manometer, or an obstructed air inlet. If bubbling does not resume when a new suction machine is applied, notify the physician.

- "Milking" the chest tubes routinely is now considered questionable because of the rise in chest pressure. It is recommended that milking be done only if clots are present after the first 4 hr. To do this, squeeze and release along the entire length of the tubing. An MD order must be obtained.

- Keep two padded clamps taped to the head of the bed at all times to be used in an emergency situation to prevent outside air from entering the pleural space (check your hospital policy as some hospitals are no longer recommending this). They are clamped as close to the chest as possible, and only for a few moments until the drainage system is restored. If there is extensive pneumothorax, do not clamp the chest tube, but instead submerge the end of the tubing in water or saline while someone else sets up a new system. Air buildup in the pleural space causes tension pneumothorax.

- Prevent dependent loops in the tubing by fastening tubing to the bedding with rubber bands and safety pins. Excess tubing can be coiled on the bed, but the client must not lie on them.

- If suction is not ordered, maintain an open air vent.

- Maintain level of suction as ordered by the physician, checking fluid level q 4 hr and adjusting if needed.

- Mark drainage level on drainage container with date, time, and your initials every hour for the first 24 hr, then a minimum of every shift. Drainage will be bloody at first, and then serosanguinous. Notify physician if there is an excess of 150 ml/hr of drainage.

- Auscultate chest for breath sounds q 4 hr with vital signs, or more frequently as needed. Help client cough out secretions and deep breathe q 2 hr or as ordered. Assist client to sitting position if possible and splint with a pillow. Assist with range-of-motion exercises, especially upper extremities to maintain joint mobility. Maintain comfort by giving analgesics as required, especially before deep breathing.

GUIDELINES

- Review pulmonary anatomy and physiology and become familiar with closed-chest drainage systems and suction equipment.

- *Drainage systems are never emptied unless specifically ordered by the physician.*

- Transport or ambulate a client with chest tubes keeping the water-seal unit below chest level and upright at all times. Nursing staff should accompany the client. Clamps should accompany the client for emergency use.

- Always keep an extra drainage set and tubing in the client's room in case of breakage, or damage to the system.

- When the client's lungs are fully expanded drainage will become minimal. With minimal drainage for 8–24 hr and the presence of normal breath sounds, the chest tubes will probably be removed. Sometimes the physician orders the tubes clamped for 24 hr before removal. Once the tube has been removed, the wound is covered with petroleum gauze and sterile dressing; this remains for 48 hr to allow the wound to heal.

REFERENCES

Bean MK. Preparation for surgery in an ambulatory surgery unit. J Post Anesthesia Nursing 1990; 5:42–47.

Beck C, Paulos L, Rosenburg T. Postsurgical care for arthroscopic surgery of the knee and shoulder. Orthopaedic Clinics of North America. 1988; 19:715–723.

Bryant R. Acute and chronic wounds: nursing management. St. Louis: Mosby Year Book, 1992.

Burden N. Ambulatory surgical nursing. Philadelphia: W B Saunders, 1993.

Carroll P. What's new in chest tube management. RN 1991; 54(5):34–40.

Carroll P. Technical update brief: the child with a chest tube. Pediatric Nursing 1993; 19(4):370–371.

Gauwitz D. Endoscopic cholecystectomy: the patient-friendly alternative. Nursing 90. 1990; December:58–59.

Glass E. Informed consent: the nurse's role. Cancer Nursing News 1990; 8(1):3.

Haicken B. Laser laparoscopic cholecystectomy in the ambulatory setting. J Post Anesthesia Nursing 1991; 6:33–39.

Ignatavicius D and Bayne M. Medical-surgical nursing: a nursing process approach. Philadelphia: WB Saunders, 1991.

Illustrated manual of nursing practice. 2nd ed. Springhouse, PA: Springhouse Corporation, 1994.

Levin DH. Introduction to surgery. 2nd ed. Philadelphia: WB Saunders, 1993.

Matthews K. Endoscopic cholecystectomy. Gastroenterology Nursing 1990; 13:13–17.

Morris P, Piper R, Reinke B, Young J. Outpatient carbon dioxide laser mastectomy. AORN Journal 1992; 55(4):984–992.

Musgrave C. Acute postoperative pain: the causes and the care. J Post Anesthesia Nursing 1990; 5:329–337.

Smith S, Duell D. Clinical nursing skills: nursing process model basic to advanced skills. 3rd ed. Appleton & Lange, Norwalk, CT: 1992.

Teplitz L. Update: are milking and stripping chest tubes necessary? Focus on Critical Care 1991; 18(6):506–511.

THE CLIENT WITH CANCER

About 85 million Americans now living, or about 30%, will be diagnosed as having cancer at some point during their lifetime. Over 8 million Americans alive today have a history of cancer, 5 million diagnosed 5 or more years ago. It will affect three out of four families. Cancer is second only to heart disease as the leading cause of death.

Though the incidence of cancer is not declining, treatment modalities are continually being improved. Except in the case of lung cancer, there has been a steady decline in the cancer mortality rate over the last decade. Now 4 of 10 cancer clients are alive 5 yr and longer after diagnosis. Many authorities consider the person cured if there is no evidence of disease 5 yr after the initial diagnosis.

11-1   HEALTH TEACHING FOR PREVENTION

Health officials now more than ever are stressing the importance of prevention. All health professionals must help educate the public about how to reduce the risk of cancer. The most important actions are:

- Avoid tobacco and alcohol and other known cancer-causing agents (see Section 11-2).

- Avoid obesity.

- Eat a balanced diet with foods low in fat, high in fiber, and high in vitamins and minerals. Eat cruciferous vegetables: broccoli, cabbage, brussels sprouts, and cauliflower. Avoid smoked foods, salt-cured or nitrite-cured foods (see also Chapter 8, Nutrition and Medical Nutrition Therapy).

- Avoid overexposure to the sun. Use a sunscreen of SPF > 15.

- Perform monthly self-examination for detection of breast and testicular cancer. Follow recommendations (Table 11-1) for other screening procedures.

- Know the seven warning signals of cancer and see a physician immediately if one occurs (Table 11-2).

11-2 CAUSES

Scientists are considering many theories in researching the causes of cancer. Two leading hypothesis related to cancer development are:

- Healthy cells are transformed into malignant cells upon exposure to causative agents

- Malignant cells are not destroyed as normal because of failure of the immune response

Carcinogenic Agents

Though the exact cause of cancer remains undetermined, certain agents are known to be carcinogenic. Carcinogenic agents are either chemical, viral, or associated with radiation exposure. Of these three, chemical agents have been found to be the most significant in the induction of human cancers (less than 1% of all cancers are attributable to radiation exposure).

TABLE 11–1. PROTOCOL FOR EARLY DETECTION OF CANCER IN ASYMPTOMATIC PERSONS

	RECOMMENDATION		
	SEX	**AGE/RISK**	**FREQUENCY**
Chest x-ray		Not recommended	
Sputum cytology		Not recommended	
Sigmoidoscopy	M&F	Over 50	Every 3–5 yr†
Stool guaiac slide test	M&F	Over 50	Every year
Digital rectal examination	M&F	Over 40	Every year
Pap test	F	20–40‡	Every 3 yr§
		Over 40	Every year
Pelvic examination	F	20–40	Every 3 yr
		Over 40	Every year
Endometrial tissue sample	F	At high risk ‖ Menopause	At menopause
Breast self-examination	F	Over 20	Every month
Breast physical examination	F	20–40	Every 3 yr
		Over 40	Every year
Mammography	F	Between 35–40	Baseline
		40–50	Every 1–2 yr
		Over 50	Every year
Health counseling and cancer checkup**	M&F	Over 20	Every 3 yr
	M&F	Over 40	Every year

†After two initial negative examinations a year apart.

‡Pap test should also be done on women under 20 who are sexually active.

§After two initial Pap tests done a year apart are negative.

‖ History of infertility, obesity, failure to ovulate, abnormal uterine bleeding, or estogren therapy.

**To include examination for cancers of the thyroid, testicles, prostate, ovaries, lymph nodes, oral region, and skin.

Data from Holleb AI et al. American Cancer Society Textbook of Clinical Oncology, ACS 1991 and Cancer Facts and Figures. Rochester, NY: American Cancer Society, 1993.

**TABLE 11–2. CANCER'S SEVEN
WARNING SIGNALS**

Change in bowel or bladder habits
A sore that does not heal
Unusual bleeding or discharge
Thickening or lump in breast or elsewhere
Indigestion or difficulty in swallowing
Obvious change in wart or mole
Nagging cough or hoarseness
If you have a warning signal, see your doctor!

Courtesy of the American Cancer Society, Rochester, NY.

Cigarette smoke and alcohol consumption are high on the list of those substances known to cause lung cancer and upper aerodigestive tract malignancies, such as oral cavity, oropharyngeal, laryngeal, and esophageal cancers. These agents are also associated with bladder cancer. Other chemical irritants include the industrial compounds asbestos, asphalt, vinyl chloride, ethylene oxide, uranium, chromium, nickel, and benzene. Also, air pollutants, water contaminants, and food additives such as nitrites, nitrosamines, and saccharine are all being carefully watched as potential carcinogens. Drugs have also been implicated, e.g., diethylstilbesterol (DES), certain chemotherapeutic agents, and immunosuppressive drugs.

Viral agents associated with the development of cancer include human papilloma virus (HPV) and Epstein-Barr virus (EBV) among others.

Predisposing Factors

Factors that contribute to the development of neoplasia include:

Age Incidence increases steadily after age 40.
Sex Women are more susceptible to breast cancer and cancer of the intestines. Men get more lung cancer and stomach cancer, however there is a steady increase in the

number of women being diagnosed with lung cancer. More men die of cancer than women.

Urban environment Cancer is more common in urban areas than rural.

Geographic location Some cancers are more prevalent in certain areas, e.g., stomach cancer is more prevalent in Japan than the United States.

Occupation Some occupations require greater exposure to carcinogens.

Familial susceptibility Evidence suggests that certain types of malignancies (breast cancer, malignant melanoma) run in families.

Precancerous lesions Pigmented moles, burn scars, senile keratosis, leukoplasia, benign adenomas, or polyps of the intestinal tract need to be carefully and periodically observed for malignant changes.

11-3 PATHOLOGY

Neoplasia is abnormal new growth of tissue that serves no purpose and can be highly damaging. Neoplasms are either benign or malignant and can arise from any body tissue (Table 11-3). Benign neoplastic cells are confined to a local area, do not tend to metastasize, and are usually treated with a local treatment such as surgery or radiation therapy. Malignant neoplastic cells grow rapidly, become invasive, impinge on healthy tissues, and cause widespread metabolic disturbances. Pathophysiologic changes include anemia, infection of the surface of the tumor, serous effusions, pain, and cachexia syndrome. How cancer affects an individual is influenced by the rate of tumor growth and the host's physiologic response. In many cancers, if the cancer is detected early, chances are strong the lesion will be localized; small localized lesions (<2 cm) are highly curable by current treatment methods. In advanced stages of malignancy, death typically results from metastasis to the brain, uremia from obstruction of ureters, uncontrolled hemorrhage, intestinal obstruction, obstruction of a bronchus, or pneumonia. See Table 11-4 for definitions of cancer terminology.

TABLE 11–3. COMPARISON OF BENIGN AND MALIGNANT NEOPLASMS

	BENIGN	**MALIGNANT**
Rate of growth	Slow	Rapid
Mode of growth	Does not infiltrate	Infiltrates into normal tissues, expands
Encapsulated	Usually	Rarely
Cell maturity	Well-differentiated, adult	Poorly differentiated, young, embryonic
Metastasis	Absent	Frequently present
Harmful to host	Only if impinging on vital organs	Always harmful to host, producing disrupted organ function, cachexia, nutritional imbalances, many other aberrations
Prognosis	Good	Dependent on when cancer is diagnosed

TABLE 11–4. GLOSSARY OF CANCER TERMS

Adjuvant chemotherapy: The use of drugs in addition to surgery and/or radiation to treat cancer.

Alopecia: Hair loss

Anemia: Low red blood cell count; symptoms include shortness of breath, lack of energy, and fatigue.

Anorexia: Absence or loss of appetite for food.

Antiemetic: A medicine that prevents or controls nausea/vomiting.

Benign: A tumor that is usually encapsulated, and does not infiltrate into surrounding tissues.

Biopsy: The removal and microscopic examination of living tissue for purposes of diagnosis.

Blood counts: The number of red blood cells, white cells, and platelets in a given sample of blood.

Bone marrow: The spongy inner tissue of a bone where red blood cells, white cells, and platelets are formed.

Cancer: A general name for over 100 diseases in which abnormal cells grow out of control; a malignant tumor.

Table continued on following page

TABLE 11–4. GLOSSARY OF CANCER TERMS
Continued

Carcinoma: A malignancy of epithelial origin.

Carcinoma in situ: An epithelial neoplasm that remains confined to site of origin, e.g., the cervix.

Dosimeter: A small device worn by nursing and radiation personnel to monitor their exposure to radiation while they provide direct care to clients.

Catheter: A tube used for injection or withdrawal of fluid.

Chemotherapy: The treatment of disease with anticancer drugs.

Combination chemotherapy: The use of several drugs at the same time or in a particular order to treat cancer.

Immunotherapy: Treatment by stimulation of the body's immune defense system. Immunotherapy as a treatment for cancer is still largely experimental.

Immunosuppressed: A condition that renders a person's immune system less able to fight infections.

Intramuscular (IM): Into a muscle; some anticancer drugs are given by IM injection.

Intravenous (IV): Into a vein; anticancer drugs are often given by IV injection or infusion.

Malignant: A nonencapsulated tumor made up of cancerous cells that infiltrates chaotically into surrounding tissues.

Metastasis: Action during which cancer cells break from their original site and spread through the body.

Neoplasm: Growth of new tissue.

Neutropenia: Low white blood cell count; symptoms include an increased susceptibility to infection.

Oncologist: A physician trained to treat clients who have cancer.

Palliative care: A treatment that may relieve symptoms without curing the disease.

Pathologist: A doctor who studies cells and tissues to determine if disease is present.

Platelets: A type of blood cell that helps the blood clot when a cut occurs. Clients with low platelet counts are at a somewhat increased risk for bleeding.

RAD (radiation absorbed dose): A unit of measurement of the absorbed radiation dose.

Radiation therapy: Cancer treatment with radiation (high energy rays).

Remission: The disappearance of signs and symptoms of disease.

Stomatitis: Sores on the inside lining of the mouth.

TABLE 11–4. GLOSSARY OF CANCER TERMS
Continued

Thrombocytopenia: Low platelet count; symptoms include inability to stop bleeding, increased bleeding and bruising.
Tumor: An abnormal growth of cells or tissues; tumors may be benign (noncancerous) or malignant (cancerous).

11-4 DIAGNOSIS, CLASSIFICATION, AND STAGING

When cancer is suspected, the client will have to have a thorough diagnostic workup, which could include any or several of the procedures explained in Chapter 4, Diagnostic Procedures. Proper preparation and emotional support from the nurse is essential for clients faced with this necessity.

An exploratory laparotomy or staging laparotomy may be performed in order to locate the primary tumor and determine the extent of its involvement. In addition to histologic determination of the type of cancer cell, tumors are staged and graded.

The stage of tumor growth refers to the maturity of the cancer cell and its differentiation. The International Classification System for Staging is as follows:

O = carcinoma in situ
I = limited to tumor
II = tumor with local lymph-node metastasis
III = tumor with metastasis beyond primary site or organ
IV = metastasis to distant body regions.

Though various specialty medical groups use different classification systems, the TNM (tumor, node, metastasis) system, developed jointly by the American Joint Committee for Cancer Staging and End Results Reporting (AJC) and the International Union Against Cancer (IUCC) in 1978 is an attempt at a consistent way of designating the extension of metastasis for many primary site tumors (Table 11-5). There are also staging and grading systems for specific can-

---

**TABLE 11–5. THE TNM SYSTEM: STAGING AND
GRADING CANCERS**

T = primary tumor **N** = regional lymph node involvement
M = distant metastases

Stage 1 T_1, N_0, M_0
Mass is limited to organ of origin. The lesion is operable and
resectable. Local involvement only with no nodal or vascular
spread.
Stage II T_2, N_1, M_0
Clinical evidence of local spread into surrounding tissue and
first-station lymph nodes. The lesion is operable and resectable
but completeness of removal is uncertain. The specimen shows
evidene of microinvasion into capsule and lymphatics.
Stage III T_3, N_2, M_0
Extensive primary tumor with fixation to deeper structures,
bone invasion, and lymph nodes of a similar nature. The lesion
is operable but not resectable and gross disease is left behind.
Stage IV T_4, N_3, M_+
Evidence of distant metastasis beyond the local site or organ.
The primary lesion is inoperable.

From Clinical oncology for medical students and physicians: a
multidisciplinary approach. 6th ed. Rochester, NY: University of
Rochester School of Medicine/Dentistry, American Cancer Society,
1983.

cers. Consult a source such as *The Cancer Manual* (8th
ed.), American Cancer Society, or *The Manual for Staging
of Cancer* (3rd ed.), American Joint Committee on Cancer,
for the staging systems for specific cancers.

Table 11-6 shows the 10 body systems and the types of
neoplasms that tend to arise within these systems.

11-5 CARE OF THE CLIENT WITH CANCER

The treatment plan for the client diagnosed with cancer
is individualized based on the type of cancer, the extent of
the disease, and the desires of the client and the family. The

Text continued on page 516

TABLE 11–6. NEOPLASMS CLASSIFIED BY BODY SYSTEMS

CIRCULATORY

Leukemias
  Acute
    Lymphoblastic (ALL)
    Myeloid (AMC)
  Chronic
    Lymphocytic (CLL)
    Myelocytic (CML)
    Hairy cell (HCL)
    Myelodysplastic syndrome
Lymphomas
  Hodgkin's disease
  Non-Hodgkin's lymphoma
    (NHL)
  Noncleaved-cell
    Burkitt's
    Mycosis fungoides
Plasma-cell dyscrasias
  Macroglobulinemia
  Primary systemic amyloidosis
  Heavy-chain diseases
  Multiple myeloma

RESPIRATORY

Primary bronchogenic
    carcinomas
  Squamous cell
  Undifferentiated small (oat)-
    cell
  Undifferentiated large-cell
  Adenocarcinoma
Other primary tumors
  Alveolar cell (bronchiolar)
  Bronchial adenoma
    (sometimes malignant)
  Chondromatous hamartoma
    (benign)
  Solitary lymphoma
  Sarcoma (malignant)

NERVOUS

Intracranial neoplasms
  Skull
    Osteoma
    Hemangioma
    Granuloma
    Xanthoma
    Osteitis
  Meninges
    Meningioma
    Sarcoma
    Gliomatosis
  Cranial nerves
    Glioma of optic nerve
    Schwannoma
  Supportive tissue
    Glioma
  Pituitary or pineal bodies
    Pituitary
      Chromophobic
      Acidophilic
      Basophilic
    Pinealoma
  Brain stem
    Glioma
  Neuroblastoma
  Congenital origin
    Craniopharyngioma
    Chordoma
    Germinoma
    Teratoma
    Dermoid cyst
    Angioma
    Hemangioblastoma
  Tumors of the cerebral
    hemisphere
    Locations
      Frontal lobe
      Parietal lobe
      Temporal lobe
      Occipital lobe
      Subcortical lobe
      Cranial
      Extradural
      Subdural
    Types
      Gliomas
        Glioblastoma

Table continued on following page

**TABLE 11–6. NEOPLASMS CLASSIFIED BY
BODY SYSTEMS** *Continued*

SKELETAL

Benign tumors
  Osteochondromas
  Chondromas
  Chondromyxofibromas
  Osteoid osteomas
  Chondroblastoma
  Giant-cell tumor
  Fibromatous lesions
Primary malignant tumors
  Osteogenic sarcoma
    (osteosarcoma)
  Fibrosarcomas
  Malignant fibrous histiocytoma
  Chondrosarcoma
  Mesenchymal chondrosarcoma
  Ewing's tumor
  Malignant lymphoma
    (marrow)
  Malignant giant-cell tumor

INTEGUMENTARY

Benign tumors
  Warts
  Sebaceous cysts
  Moles
  Dysplastic nevi
  Skin tags
  Angiomas
    Congenital hemangiomas
    Spider angiomas (vascular
      spider)
    Lymphangiomas
  Lipomas
  Pyrogenic granulomas
  Seborrheic keratoses
  Dermatofibroma (fibrous
    histiocytoma)
  Keratocanthoma
  Keloid
Malignant tumors
  Basal-cell carcinoma (rodent
    ulcer)
  Squamous-cell carcinoma
    (Bowen's disease)
  Malignant melanoma

EAR, NOSE, THROAT

Ear
  Sebaceous cysts
  Osteomas
  Keloids
  Ceruminomas
  Basal-cell and squamous-cell
    carcinomas
Nose
  Exophytic
  Inverted papillomas
  Fibromas
  Squamous cell carcinoma
Nasopharynx
  Juvenile angiofibroma
  Nasopharyngeal carcinoma
Larynx
  Polyps, nodules
  Juvenile papillomas
  Squamous-cell carcinoma
Oral cavity
  Epidemoid carcinoma
  Lymphoepithelioma
  Ameloblastoma
  Odontomas
  Squamous carcinoma of the
    tonsil

ENDOCRINE

Pituitary adenoma
  Chromophobic
  Acidophilic
  Basophilic
Thyroid
  Papillary
  Follicular
  Mixed
  Medullary
  Anaplastic
Adrenal
  Adenoma
  Adenocarcinoma
Parathyroid carcinoma
Pheochromocytoma
Multiple endocrine neoplasia
  Type I

TABLE 11–6. NEOPLASMS CLASSIFIED BY BODY SYSTEMS *Continued*

INTEGUMENTARY

Lentigo-malignant melanoma
Superficial spreading
melanoma
Nodular melanoma
Acrolentiginous melanoma
Paget's disease of the nipple
Mycosis fungoides
Kaposi's hemorrhagic sarcoma
(multiple idiopathic
hemorrhagic sarcoma)

GASTROINTESTINAL

Malignant neoplasms of the
stomach
Adenocarcinoma
Lymphoma
Leiomyosarcoma
Cancer of the pancreas
Nonendocrine tumors
Adenocarcinomas
Cystadenocarcinoma
Endocrine tumors
Nonfunctioning tumors
Functioning tumors
Insulinoma
Gastrinoma
Glucagonoma
Vipomas
Somatostatinoma
Neoplasms of the bowel
Benign tumors of the small
intestine
Leiomyomas
Lipomas
Neurofibromas
Fibromas
Polyps
Malignant tumors of the small
intestine
Adenocarcinoma
Primary malignant
lymphoma
Carcinoid tumors
Tumors of the large bowel
Polyps

ENDOCRINE

Type II
Type III
Carcinoid syndrome

REPRODUCTIVE

Breast tumors
Benign
Fibroepithelial tumors
Fibroadenomas
Cystosarcoma phyllodes
Lipomas
Fibrocystic disease
Intraductal papillomas
Carcinoma of the breast
Inflammatory carcinoma
Lobular
Scirrhous
Infiltrative
Papillary
Ductal
Paget's disease
Male reproductive malignancies
Prostate tumors
Adenocarcinoma
Sarcoma
Carcinoma of the penis
Testicular tumors
Benign
Malignant
Gynecologic neoplasms
Endometrial carcinoma
Cervical carcinoma
Invasive squamous cell
carcinoma
Carcinoma in situ
Ovarian carcinoma
Carcinoma of the vulva
Vaginal carcinoma
Carcinoma of the fallopian
tube
Trophoblastic disease
(hydatidiform mole,
chorioadenoma
destruens,
choriocarcinoma)

Table continued on following page

**TABLE 11–6. NEOPLASMS CLASSIFIED BY
BODY SYSTEMS** *Continued*

GASTROINTESTINAL

Familial polyposis
Other polyps
Cancer of the colon
Cancer of the rectum
Squamous cell carcinoma of
the anus

URINARY

Kidney neoplasms	Malignancies
Tubulointerstitial disease	Of the renal pelvis
Wilm's tumor	Of the ureter
(nephroblastoma)	Of the urinary bladder
Carcinoma of the kidney	Carcinoma of the urethra
(adenocarcinoma,	
hypernephroma)	

Data from Berkow R et al. The merck manual of diagnosis and therapy. 16th ed. Rahway, NJ: Merck, Sharp & Dohme Research Laboratories, 1992.

goals of cancer treatment include cure, control, or palliation.

Surgery is still the primary form of treatment in many types of cancer, particularly those arising from tissue with a slow rate of cellular replication (Table 11-7). Radiation treatments are received by over 50% of clients diagnosed as having cancer. Chemotherapy is used to cure acute lymphocytic leukemia (in children), Hodgkin's disease, Burkitt's lymphoma, Wilms' tumor, and neuroblastoma; and to control breast cancer, oat-cell carcinoma of the lung, gastrointestinal cancer, and other cancers. Immunotherapy is used as an adjuvant therapy with surgery, radiation, or chemotherapy.

Nursing care corresponds to the medical treatment program being administered, but must also attend to needs that are similar for all cancer clients. Using the nursing process, nurses will be able to determine unmet needs and help clients to meet them. The following are some of the

TABLE 11–7. TREATMENT MODALITIES USED IN CANCER

Initial treatment of localized (Stage I or II) disease, not advanced or metastatic cancer

ORIGINAL CANCER	SUR-GERY	RADIO-THERAPY	CHEMO-THERAPY	IMMUNO-THERAPY	HOR-MONE
Head and neck	P	P	Adj.,E	ND	
Brain	P	Adj.	Adj.	E	
Lung					
Small (oat)-cell	Alt.*	Adj.E	P	E	
Adenocar-cinoma	P	Adj.	Adj.E	E	
Hodgkin's disease					
Stage I	NU	P	Alt.	ND	
Stage III	NU	Alt.	P	ND	
Melanoma					
Stage I	P	E	E	NU	
Breast (stage I)	P	Alt.	E	ND	Adj.
Ovary (stage I)	P	Adj.E	E	ND	
Uterine cervix					
In situ	P	Alt.	NU	NU	
Stage II	P	P	E	ND	
Colon	P	Adj.	Adj.,E	E	
Stomach	P	NU	Adj.,E	ND	
Kidney	P	Adj.	NU	NU	NU
Prostate	P	Adj.	NU	ND	
Testes					
Seminoma (stage I)	P	P	NU	ND	

P = primary form of treatment;

Alt. = alternate, though less commonly used, method of primary treatment;

Adj. = used as an adjunctive therapy after localized tumor is treated by a primary method; routine use not considered essential;

E = experimental role in treatment is being evaluated in controlled clinical trials;

Alt.E = an older approach that, in the absence of sufficient data to support its frequent use, is being evaluated in controlled clinical trials;

NU = not used in primary treatment program; control rate of tumor with other modalities may be high enough that testing is not warranted;

ND = no data is available to evaluate this form of treatment.

*For limited Stage I or II only.

Data from Braunwauld E et al., eds. Harrison's principles of internal medicine. 12th ed. New York: McGraw-Hill, 1991.

major problems in cancer (see also Table 11-8 and specific problems in Chapter 2.)

Inadequate nutrition (cancer has been called a nutritional disease). This is true not only because of gastrointestinal neoplasms, advanced malignancy, and cachexia syndrome, but because the three main treatment methods (surgery, radiation, and chemotherapy) all can potentially cause nausea, vomiting, and/or other GI disturbances.

Fluid and electrolyte imbalances (see Chapter 5)

Immobility (see Impaired Physical Mobility, Section 2-11)

Pain with advanced cancer If pain is present it tends to be continuous and chronic. (See Pain, Section 2-3.)

Side effects of radiation and/or chemotherapy (see Table 11-8)

Psychosocial and emotional adjustment (see end of this section)

I. **Surgery.** The primary treatment for cancer is sometimes combined with the other treatment modalities for the most beneficial therapeutic effect. Refer to Chapter 10 for a brief review of principles of preoperative and postoperative care and selected types of surgeries.

II. **Radiation therapy.** The emission of tiny particles or waves of energy from radioactive sources to effect physical and chemical changes within cells. It may be administered externally (teletherapy) or internally (brachytherapy). The route of administration will depend on the cell type, location, size and age of the cancer, the client being treated, and the current thinking regarding the most effective treatment plan for the specific cancer.

A. **External radiation therapy**

Nursing interventions:

- Help prepare client by collaborating with physician on treatment plan and reinforcing explanations as to what client can expect. Explain that receiving external radiation treatments is painless and similar to having x-rays taken.

Text continued on page 527

TABLE 11–8. PROBLEMS ASSOCIATED WITH CANCER

PROBLEM	EXPECTED OUTCOME	NURSING INTERVENTIONS
Anorexia and Weight Loss	Maintenance or improvement of adequate intake and body weight	• See Altered Nutrition: Less than Body Requirements Related to Anorexia, Section 2-4, and Potential for Fluid Volume Deficit Related to Nausea and Vomiting, Section 2-5 • Stress nonspicy, high protein foods. • Assess for and treat stomatitis if present. • Assess for alteration in taste sensation. • Encourage intake, but do not nag. • Allow sufficient time for meals.
Nausea and Vomiting	Decreased symptoms; adequate intake	• See Potential for Fluid Volume Deficit Related to Nausea and Vomiting, Section 2-4, for control of symptoms. • Give antiemetics routinely q 4–6 hr as well as right before chemotherapy.

Table continued on following page

TABLE 11–8. PROBLEMS ASSOCIATED WITH CANCER *Continued*

PROBLEM	EXPECTED OUTCOME	NURSING INTERVENTIONS
		• Use relaxation techniques (see Stress Reduction, Section 12-3)
Stomatitis, Mucositis, Mouth	Integrity of mucous membranes; no infections	• Assess oral mucosa every day. Teach client to inspect oral cavity. Look for small oral ulcers, breaks in tissue integrity.
		• Maintain good oral hygiene. Use mouthwashes of baking soda, normal saline, or elixir of Benadryl every 2 hr. Use soft toothbrushes, toothettes, or an irrigating syringe to cleanse. Do not use lemon glycerine swabs.
		• Apply topical anesthetics such as viscous xylocaine, chloraseptic prior to meals to reduce discomfort.
		• Encourage water or other liquid intake frequently throughout the

TABLE 11–8. PROBLEMS ASSOCIATED WITH CANCER *Continued*

PROBLEM	EXPECTED OUTCOME	NURSING INTERVENTIONS
		day. Popsicles give moisture and numbness to the mouth while providing needed calories. • Moisten lips with petroleum jelly, baby oil, or cocoa butter.
Diarrhea	Normal bowel elimination	• See Diarrhea, Section 2-6.
Chronic Pain	Maintain maximal level of mental and physical functioning. Gain control of pain.	• Discuss pain control methods with physician and develop alternatives based on efficacy of therapies. • Create a calm environment, which will help the client relax. • Move, touch, and talk to the client calmly and gently. • Assess client's pain level on "0–10" scale at routine intervals. • Notify physician if analgesics lose their effectiveness (usual analgesics ordered

Table continued on following page

TABLE 11–8. PROBLEMS ASSOCIATED WITH CANCER *Continued*

PROBLEM	EXPECTED OUTCOME	NURSING INTERVENTIONS
		include oral analgesics, IV morphine sulfate, Brompton's cocktail, and methadone. Compazine or thorazine are frequently given with analgesics to potentiate their action). • Continuous intraspinal or IV morphine infusion therapy may be considered for intractable cancer pain. • See Pain, Section 2-3.
Fatigue	Undertand the causes of fatigue. Make adjustments to obtain the needed rest.	• Inform the client that fatigue occurs as an expected adjunct of therapy. It usually begins during the first week of therapy, reaches its peak in 2 wk, and subsides 2–4 wk after therapy has ended. • Encourage the client to rest when needed. Help maintain activity level in

**TABLE 11–8. PROBLEMS ASSOCIATED WITH
CANCER** *Continued*

PROBLEM	EXPECTED OUTCOME	NURSING INTERVENTIONS
		accordance with energy level. Preserve usual lifestyle patterns as much as possible.
		• Encourage high fluid intake (3000 ml/day), unless contraindicated, and high nutritional status.
Alopecia	Cope with hair loss. Maintain usual lifestyle pattern.	• Provide psychological support. Inform client of expected hair loss.
		• Encourage client to select a wig, scarf, or turban before time of hair loss and if client is interested, to wear it before time of hair loss.
		• Use mild shampoo and hair conditioner every 4–7 days. Avoid excessive shampooing or brushing of hair. Dry shampoo can be used.
Anemia	Blood counts normal, adequate oxy-	• Attend to nutritional needs.

Table continued on following page

TABLE 11–8. PROBLEMS ASSOCIATED WITH CANCER *Continued*

PROBLEM	EXPECTED OUTCOME	NURSING INTERVENTIONS
	genation of tissues.	Intervene as needed for anorexia, nausea, and vomiting as listed above.
		• Intervene for fatigue as listed above.
		• Protect from infection (good handwashing, seclusion from infected persons, oral temp. q 4 hr)
		• Prevent complications of immobility (see Impaired Physical Mobility, Section 2-11).
		• Administer blood products as needed (see Blood Transfusions, Section 6-7).
		• Closely monitor lab reports—complete blood count, blood studies.
Leukopenia	White-cell count normal; no signs of infection	• Private room, isolation precautions. Limit visitors.
		• Good handwashing technique

TABLE 11–8. PROBLEMS ASSOCIATED WITH CANCER *Continued*

PROBLEM	EXPECTED OUTCOME	NURSING INTERVENTIONS
		with antiseptic solution.
		• Restrict fresh fruits and vegetables and plants. Food must be cooked, pasteurized, or sterilized.
		• Maintain skin integrity. Reduce number of venipunctures. Avoid IV catheters and other invasive procedures if at all possible.
		• Take all actions to prevent skin breakdown (see Impaired Physical Mobility, Section 2-11).
		• Maintain scrupulous perianal care. Diarrhea and constipation can irritate bowel mucosa and perianal tissues.
		• Recognize signs of developing infection, especially fever.
		• Assess all complaints. Routinely assess mouth for infection.

Table continued on following page

TABLE 11–8. PROBLEMS ASSOCIATED WITH CANCER *Continued*

PROBLEM	EXPECTED OUTCOME	NURSING INTERVENTIONS
		• Assess vital signs q 3 hr. Report temp. >38°C. Give acetaminophen, not aspirin as antipyretic, only if ordered. • Encourage high fluid intake— 3000 ml/day.
Thrombocytopenia	Platelet count normal; not evidence of bleeding	• Protect against injury that could lead to hemorrhage. Handle client very gently. Reduce BP monitoring and alternate extremities. • Avoid venipunctures, intramuscular and subcutaneous medications as much as possible. • Do not administer aspirin. • Assess for blood loss via epistaxis, petechiae, ecchymoses. Test all body excreta and secretions for occult blood. • Evaluate complete blood count and platelet counts.

TABLE 11–8. PROBLEMS ASSOCIATED WITH CANCER *Continued*

PROBLEM	EXPECTED OUTCOME	NURSING INTERVENTIONS
		• Use ice and direct pressure to control active bleeding.
		• Administer platelets as ordered (see Table 6-10, Platelets).

- Teach client to avoid sun, as skin is especially prone to severe sunburn during radiation therapy.

- If lying immobile on the hard, flat, treatment table will cause the client discomfort or pain, administer pain medications 1 hr before treatment to assure comfort.

- *See that marks applied by radiologist are not removed between treatments.*

- Assess for problems listed in Table 11-8 and carry out nursing interventions as needed.

- Observe skin in area of radiotherapy for redness, desquamation, or telangiectasis (hyperemic spot similar to a birthmark) and notify physician if present.

- Teach client to provide gentle skin care to affected area. Use only water to cleanse. Avoid powder, lotions, and ointments unless prescribed. Avoid shaving or rubbing the area.

- Observe lab data for bone-marrow depression.

B. **Internal radiation implants** are placed within a particular body cavity in the operating room and usually remain in place for 24–72 hr. Special precautions must be taken.

Nursing interventions:

- Place the client in a private lead-lined room, preferably at the farthest end of the hall, adjacent to an empty room, and away from clients of childbearing age.

- Post "Radiation precaution" sign.

- Prevent pregnant women and people under age 18 from being in the same room as client.

- Limit time spent in the room by nurses and visitors according to physician and hospital policy.

- All health personnel caring directly for these clients must *wear a dosimeter* to monitor radiation exposure.

- Maintain as much distance as possible from the site. Limit time spent in close proximity to the source. Utilize lead shield as much as possible when dealing with client.

- Keep a sealed lead-lined container in the client's room at all times for immediate use in the event of a dislodgement. The radiation source should be picked up with a pair of long-handled forceps or tongs and placed in the lead container. *Never pick it up with bare hands or place it in the sewage system via the sink or toilet.*

III. **Chemotherapy.** The use of drugs to destroy cancer cells with the goal of minimal toxicity to healthy cells. The goals of treatment may be cure, control, palliation, and/or prevention of recurrence. The medications may be administered intravenously, intra-arterially, intramuscularly, intraperitoneally, intrathecally (into the cerebrospinal fluid by lumbar puncture or through an Omaya reservoir), intracavitarily (directly into a cavity, such as the bladder), subcutaneously, orally, topically, or with an implantable infusion device.

Nursing interventions:

- Be aware of side effects and problems which can be severe with these drugs. Know all the effects of the specific drug you are giving by referring to the package insert or the PDR. Some of the major problems to be anticipated are listed in Tables 11-8, 11-9 and 11-10. Prepare client accordingly, i.e., for alopecia, neutropenia, stomatitis, and other side effects but reassure that side effects are temporary.

- Monitor lab reports for electrolyte imbalance, thrombocytopenia, leukopenia, anemia. Notify the physician of all abnormalities.

- Protect client from bleeding.

- Protect client from infection. Require that all people entering client room be infection-free (no colds, flus, or other communicable diseases) and that they wash their hands.

- Monitor intake and output.

- Ensure IV medication compatibility before administering multiple IV piggybacks (see Parenteral Drug Administration, Section 7-3). Flush IV line prior to readministration.

- Be knowledgeable and trained in extravasation management technique and have antidotes and extravasation tray readily available. Be prepared to administer antidotes to particular drugs as appropriate (See Section 7-3).

- Use only a patent, infection-free IV line. Avoid veins in the hands and the antecubital space if possible (extravasation into these areas could cause loss of function).

- Leave the insertion site exposed so that you can observe it continuously for signs of extravasation. Stabilize the catheter with one or two V-shaped patches of tape below the insertion site.

- Protect yourself from the hazards of anticancer drugs. Wear gloves and a barrier gown when dealing with chemotherapy. If your skin does come in

Text continued on page 538

TABLE 11–9. ADVERSE REACTIONS TO COMMONLY USED INTRAVENOUS CHEMOTHERAPY DRUGS

ALKYLATING AGENTS

Carmustine (BCNU, BiCNU):
  Nausea and vomiting
  Facial flushing
  Pain at injection site on administration
  Bone marrow depression
  Hyperpigmentation
  Hepatotoxicity
  Skin necrosis
  Pulmonary fibrosis
  Stomatitis
Cisplatin (Platinol):
  Severe nausea and vomiting
  Nephrotoxicity
  Ototoxicity
  Hyperuricemia
  Bone marrow depression
  Neurotoxicity
  Abnormal liver function
  Cardiac toxicity
  Hypocalcemia
  Hypokalemia
  Hypomagnesemia
  Anaphylaxis-like reactions
Cyclophosphamide (Cytoxan, Endoxan):
  Nausea and vomiting
  Alopecia (reversible)
  Hemorrhagic cystitis
  Metallic taste
  Leukopenia
  Cardiotoxicity
Decarbazine (DTIC Dome):
  Nausea and vomiting
  Facial flushing
  Pain at injection site on administration
  Tissue damage and severe pain with infiltration
  Bone marrow depression
  Flu-like syndrome
  Alopecia
  Metallic taste
  Elevated liver enzyme levels

**TABLE 11–9. ADVERSE REACTIONS TO
COMMONLY USED INTRAVENOUS
CHEMOTHERAPY DRUGS** *Continued*

ALKYLATING AGENTS

Mechlorethamine (Mustargen, nitrogen mustard):
Severe nausea and vomiting
Skin necrosis
Diarrhea
Anorexia
Myelosuppression
Alopecia
Thrombophlebitis
Sperm depression
Streptozocin (Zanosar):
Nausea and vomiting
Nephrotoxicity
Hepatotoxicity
Diarrhea
Bone marrow depression
Skin necrosis
Anorexia
Sudden hypoglycemia
Thiotepa:
Pain at injection site on administration
Nausea and vomiting
Myelosupression

ANTIMETABOLITES

Cytarabine (Cytosar-U):
Bone marrow depression
Nausea and vomiting
Alopecia
Stomatitis
Hepatic dysfunction
Neurotoxicity
Fluorouracil (5-FU, Adrucil):
Bone marrow depression
Nausea and vomiting
Diarrhea
Stomatitis
Gastrointestinal (GI) ulceration
Photosensitivity
Hyperpigmentation

Table continued on following page

TABLE 11–9. ADVERSE REACTIONS TO COMMONLY USED INTRAVENOUS CHEMOTHERAPY DRUGS *Continued*

ANTIMETABOLITES

Methotrexate (MTX, amethopterin, Mexate):
 Bone marrow depression
 Stomatitis
 GI ulceration
 Nausea and vomiting
 Diarrhea
 Menopausal symptoms
 Photosensitivity
 Hepatic dysfunction
 Nephrotoxicity with high dose

ANTIBIOTIC ANTINEOPLASTIC AGENTS

Actinomycin (Cosmegen, Lyovac Cosmegen):
 Severe nausea and vomiting
 Bone marrow depression
 Alopecia
 Stomatitis
 Occasional skin eruptions: radiation recall, skin erythema,
  hyperpigmentation
 Photosensitivity
 Skin necrosis
 Diarrhea
Bleomycin (Blenoxane):
 Nausea and vomiting
 Pulmonary fibrosis
 Interstitial pneumonitis
 Skin lesions, desquamation of hands and feet, ridging of nails,
  and so forth
 Potential anaphylaxis
Daunorubicin (Daunomycin, Cerubidine, Cerubidin):
 Cardiac toxicity: both transient (tachycardia,
  electrocardiogram changes) and delayed (cardiomyopathy
  and congestive heart failure)
 Bone marrow depression
 Nausea and vomiting
 Fever
 Alopecia
 Diarrhea
 Skin necrosis

**TABLE 11–9. ADVERSE REACTIONS TO
COMMONLY USED INTRAVENOUS
CHEMOTHERAPY DRUGS** *Continued*

ANTIBIOTIC ANTINEOPLASTIC AGENTS

Radiation recall
Doxorubicin (Adriamycin):
Radiation recall
Nausea and vomiting
Alopecia
Stomatitis and mouth ulcers
Bone marrow depression
Cardiac toxicity: both transient (tachycardia,
    electrocardiogram changes) and delayed (cardiomyopathy
    and congestive heart failure)
Skin necrosis
Diarrhea
Thrombophlebitis at injection site
Vein discoloration
Discoloration of urine (pink)
Mithramycin (Mithracin):
Nausea and vomiting
Fever
Alopecia
Stomatitis
Hyperpigmentation
Bone marrow depression
Tendency to bleed
Mitomycin C (Mutamycin):
Nausea and vomiting
Anorexia
Bone marrow depression
Diarrhea
Thrombophlebitis at injection site
Skin necrosis
Alopecia
Microangiopathic hemolytic anemia (after long-term
    therapy: 6–12 mo)

VINCA ALKALOIDS

Vinblastine (VLB, Velban, Velbe):
Nausea and vomiting
Constipation

Table continued on following page

**TABLE 11–9. ADVERSE REACTIONS TO
COMMONLY USED INTRAVENOUS
CHEMOTHERAPY DRUGS** *Continued*

VINCA ALKALOIDS

Peripheral neuropathies
Stomatitis
Bone marrow depression
Alopecia
Skin necrosis

Vincristine (VCR, Oncovin):

Constipation
Peripheral neuropathies
Alopecia
Nausea and vomiting
Intestinal necrosis
Muscle weakness and cramps
Skin necrosis
Red blood cell depression

MISCELLANEOUS AGENTS

Etoposide (VP-16):

Nausea and vomiting
Alopecia
Myelosuppression
Skin necrosis
Severe hypotension

L-Asparaginase (Elspar, Leunase):

Nausea and vomiting
Fever
Hypersensitivity reactions
Confusion
Hypatotoxicity
Potential anaphylaxis

Data from Petton S. Easing the complications of chemotherapy.
Nursing '84 1984; February, p. 80. and Nursing '94 Drug Handbook,
Springhouse, PA: Springhouse Corp., 1994.

TABLE 11–10. ADVERSE REACTIONS TO COMMONLY USED ORAL CHEMOTHERAPY DRUGS

ALKYLATING AGENTS

Busulfan (Myleran):
Interstitial pulmonary fibrosis
Bone marrow depression (mostly white blood cells)
Sterility
Fetal death
Nausea and vomiting

Chlorambucil (Leukeran):
Bone marrow depression
Nausea and vomiting (especially with high dosages)
Alopecia
Nephrotoxicity
Stomatitis
Diarrhea
Hepatotoxicity

Cyclophosphamide (Cytoxan, Endoxan):
Hemorrhagic cystitis
Bone marrow depression
Diarrhea
Anorexia
Stomatitis
Alopecia
Nasal congestion
Headache
Nausea and vomiting
Liver dysfunction
Metallic taste
Birth defects (if taken during pregnancy)

Lomustine (CeeNU):
Bone marrow depression
Nausea and vomiting
Anorexia
Stomatitis
Alopecia
Hepatotoxicity

Melphalan (Alkeran):
Bone marrow depression
Nausea and vomiting
Hair thinning
Pulmonary fibrosis

Table continued on following page

**TABLE 11–10. ADVERSE REACTIONS TO
COMMONLY USED ORAL CHEMOTHERAPY
DRUGS** *Continued*

ALKYLATING AGENTS

Hydroxyurea (Hydrea):
  Bone marrow depression
  Drowsiness
  Anorexia
  Stomatitis
  Alopecia
  Dermatitis
Mercaptopurine (Purinethol):
  Bone marrow depression
  Hepatotoxicity
  Nausea and vomiting
  Anorexia
  Diarrhea
  Stomatitis
Methotrexate (Amethopterin, Mexate):
  Bone marrow depression
  Nausea and vomiting
  Alopecia
  Menopausal symptoms
  Nephrotoxicity
  Stomatitis
  Diarrhea
  Hepatotoxicity
Thioguanine (6-TG, 6-Thioguanine, Lanvis):
  Bone marrow depression
  Anorexia
  Diarrhea
  Nausea and vomiting
  Stomatitis
  Hepatotoxicity

HORMONAL AGENTS

Chlorotrianisene (Tace):
  Nausea and vomiting
  Fluid retention
  Tender breasts (women only)
  Increased serum calcium
  Uterine bleeding
  Gynecomastia

TABLE 11–10. ADVERSE REACTIONS TO COMMONLY USED ORAL CHEMOTHERAPY DRUGS *Continued*

HORMONAL AGENTS

Diethylstilbestrol (DES, Stilboestrol, Stibilium):
  Nausea and vomiting
  Fluid retention
  Tender breasts (women only)
  Increased serum calcium
  Uterine bleeding
  Gynecomastia
Fluoxymesterone (Halotestin):
  Lowering of voice
  Hair growth
  Fluid retention
  Nausea and vomiting
  Liver damage
  Jaundice
Megestrol Acetate (Megace):
  Hypercalcemia (in patients with breast cancer and bony
    metastases)
  Minimal fluid retention
Prednisone (Deltasone):
  Behavior changes
  Epigastric distress
  Fluid and sodium retention
  Hypertension
  Osteoporosis
  Increased susceptibility to infections
  Prolonged or delayed healing
  Body changes: moon face, purpura, abdominal striae, acne,
    truncal obesity, buffalo hump (with long-term use)
Tamoxifen (Nolvadex):
  Headache
  Dizziness
  Nausea and vomiting
  Vaginal bleeding
  Menopausal symptoms (hot flashes)
  Light-headedness
  Mild leukopenia and thrombocytopenia
  Menstrual irregularies
  Hypercalcemia

Data from Petton S. Easing the complications of chemotherpy. Nursing '84 1984; February, p. 80. and Loeb S et al. Nursing '94, Drug Handbook. Springhouse, PA: Springhouse Corp., 1994.

contact with anticancer drugs, wash area immediately with water for 5–10 min.

- Be aware that for 48 hrs after chemotherapy drug administration, all blood and body fluids are considered cytotoxic and appropriate precautions should be taken (i.e., gown and gloves).

- Bag and label used chemotherapy bottles, tubing, and linen per hospital policy (usually the same as those for infective materials).

- Flush IV line with 50–100 ml of plain solution after giving entire dose of medication.

- Carefully observe client and thoroughly document client's treatment experience.

IV. **Immunotherapy.** Usually given in combination with other treatments to bolster the immune response. Some species of genetically engineered substances such as Interferon have had appreciable antitumor effects against tumors and some malignancies. Monoclonal antibodies have provided another major approach for the treatment of metastatic cancer. Because it is still in the experimental stage, nursing assessment and observation is of major importance in caring for cancer clients undergoing treatment. Observe particularly for allergic reaction: fever, urticaria, shortness of breath, dyspnea, swelling of lymph nodes, malaise, local abscess. Also be alert for signs of infection and general changes in client condition. Be very familiar with all related drug information including indications, side effects, and dosages before administering this type of therapy.

V. **Psychosocial adjustment to cancer.** Helping the cancer client cope with the illness as positively as possible is one of the most challenging aspects of nursing care. Psychological support from the health care team is essential in bringing about desired results of treatment. The client with newly diagnosed cancer may experience the various stages of grieving: denial, anger, bargaining, depression, and finally acceptance (see Grieving, Section 12-7). Fear of pain, bodily mutilation, dependency, and death may arise and the client must be supported through these fears.

Nursing interventions:

- Be available to listen to client and family members. Recognize that they may not be ready to express feelings at certain times and may need to at other times. Recognize the stages of grieving.

- Use good communication techniques (see Communication and the Therapeutic Relationship, Section 12-1) including active listening, paraphrasing, nonverbal communication, etc.

- Prepare client for treatment programs so that they know what may be expected and feel a measure of control.

- Include client, family, and all members of the health care team in all aspects of the health care plan.

- Be available to answer questions posed by the client or family, and clarify misconceptions about disease process, treatment, etc. Answer questions honestly and acknowledge that at times we do not have "adequate" answers to their questions.

- Help the client preserve normal lifestyle patterns as much as possible.

- Help the client think of cancer as a chronic illness as opposed to a terminal one.

- Involve social services, chaplaincy and/or psychologist as needed.

- Refer family and client to hospital and community support groups when possible.

- Refer client to American Cancer Society and local agencies for client's specific type of cancer.

REFERENCES

Braunwald E et al., eds. Harrison's principles of internal medicine. 12th ed. New York: McGraw-Hill, 1991.

Cancer facts and figures. Rochester, NY: American Cancer Society, 1993.

Cancer Manual. 8th ed. Boston: American Cancer Society, 1990.

Crosely M. Watch out for the nutritional complications of cancer. RN 1985;46:22–27.

Gregory-Addesa G. Helping your patient when nausea goes with the treatment. RN 1986; April: 43–44.

Groenwald SL, Frogge MH, Goodman M, Yarbro CH, eds. Comprehensive cancer nursing review. Boston: Jones and Bartlett Publishers, 1992.

Haskell CM. Cancer treatment. Philadelphia: WB Saunders, 1990.

Holleb AI, Fink DJ, Murphy GP, eds. American Cancer Society textbook of clinical oncology. Atlanta, GA: American Cancer Society, 1991.

Kushner R. If you've thought about breast cancer. Kensington, MD: Women's Breast Cancer Advisory Center, 1985.

LaFond RE, ed. Cancer: the outlaw cell. Washington, D.C.: American Chemical Society, 1988.

Loeb S et al. Drug handbook, Nursing '94. Springhouse, PA: Springhouse Corp., 1994.

Pageau MG et al. New analgesic therapy relieves cancer pain without oversedation. Nursing 85 1985; April: 46–49.

Petton S. Easing the complications of chemotherapy. Nursing 84 1984; February: 58–62.

Rubin P et al. Clinical oncology for medical students and physicians: a multidisciplinary approach. 6th ed. Rochester, NY: The American Cancer Society, 1983.

Suppers VJ, McClamrock EA. Biologicals in cancer treatment: future effects on nursing practice. Oncol Nurs Forum 1985; 12:27–31.

What foods may reduce your cancer risk? Rochester, NY: American Cancer Society, 1985.

PSYCHOSOCIAL CONSIDERATIONS IN CLIENT CARE

Because nursing focuses on client response to illness, psychosocial and emotional considerations are of prime importance in assessing client health and well-being. Because of their close interrelatedness, physiological states can affect mental function, and emotional states can produce physiologic symptoms. The goal in nursing is always to

---

*NANDA approved nursing diagnosis

restore the system that is malfunctioning and increase the client's self-care abilities.

Stress is almost always a factor in major illness. Anxiety and depression are very common and can be primary states or secondary to many diseases. Grief is a normal response that almost always accompanies illness and loss. Much progress has been made in the understanding of these and other biopsychosocial phenomenon in recent years. Health professionals must keep abreast of new knowledge and scientific developments (such as new chemotherapeutic treatments), which assist in better management of these and related nursing challenges.

Along with the stress response and the common reactions of anxiety, depression, and grief, the nurse must be readily familiar with the major psychiatric disorders as classified by the American Psychiatric Association, and the most commonly used psychotropic medications. The nurse must be able to recognize and describe clearly abnormal or bizarre behavior (Table 12-1). Table 12-2 briefly reviews the characteristics of the major disorders along with examples and treatment. Table 12-3 lists commonly used psychotropic medications with recommended dosages. Table 12-4 lists the defense mechanisms that normally function to facilitate coping with stress.

The nursing diagnoses and other problems in this chapter are encountered frequently in general nursing practice. The assessment, treatment, and education of the client experiencing mental/emotional difficulties are primary nursing responsibilities.

12-1 COMMUNICATION AND THE THERAPEUTIC RELATIONSHIP

The basic principles of therapeutic communication are described below.

Establish Trust

- Offer client clear understanding of the purpose of nurse-client relationship.

- Be consistent, reliable, and open. Be available.

TABLE 12–1. PSYCHIATRIC DEFINITIONS

Observing and describing the behavior of the client is one of the most essential parts of psychiatric assessment. Watch for the following:

Motor Behaviors

Automatism—unconsciously controlled, automatic, undirected motor activity

Catalepsy—a trance-like state with diminished responsiveness and loss of voluntary motion

Catatonic stupor—extreme underactivity

Choreiform movements—irregular, involuntary actions of muscles of face and extremities

Compulsion—undesirable urge to perform repetitive actions

Hyperkinesia—abnormally increased motor activity

Psychomotor retardation—decreased, slowed activity

Speech Patterns

Aphasia—partial or total loss of the ability to express self through language

Echolalia—Repetitive imitation of another's speech

Mutism—inability or refusal to speak

Rhyming—interjecting rhyming words at the ends of phrases or sentences as in poetry

Verbigeration—repetitive, meaningless expression of sentences, phrases, or words

Perceptions

Illusion—misinterpretation of actual sensory stimuli by the senses

Hallucination—sensory perceptions for which there are no external stimuli

Thought Processes and Content

Blocking—obstruction to thought or memory, frequently produced by strong emotion

Circumstantiality—detailed, incidental material that has no significance to the central idea

Condensation—reducing several ideas into one symbol

Delusion—a false belief kept despite nonsupportive evidence

Hypochondriasis—morbid concern over one's health and feeling ill with no medical basis

Ideas of reference—the incorrect belief that others' words and actions refer to one's self

Flight of ideas—rapid conversation with logically unconnected shifting of topics

Neologisms—using new or made up expressions, phrases, or words instead of accepted ones

Obsession—persistent, unwanted, recurring thought

TABLE 12–1. PSYCHIATRIC DEFINITIONS
Continued

Phobia—a strong, persistent, abnormal fear of a situation or object

Perseveration—pathologic repetition of a sentence, phrase, or word

Poverty of ideas—cliches and set phrases repeated

Word salad—sentences, phrases, and words combined in a disconnected and incoherent fashion

Emotional (Affective) State

Ambivalence—the existence of two opposing emotions at the same time

Anxiety—apprehensive, uneasy feeling not based on external stimuli

Blunting—loss of affective capacity

Depersonalization—feeling unreal about oneself or the environment

Ecstasy—an overpowering feeling of joy and rapture

Elation—a high degree of confidence, boastfulness, uncritical optimism, and joy

Euphoria—excessive feeling of emotional and physical well-being inappropriate for actual environmental stimuli

Fear—apprehensive, uneasy feeling related to a known source of danger, usually externally based

Flat affect—less than normal expression of feelings

Lability—quick changing expression of mood or feelings

Rage—furious, uncontrolled anger

- Demonstrate interest in and commitment to client over a period of time.

- Listen to the client in a way that encourages expression of whatever feelings he or she has.

- Convey acceptance and understanding.

Employ Specific Techniques to Facilitate Communication, Healing, and Growth

ACTIVE LISTENING

The most important aspect of active listening is paying very close attention to the client. As someone else listens empathetically to their feelings, the client can slowly

TABLE 12–2. MAJOR PSYCHIATRIC DISORDERS (DSM IV-R)

These disorders are among those most likely to be encountered in the general hospital.

CATEGORY	MAJOR CHARAC- TERISTIC	EXAMPLES	TREATMENT
Delirium, Dementia, Amnestic, and Other Cognitive Disorders	Breakdown in intellec- tual func- tioning due to physical pathology	Delirium Dementia of the Alzeimer's type Disorder in- duced by drugs or poi- sons	Correction of underlying pa- thology if pos- sible, symptom relief, medica- tions to relieve anxiety, depression, or agitation, psy- chotherapy, safety precau- tions, custodial care.
Substance- related Disorders	Impairment in social and occupa- tional func- tions re- lated to drugs or al- cohol	Alcoholism Narcotics de- pendence Amphetamine abuse Barbiturate abuse Cocaine abuse	Treatment tai- lored to indi- vidual, detoxi- fication programs, AA, maintenance programs for addicts, deter- rents such as Antabuse. Treatment of physical com- plications, i.e., malnutrition, liver damage, infections, heart disease
Schizophre- nia and Other Psychotic Disorders*	Disordered thinking; bi- zarre social behaviors, withdrawal from others	Undifferen- tiated schizo- phrenia Paranoid schizophrenia Delusional dis- order Brief psychotic disorder	Tailored to in- dividual. Psy- chotherapeutic agents, psycho- therapy, group therapy, OT, RT

Table continued on following page

TABLE 12–2. MAJOR PSYCHIATRIC DISORDERS (DSM IV-R) *Continued*

CATEGORY	MAJOR CHARAC-TERISTIC	EXAMPLES	TREATMENT
Mood Disorders	Mood disturbance with associate changes in thinking and feeling	Major depressive disorder Bipolar disorders Dysthymic disorder	Antidepressants, lithium, psychotherapy, OT, RT, electroconvulsive therapy
Anxiety Disorders	Exaggerated feelings of apprehension	Panic disorder Phobic disorders Obsessive-compulsive disorder	Anxiolytics, behavioral therapy relaxation techniques, psychotherapy, OT, RT
Somatoform Disorders	Multiple somatic complaints with no physical illness	Hypochondriasis Conversion disorder Somatization disorder	Rule out physical pathology, psychotherapy, antianxiety drugs, OT, RT
Adjustment Disorder	Difficult adapting to life situation	Adjustment disorder with depressed mood	Psychotherapy, group therapy chemotherapy appropriate to mood
Personality Disorders	Lifelong patterns of maladaptive behaviors	Paranoid personality Schizoid personality Dependent personality	Sedatives, hypnotics, psychotherapy, set firm limits.

*Data from diagnostic and statistical manual of mental disorders. DSM IV. 4th ed. Washington, DC: American Psychiatric Association, 1994.

become more accepting of themselves and their emotional responses, thus moving towards positive growth and change.

- Listen for feeling tones and nonverbal communication. What is the emotion behind the words?

TABLE 12–3. PSYCHOTROPIC MEDICATIONS

GENERIC NAME/ TRADE NAME	USUAL DAILY DOSE (mg)
Antipsychotics and Neuroleptics	
Chlorpromazine (Thorazine)	25–1,000
Thioridazine (Mellaril)	10–800
Trifluoperazine (Stelazine)	2–40
Triflupromazine (Vesprin)	100–150
Perphenazine (Trilafon)	4–64
Acetophenzine (Tindal)	80–120
Prochlorperazine (Compazine)	15–150
Fluphenazine (Prolixin)	1–4
Chlorprothixene (Taractan)	30–600
Thiothixine (Navane)	6–60
Haloperidol (Haldol)	1–100
Pimozide (Orap)	1–2
Molindone (Moban)	20–225
Loxapine (Loxitane)	20–250
Clozapine (Clozaril)	<300–900
Droperidol (Inapsine)	2.5–10
Barbiturates	
Phenobarbital (Luminal)	100–200
Pentobarbital (Nembutal)	100–200
Secobarbital (Seconal)	100–200
Amobarbital (Amytal)	100–200
Hypnotics	
Chloral hydrate (Noctec)	500–2000
Glutethimide (Doriden)	250–500
Methylprylon (Noludar)	200–400
Flurazepam (Dalmane)	15–30
Temazepam (Restoril)	30
Triazolam (Halcion)	0.25–0.5
Anxiolytics, Minor Tranquilizers	
Alprazolam (Xanax)	0.25–10
Diazepam (Valium)	2–40
Lorazepam (Ativan)	0.5–6
Oxazepam (Serax)	30–60
Chlordiazepoxide (Librium)	5–80
Chlorazepate (Tranxene)	3.75–60
Hydroxyzine (Atarax, Vistiril)	50–400
Meprobamate (Equanil, Miltown)	800
Buspirone (BuSpar)	15–60
Clonazepam (Klonopin)	0.5–2

Table continued on following page

TABLE 12–3. PSYCHOTROPIC MEDICATIONS
Continued

GENERIC NAME/ TRADE NAME	USUAL DAILY DOSE (mg)
Tricyclic Antidepressants	
Amitriptyline (Elavil)	75–200
Nortriptyline (Aventyl, Pamelor)	75–200
Protriptyline (Vivactil)	15–40
Imipramine (Tofranil)	100–200
Despramine (Norpramin)	100–200
Triimipramine (Surmontil)	75–200
Doxepin (Sinequan, Adapin)	75–150
Clomipramine (Anafranil)	100–250
Monoamine Oxidase Inhibitors	
Isocarboxazid (Marplan)	10–30
Phenelazine (Nardil)	15–60
Tranylcypromine (Parnate)	20–30
Other Antidepressants	
Trazodone (Desyrel)	50–400
Fluoxetine (Prozac)	20–80
Maprotiline (Ludiomil)	75–300
Amoxapine (Asendin)	150–300
Bupropion (Wellbutrin)	225–450
Sertraline (Zoloft)	50–150

- Observe body posture, facial expression, breathing rate, tone of voice, volume of voice, speed of talking, lack of noticeable emotion, silence, and improper laughing or crying. Do nonverbal cues match the verbal ones?

EXPRESSION OF INTEREST

Convey interest by leaning forward, making eye contact, maintaining an alert facial expression, nodding your head, saying "uh-huh," and being appropriately silent when the client is talking. Not interrupting tells the client you want to hear more.

TABLE 12–4. DEFENSE MECHANISMS

Healthy use of coping (defense) mechanisms can minimize anxiety and mental illness; inappropriate or exclusive use can increase anxiety and maladaption.

Denial—blocking out a painful reality

Displacement—redirecting feelings from original object or person to safer substitute

Compensation—covering up inadequate aspects of character by overemphasizing other aspects

Conversion—unconscious expression of emotional distress in physical symptoms

Identification—imiating a person who has attributes the client considers admirable

Introjection—internalizing the feelings, values, and attitudes of another person

Isolation—blocking the feelings associated with an unpleasant, threatening situation or thought

Projection—attributing one's own unacceptable feelings to someone else

Rationalization—attempting to justify rationally and logically unacceptable feelings or behavior

Reaction formation—expressing the opposite of what one really feels

Regression—behaving at a level more appropriate to an earlier age

Repression—unconsciously keeping painful thoughts, feelings, and impulses out of awareness

Suppression—consciously keeping certain ideas out of awareness

Sublimation—substituting a more socially acceptable activity for an unacceptable one

Freud A. The ego and the mechanisms for defense. Rev. ed. New York: International Universities Press, 1966.

ONGOING FEEDBACK AND CLARIFICATION

Clarifying what is said, heard, and understood in an ongoing process helps to facilitate therapeutic communication.

- Reflect what you perceive to be the feeling tone back to the client, i.e., say "I sense that you feel disappointed about this. Am I right?" Reflection lets clients know you are actively listening and fully understanding, which will help them express emotions more freely.

- Paraphrase client's words to let them know you understand what they said, and also perhaps see what they said in a different light, i.e., "so what you are saying is that you don't like the food here?"

- Ask directed questions when appropriate. "Yes" or "no" questions are sometimes best, i.e., "Are you in pain?" or "Are you allergic to any medications that you know of?"

- Ask open-ended questions to encourage more expression of what clients are thinking or feeling. Questions that start with "who, what, where or how" encourage clients to expand their answers and define problems in thier own ways.

- Summarize the client's thoughts and feelings in order to highlight main ideas, recall important points, and review progress. If you have any incorrect information, it can then be corrected.

- Give support and reassurance often. Comforting words, gestures, facial expressions, and your mere presence can be highly effective in allaying anxiety and facilitating therapy.

BARRIERS TO COMMUNICATION

- If language is a barrier, use an interpreter, a friend, or relative, or family member to interpret for you. Use facial and hand gestures and body language to get ideas across. Also use pictures and graphs, or chalkboards to convey ideas. (See also Appendices F and G.)

- Be aware of cultural issues that may impede communication, i.e., different meanings ascribed to symbols, attitudes, facial expressions, pain. Talk openly with clients about what might appear strange or what would make them feel more comfortable.

- Avoid rejecting, disapproving phrases that close communication. The following are examples:
  That's wrong.
  Don't tell me that.
  You can't be mad.
  Don't get so upset about it!
  You don't see pink elephants.
  I don't believe you.
  There are no loud voices. You can't be hearing them.
  How can you say that? This is the best hospital!
  You are not using drugs are you?

- Pain, lethargy, anxiety, confusion, or disordered thought processes can make communication very difficult. These conditions need to be assessed and treated in order to enhance communication possibilities.

PROBLEM SOLVING

- Problem solving should take place only after the nurse has fully explored the client's feelings about the situation being discussed, perhaps after several encounters. The problem-solving method is the process whereby clients are empowered to help themselves (see Sec. 12-3 for steps).

- Let the client do the work! Do not give advice or opinions, but let client come to see his or her own solutions.

- Let client eliminate those alternatives that are not appealing from a list that you make together.

- End the interaction with positive feelings, whether or not the problem(s) are solved. Some problems require years of work.

12-2 PSYCHOSOCIAL, MENTAL STATUS ASSESSMENT

The mental and emotional responses of every client should be assessed and observed for strengths and potential or actual problems. Complete psychosocial assessments are done on admission for clients with psychiatric diagnoses only. However, mental status assessments are necessary for all clients in the hospital, especially when the physical diagnosis is psychologically sensitive, i.e., if cancer, cerebrovascular accident, heart disease, or severe injuries are present. In addition to the physical and neurological exams outlined in Chapter 1, use the following tool to assess mental/emotional status.

Mental Status Assessment

GENERAL APPEARANCE

- Apparent age
- Grooming, hygiene

MOTOR STATUS

- Body language, posture, gait, gestures, mannerisms, facial expressions
- Movements (agitated, restless, tremors)
  - Hyperkinesia (abnormally increased motor activity)
  - Psychomotor retardation (decreased, slowed activity)

ORIENTATION

- Client is oriented to time, place, person

LEVEL OF CONSCIOUSNESS

- Sensorium (i.e., clear, clouded, confused)

BEHAVIOR/ATTITUDE TOWARD INTERVIEWER

- Client's attitude (i.e., friendly, angry, dramatic or muted, cooperative, hostile, passive, dependent, indifferent)

LANGUAGE AND SPEECH

- Speed, number of words, tone, pressured speech, strange usage (i.e., echolalia, verbigeration)

AFFECT AND MOOD

- Affect is range of feeling based on objective and subjective data, i.e., range may be full, blunted, flat, constricted, labile.
- Mood may be sad, angry, happy, depressed, worried, nervous, suspicious, dull, hostile, elated, apathetic.

THOUGHT CONTENT

- Assess for disturbed thought processes, difficulty and strangeness in thinking, delusions (false fixed beliefs), hallucinations (perceptions not perceived by others), illusions (misperceptions of real stimuli), suicidal ideation, irrelevant responses, incoherent tangential responses, conceptual disorganization, grandiosity, blocking of significant memories or events, or ideas of reference.

MEMORY

- Immediate: Ask the client to remember three items, such as a key, a lamp, and a book for a few minutes. Move on to other questions and then ask if client remembers the three items.
- Recent: Ask the client to tell you, with considerable detail and accuracy, the events that led to the hospitalization.
- Remote: Ask where client grew up, went to school, etc. (may be difficult to check for accuracy).

GENERAL FUND OF KNOWLEDGE

- Ask the name of the president of the United States, the name of the biggest city in the state where the client lives, and/or answers to simple mathematical calculations.

REASONING AND JUDGMENT

- Ask what the client would do if they were at work and there was a fire. Check for appropriate response.

INSIGHT

- Check insight by asking the client to verbalize his or her perception of their illness or of what is happening to them at the present time.

Complete Psychosocial Assessment

A complete psychosocial assessment is warranted when there is a psychiatric diagnosis, such as depression, which may be secondary to another disease. Hospitals usually use their own assessment tools, which usually include an extensive history of the client's background, support systems, lifestyle, socioeconomic circumstances, sexual history, level of stress during year before admission, development of current problem, normal coping strategies, developmental history, drugs taken, and significant life events.

Mini-Mental Status Exam

A mini-mental status exam can involve simply determining whether the client is oriented to time, place, and person, neuro checks (see neuro exam section 1-5) or elicit some of the more detailed information as outlined in the above mental status exam. It can be used when time is limited but deviations from baseline may be significant.

12-3 STRESS REDUCTION

Stress is inevitable and necessary in all of our lives. It cannot be eliminated, only reduced or more successfully managed. Hospitalization itself is usually stressful. Developing adaptive responses to stressors and successful management strategies are essential in reducing illness and promoting health. General health principles, such as maintaining sound nutrition, adequate rest, regular exercise, meaningful work, and supportive relationships will bolster strength and help the body deal with stress. Four other strategies you can recommend to client are regular use of relaxation techniques and visualization, controlling and coping with significant life changes, development of problem-solving and coping skills, and one or more alternative therapies. Help client find out what works well.

Relaxation Techniques

Many relaxation techniques are available that result in integrated physiologic changes such as lowered vital signs and act to reduce the damaging psychophysiologic effects of stress. Teach client to use one of these and/or other techniques daily. The four elements that facilitate the relaxation response are:

1. A calm, quiet environment with minimal distractions

2. A comfortable position, which reduces the need for muscular effort (ideally head and arms are supported, clothing is loose, shoes are off)

3. A mental device such as mantra or syllable repeated over and over; mental imagery

4. A passive attitude wherein the individual simply allows the relaxation to happen

QUIET BREATHING

Close your eyes. Become aware of your breathing pattern. Breathe normally but focus the attention on the air going in and out of your respiratory passages. With each expiration say mentally "one" or "calm" or "peace." See in your mind's eye the air entering the nostrils, going down the throat, through the larynx, trachea, bronchi, filling the alveoli to exchange oxygen for carbon dioxide, and leaving the body. Fill your mind with the sensation of breathing. Let other thoughts drift away. Continue for 2–20 min.

PROGRESSIVE MUSCLE TENSION AND RELAXATION

Close your eyes and focus your attention on your feet. Completely tense all the muscles in your feet and toes for about 5 sec. then completely relax all your muscles. See in your mind's eye all tension and stress leave your feet as you tell your feet to relax. Move up to your ankles; tense and relax your ankles. Progress to the calves, knees, thighs, pelvis, abdomen, chest, back, and shoulders. Pay particular attention to the shoulders, which are usually in a perennial state of tension. Continue with the upper arms, elbows, lower arms, wrists, hands, and fingers. Move at any time to facilitate better relaxation. Return to the shoulders and move the relaxation up to the neck, the chin, the facial muscles, and scalp. Experience for 1–2 min what it feels like to be completely relaxed all over. Repeat a positive health affirmation such as "I feel calm, confident, and pain-free." When you feel ready, count backward from 5 to 1, awakening renewed and fresh. If using to promote sleep, use the affirmation at the end, "I feel totally relaxed and am drifting off to sleep."

Controlling Significant Life Changes

Studies show that both the number and the severity of significant life changes within a given amount of time in an individual's life affect predisposition to disease. Use the Holmes and Rahe Social Readjustment Rating Scale (Table 12-5) to help client see how multiple life changes might be increasing the risk of illness and how risk might be reduced by reducing major changes. For example, the newly widowed or divorced might be counseled to wait a year or so before moving, changing jobs, going on a radical diet, or seeking new friends. The family of a suicidal teenager can be assisted to stabilize their child's life in order to reduce the risk of suicide.

Development of Problem-Solving Skills

Many people resort to such short-term coping measures as illness (hypochondria), overeating, drinking alcohol excessively, taking drugs, or sleeping too much in an attempt to deal with stressful life problems. These may relieve tension for short periods, but actually exacerbate difficulties and are dangerous. On the other hand, the problem-solving approach offers the client constructive ways to handle stressful situations.

All problem solving involves these essential steps:

1. Identify the problem.
2. Assess the cause of the problem, including personal behavior patterns that contribute to it.
3. Generate possible solutions.

TABLE 12–5. SOCIAL READJUSTMENT RATING SCALE

RANK	LIFE EVENT	LIFE CHANGE UNITS	RANK	LIFE EVENT	LIFE CHANGE UNITS
1	Death of spouse	100	16	Change in financial state	38
2	Divorce	73			
3	Marital separation	65	17	Death of close friend	37
4	Jail term	63			
5	Death of close family member	63	18	Change to different line of work	36
6	Personal injury or illness	53	19	Change in number of arguments with spouse	35
7	Marriage	50			
8	Fired from job	47			
9	Marital reconciliation	45	20	Morgage over $10,000	31
10	Retirement	45	21	Foreclosure of mortgage or loan	30
11	Change in health of family member	44			
12	Pregnancy	40	22	Change in responsibilities at work	29
13	Sexual difficulties	39			
14	Gain of new family member	39	23	Son or daughter leaving home	29
15	Business readjustment	39	24	Trouble with in-laws	29

Table continued on following page

TABLE 12–5. SOCIAL READJUSTMENT RATING SCALE *Continued*

RANK	LIFE EVENT	LIFE CHANGE UNITS	RANK	LIFE EVENT	LIFE CHANGE UNITS
25	Outstanding personal achievement	28	34	Change in recreation	19
			35	Change in church activities	19
26	Spouse begins or stops work	26	36	Change in social activities	18
27	Begin or end school	26	37	Morgage or loan less than $10,000	17
28	Change in living conditions	25			
			38	Change in sleeping habits	16
29	Revision of personal habits	24	39	Change in number of family get-togethers	15
30	Trouble with boss	23			
31	Change in work hours or conditions	20	40	Change in eating habits	15
			41	Vacation	13
32	Change in residence	20	42	Christmas	12
			43	Minor violations of the law	11
33	Change in school	20			

1–149 = no significant life change; 150–199 = mild life change (33% chance of illness); 200–299 = moderate life change (50% chance of illness), 300+ = major life change (80% chance of illness)

Reprinted with permission from Journal of Psychosomatic Research. Holmes TH, Rahe RH. 2:214. © 1967, Pergamon Journals, Ltd.

4. Select solution, develop plan of action.

5. Implement plan.

6. Evaluate results.

7. Repeat steps as necessary.

Alternative Therapies

Many therapies have become available to aid in stress reduction and relaxation. Nurses are increasingly becoming involved in administering these therapies, in hospitals and in private practice. Many require special training and/or certification. These therapies include biofeedback, cognitive reappraisal, decisional control, therapeutic touch, massage, humor, animal companion therapy, music therapy, art therapy, bibliotherapy (reading books, poetry), hypnotherapy, visualization therapy, Reike healing, and light therapy (for seasonal affective disorder). For more information, one organization to contact is the American Holistic Nurses Association, 4101 Lake Boone Trail, Suite 210, Raleigh, NC 27607, (919) 787-5181. Perhaps a clinical nurse specialist or other therapist in your area can be referred.

12-4 ANXIETY

Anxiety is a feeling of dread or apprehension in response to actual or perceived threats to the self and lack of confidence in ability to cope with the threats. Every client will have some anxiety associated with illness, hospitalization, surgery or invasive procedures. The severity of anxiety that is experienced is individual to the client. Anxiety can be very mild and easily controlled or can be severe and completely debilitating.

Nursing Assessment of Client with Anxiety

- Symptoms include restlessness, sleeplessness, irritability, repetitive questioning, pacing, constant seeking of attention and reassurance, dizziness, difficulty breathing, palpitations, flushing or pallor of the face, tachycardia, jitteriness, tremulousness, dry mouth, lack of concentration, headache, muscle spasms in the neck or back, excessive perspiration, hyperventilation, pain, and change in appetite.

Nursing Interventions to Reduce Anxiety

- Provide a quiet, comfortable environment.
- Begin to establish a supportive, safe relationship.
- Control your own anxiety and protect the client from others who may increase the panic, as anxiety is contagious.
- Use a calm, firm tone of voice.
- Use active listening skills. Answer questions, and provide needed information. Educate client about upcoming tests, procedures, and treatments so client knows what to expect.
- Acknowledge the client's feelings. Help to identify the actual or perceived threat. Reality test the potential danger. Reassure client of safety and security.
- Stay with client during episodes of acute anxiety.
- Avoid asking client to make decisions during episodes of acute anxiety.
- Instruct client to breathe slowly and deeply. Breathe with client as needed to demonstrate. Explain that breathing slowly may help the client become more comfortable.
- Help the client to develop constructive coping strategies for anxiety-producing situations:
  1. Specific repertoire of anxiety-reducing activities that work for him/her
  2. Alternative responses to anxiety producing stimuli
  3. Strengthened problem-solving skills
- Teach client to monitor restlessness by rating it on a scale of 1–10, with 10 as most severe. Ask what the anxiety level is at the beginning of an episode and then to see if it goes down after doing specific things to lessen the discomfort: deep breathing, talking, exercising, relaxing.

- If possible, engage the client in constructive, diversionary activities aimed at decreasing anxiety: walking, jogging, doing exercises, simple concrete tasks, grooming, simple games, letter writing, household chores, or organizing possessions, talking on the phone.

- Teach client one of the relaxation techniques in Section 12-3, and guide him/her through it.

- Administer tranquilizers or anxiolytics as prescribed for severe anxiety as needed. Be aware that the possible side effects are drowsiness, fatigue, ataxia, blurred vision, slurred speech, and hypotension. Alcohol or other CNS depressants may potentiate effects and must be avoided.

- For a severe anxiety or panic state, refer a clinical nurse specialist or other health team member as appropriate.

12-5 DEPRESSION

While anxiety is associated with anticipated losses, depression is more associated with actual losses or stressful events (i.e., bereavement, divorce, job loss, change in body image). Depression is a major health problem and occurs in all age groups, with a higher incidence in the aged. Physical illnesses may predispose to depression, i.e., viral infections, intraabdominal neoplasm, or any chronic disfiguring illness that leaves the client with a permanent handicap. Certain medications can induce depression, including antihypertensives such as reserpine and oral contraceptives. The most serious sequela of depression is suicide.

Nursing Assessment of Client with Depression

- Risk factors include physical illness, recent significant loss, unhappiness with job or no job at all, low socioeconomic status, lack of social networks, social isolation, pain, and substance abuse.

- Symptoms may include marked negative mood changes such as sadness, loneliness, apathy, persistent feelings of low self-esteem and self-blame; sleep disturbances; slow or agitated activity levels; and withdrawal and suicidal ideation. The depressed client has slumped, stooped posture, may cry frequently and have difficulty talking, concentrating, or making decisions. There may be decreased libido with impotence in men or amenorrhea in women.

- Assess the depressed client for suicidal potential. Intervene to stop suicide attempts (see Section 12-6), including removing potentially harmful objects from environment.

- Assess nutritional status and intake and output. The depressed client is inclined to overeat or undereat. Eating disorders such as anorexia or bulimia may be present.

Nursing Interventions to Relieve Depression

- Assist the physician in determining whether the depression is drug or illness induced. Primary depression must be differentiated from secondary depression.

- Depression may be a side effect of many medications, but the nurse should be aware that this effect is uncommon and usually occurs within days to weeks of starting the medication. Reserpine, glucocorticoids, and anabolic steroids are the main drugs clearly implicated in depression as a side effect.

- Develop a trusting relationship. Encourage client to talk. Use active listening skills. If client seems sluggish allow time for client to formulate thoughts.

- Recognize that depression is one of the stages of the grieving process (see Section 12-7).

- Accept the client's sadness and let him or her cry, but reassure client that depression will eventually lift.

- Check client frequently. Provide safe environment, removing dangerous objects in case there may be suicidal potential. Ask the client, "Do you have thoughts of hurting yourself?" if you sense the potential may be present.

- Be aware of side effects and other nursing implications if client is on anti-depressive drugs. Some common ones are listed in Table 12-3. Check the Physician's Desk Reference or Hospital Formulary for information on specific drugs. Monitor and document response to treatments.

- Observe intake. Weigh daily. Encourage good nutrition.

- Encourage physical activity such as walking, jogging, or doing exercises.

- Have client room with another client who is verbal but not intrusive to others.

- Increase interactions with client as he/she improves.

- Avoid undue cheerfulness, but continue to reinforce the worth and rights of client.

- Avoid agreement with self-deprecating statements of client.

- Avoid arguing with client or making light of self-statements.

- Reinforce positive statements about self or others.

- Reinforce grooming efforts.

- Encourage the client to engage in activities that may increase feelings of self-esteem (i.e., writing to friends, making objects for family, beginning relationships with others).

- Provide regular but not rigid schedule of activities.

12-6 VIOLENCE, HIGH RISK FOR: SELF-DIRECTED

Suicide is on the rise in the United States, especially among young people and the elderly. It is not only associated with depression, but also major life changes, illness, and drugs and alcohol.

Suicide Warning Signs

- Preoccupation with themes of death or expressing suicidal thoughts
- Expressions suggesting profound unhappiness or despair
- Changes in school performance, lowered grades, cutting classes, dropping activities
- Withdrawal from friends and family, or other major behavioral changes
- Changes in eating habits, sudden loss or gain of weight
- Changes in sleeping patterns—too much or too little
- Recent losses in close relationships
- Giving away of prized possessions, making a will or other "final arrangements"
- Personality changes such as nervousness, outbursts of anger, or apathy about appearance
- Recent suicide of friend or relative or other major loss
- Direct suicide threats or attempts
- Use of alcohol or drugs
- No joy in activities that usually are enjoyable

Nursing Interventions When Client Has a Potential for Self-Directed Violence

- The client who is thought to be suicidal needs careful monitoring. If you think a client may be suicidal, then ask the client directly "Are you thinking of ways to harm yourself?" or "Do you feel like killing yourself?" If the answer is yes, ask client if they have a plan, and if so, what it is.

- Determine seriousness of the suicidal intent. If the client has a specific, lethal, available method (i.e., a gun) and has attempted suicide before, the immediate risk is high.

- Establish trust (see Section 12-1). Spend time with the client especially during the acute phase.

- Notify the physician and ask for orders for suicide observation status (SOS).

  Level I.   Continuous 1:1 observation of actively suicidal clients by at least one staff member.

  Level II. Continuous sight observation. Client is allowed access to the day room if a staff member can view him/her at all times.

  Level III. Observation at 15-min intervals. For client whose mental status has improved.

  Level IV. Hourly checks when immediate threat has passed.

- Provide a safe environment. Remove all sharp objects, glass containers, drugs, cigarette lighters, pocket knives, scissors, nail files, belts, silverware, and other harmful items.

- Red-flag the client's chart and make sure all staff members know the client is on suicide precautions.

- Make sure the client takes prescribed medication and is not hoarding doses for a suicide attempt.

- In communicating with the client:

  - Take a positive approach. Emphasize more desirable alternatives.

  - Emphasize the temporary nature of the person's problem.

  - Be calm and understanding. Value the person's feelings (helplessness, hopelessness).

  - Help the person define the problem, in order to remove some of the confusion.

  - Help the client recall people with whom he/she could share problems and feelings. Encourage talking with staff members and other clients. Refer a clinical nurse specialist, psychiatrist, clergyman, or other support person with whom the client feels comfortable to work one-on-one with client.

- Help client look at positive aspects of living that can be anticipated in the future.

- Set limits in relation to destructive behavior toward self or others. Make a verbal contract with clients that includes the expectation that they will not harm themselves and will seek out staff members to verbalize feelings.

- Prevent isolation. Seek out client.

- Offer alternatives to self-destructive impulses and support alternative behaviors. Engage client in positive activities.

- Help client develop adaptive methods to cope with stress.

- Evaluate with team members progress and ongoing necessity for close observation and area-restriction measures.

12-7 GRIEVING

Grieving is a normal process that is experienced in connection with significant loss. The loss may be a person, object, status, function, or relationship that has been important to the client or a family member. Anticipatory grieving is when the process is started before the loss actually occurs. Dysfunctional grieving is a maladaptive response where grief work is suppressed, prolonged, or delayed. The nurse's goal in helping people adjust to loss is to facilitate normal grief by supporting the client and family through the normal stages.

Nursing Assessment of the Grieving Client

- Assess and expect client's behavioral responses. Expect denial, disbelief, anger, guilt, bargaining, depression, eventual acceptance. The client's stages of grief are likely to follow the following course:

AVOIDANCE PHASE	CONFRONTA-TION PHASE	REESTABLISH-MENT PHASE
Denial: "I don't believe it"	Depression	Acceptance of loss
Disbelief: "This can't be happening to me"	Withdrawal	Development of new interests/ attachments
	Social isolation	
	Psychomotor retardation	Restructuring lifestyle
Anger	Silence	Return to preloss level of functioning
Resentment		
Hostility		
Bargaining with higher power		
Loud complaints		
Sleep disturbances		
Altered appetite		

- Other reactions in the grief process may include crying, sorrow, feelings of worthlessness, suicidal thoughts, hallucinations about the object or person, delusions, phobias, anergia, inability to concentrate.

- Assess religious and sociocultural factors that may affect expectations. Grief reactions can be affected by personality, upbringing, support systems, importance of lost object, timing or suddenness of loss, and impact loss has on daily life.

Nursing Interventions When Client Is Grieving

- Ask client about past ways of coping or dealing with serious health problems. Religion may be significant in coping with loss. Refer client to clergy or other support groups as appropriate.

- Convey empathy and understanding throughout grief process. Simply allow feelings. Say "I know this must be very difficult for you." Ask if the client or significant others feel like talking and listen if indications are positive.

- Respect client's desire not to speak. Remember that the more intense or profound an emotion is, the harder it is to verbalize.

- If appropriate, explain the grieving process so that individuals know that what they are going through is normal. This may help them to accept their own feelings. Different people go through stages in different time frames. Clients may vascillate back and forth in the stages as they grieve, and may experience a combination of stages at the same time.

- Allow anger, but if necessary, set limits. "I know you feel very upset, but I cannot allow you to throw things."

- Identify any suicidal potential and take precautions to ensure client safety (see 12-6). Refer client to clinical nurse specialist, psychiatrist, clergy, or other support persons.

- Accept the client's sorrow. Avoid the temptation to make optimistic remarks or cheerful small talk.

- Identify physiological problems (i.e., eating or sleeping disturbances) and intervene to stabilize as much as possible.

- Normal grieving usually occurs over a period of 2–6 months, sometimes lasting longer.

Grieving, Anticipatory

The desired outcome and goal of nursing care when losses are anticipated is that client and significant other(s) will express grief, participate in decisions about the future, and communicate concerns to health care team members and to one another. Caregivers or significant others may experience the stages of loss prior to losing a loved one with chronic illness and again when death actually occurs.

Grieving, Dysfunctional

Dysfunctional grieving is characterized by sustained or prolonged detrimental response. The following morbid grief reactions may require extensive work with a psychotherapist: postponement of reaction (most common reaction, which may involve years), psychosomatic reaction, masked reaction, conspicuous alteration in relationships, (i.e., continued isolation from friends and family), hostility toward certain persons, prolonged agitated depression and/ or lack of decision and initiative, denial of death (acting and speaking as if the dead person were still alive), quick replacement of the lost object or person with another, or prolonged unresolved grief (slightest mention of the loss, even many years later, readily evokes crying). Most of these responses cannot be validated until months or years after the loss. For this reason, the nursing diagnosis of High Risk for Dysfunctional Grieving may be useful. For more information on the grieving process, see Grief Counseling and Grief Therapy (Worden, 1991).

12-8 CONFUSION

The prime characteristic of the confused client is cognitive impairment, with disorientation, memory difficulties, clouded consciousness, and problems coping with reality. The confused client may exhibit bizarre behavior, neglect functional needs, and have difficulty communicating. Physical causes of cognitive impairment are many; determining the cause is imperative for treatment. Postoperative confusion in the elderly is common.

Nursing Assessment of the Confused Client

- Perform physical, neurological, and mental status assessments of the client. Establish or refer to the client's baseline functioning status to see if confusion is a recurring pattern that exacerbates at certain times, or if confusion is a new development.

- Characteristics of confusion may include: disorientation, loss of memory, denial that any problems exist, confabulation, lack of judgment, illogical thinking, suspiciousness, paranoia, fear, bizarre speech, regression, inappropriate sexual acting out, delusions, hallucinations.

- Causes of confusion include: hypoxia, respiratory distress, electrolyte imbalances, endocrine and metabolic disturbances, chronic liver and kidney disorders, cerebrovascular diseases, cancers, tumors, systemic infections, CNS infections (i.e., meningitis, encephalitis, syphilis), neurological disorders (i.e., Parkinson's disease, epilepsy), nutritional imbalances, injury, trauma, toxicity (substance abuse), sensory overload, sensory deprivation, perceptual problems, genetic and birth defects (Down's syndrome), MS, depression, delirium, dementia, dementia of the Alzheimer's type.

Nursing Interventions to Reduce Confusion

- Help determine the cause of the confusion. If the confusion is a new development, evaluate what could have happened recently to impair cognition.

- Recognize that confusion is more common in the elderly, but this is only because the elderly are more prone to disease than the general population. When the underlying cause of the confusion is treated, cognition should improve; however, with chronic problems such as cardiovascular disease or Alzheimer's, deficits of varying degrees will continue.

- Monitor client frequently, placing near the nurse's station. Physical restraints may be required at times. Safety issues are of prime concern in a confused client. Client may wander, not knowing where they are or who they are.

- Soft restraints may be the last resort to assure client's safety in those that wander and are potentially dangerous to themselves or others. Check the restrained client's skin integrity, and musculoskeletal status frequently (every 15 min is the minimum).

- Monitor the client's level of awareness using the mental status exam or perhaps the mini-mental status exam. Identify trends and plan care accordingly. Confusion is often worse in the evening.

- For postoperative confusion, orient the client, make sure he/she is oxygenated, hydrated, nourished, and pain is relieved. Explain that confusion is understandable in light of hospitalization. Encourage ambulation as soon as possible. Assess lab values, medications, surgical factors, (i.e., blood loss, possible infection, obstruction). Remove catheters, tubes and devices as soon as it is permissible to do so, facilitating normal functioning and routines.

- Make sure the confused client has sensory aids intact (hearing aids, eyeglasses).

- Help to keep the client oriented by using clocks, calendars, newspapers, and other reminders in the client's room. Keep the room from becoming too cluttered, however, as environmental stimuli should be kept to a minimum.

- It may help to write down things the client wants to remember, such as names of people, routines, room number, times for meals, etc. Assess client's ability to use written direction. Signs can be posted on the door of client's room, bathroom, dining room, etc, to assist memory.

- Use simple communications, short sentences, simple words and frequent repetition.

- Administer psychotropic medications, but monitor judiciously, as tranquilizers or antidepressants can either decrease or increase client's confusion and comprehension.

- Offer support and reassurance to the client and family, always treating the client with dignity. Use the client's proper name. Allow client as much choice and control as possible. Give positive feedback for appropriate responses. Enhance self-esteem as much as possible.

- Provide the family with information regarding confusion and disease process. The Alzheimer's client requires tremendous altering of family patterns, and family members must be prepared. More information can be obtained from the Alzheimer's Disease and Related Disorders Association, 420 Lexington Ave., Suite 610, New York, New York, 10070, (212) 983-0700.

12-9 ALTERED THOUGHT PROCESSES

Altered thought processes is a condition in which conscious thought, reality orientation, problem solving, judgment, and comprehension related to coping are disrupted. This nursing diagnosis is related to confusion, and may be caused by some of the same pathologies, however "altered thought processes" is more associated with inaccurate interpretation of internal and external stimuli than with disorientation.

Nursing Assessment of Client with Altered Thought Processes

- Observe for evidence of verbal and nonverbal hallucinations—inappropriate laughter, delayed verbal response, talking to one's self, increased eye movements or motor movements, grinning.

- Hallucinations may be visual, auditory, olfactory, tactile or gustatory. Visual and auditory are the most common.

- Help determine cause of disordered thinking using physical, neurological, and mental status assessments. Identify violent, or bizarre thinking. Determine if cause is situational or part of chronic pathology.

PATHOPHYSIOLOGICAL ETIOLOGIES	SITUATIONAL OR PERSONAL ETIOLOGIES
Personality and mental disorders related to alteration in biochemical compounds, i.e., psychosis, schizophrenia, chronic illness, surgery	Depression or anxiety Substance abuse Fear Loss (of control, routine, income, significant others) Emotional trauma
Genetic disorder	Rejection or negative
Progressive dementia	appraisal by others
Hormonal changes	Isolation

PATHOPHYSIOLOGICAL ETIOLOGIES	SITUATIONAL OR PERSONAL ETIOLOGIES
	Unclear communication
	Abuse (physical, emotional, sexual)
	Torture
	Maturational difficulties
	Sleep deprivation
	Medications (side effects)

Nursing Interventions When the Client Has Altered Thought Process

- Plan care based on the cause. Assist in diagnostic procedures and monitor lab values particularly electrolytes, if the cause is not yet diagnosed.

- Approach calmly, establish trust.

- Assess client's ability to communicate. Identify what the person is feeling, and verify your interpretation, i.e., "I get the sense you are feeling afraid."

- Reorient the client to reality, time, place, and recent events.

- Provide a safe environment. Assess client's potential for self-harm. Persons experiencing command hallucinations (i.e., voices that tell a person to harm him- or herself) are extremely dangerous to their own safety. The client who is delusional and feels persecuted may act irrationally, violently, and unpredictably towards others.

- Decrease stimulation, and provide a calm, relaxing, restful atmosphere. Make brief but frequent contacts with the client. Approach in a nonthreatening manner.

- Do not argue with client experiencing delusional thoughts or hallucinations. Instead let them know you believe them. However, provide reality orientation by differentiating stimuli arising from their internal sources and external stimuli. Say "I know you feel afraid of aliens, but I do not see any aliens anywhere." Or, "I don't see any of the spiders that you say you see. What were you thinking about when you started seeing them?"

- Set limits on repetitively discussing delusional material (i.e., "You've told me about that. Let's talk about real things that we both can see"). Direct attention to outward stimuli.

- Assist client in communicating more effectively. Ask for clarification if unsure of meaning. Refocus the client's attention if person then changes the subject suddenly.

- Help client identify measures that increase or decrease anxiety. Anxiety can exacerbate symptoms. Use problem-solving measures to find ways to cope with anxiety, before or after (not during) an anxiety attack. Discuss alternative methods of coping (i.e., taking a walk rather than pacing, wringing hands).

- Monitor medications and check responses to treatments. Ascertain whether current medications can cause altered thought processes.

- Use physical contact cautiously, as the clients not perceiving correctly may interpret contact as threatening.

- A team effort and restraints may be required to ensure client safety if he/she is violent.

12-10   CHEMICAL DEPENDENCY

It is estimated that more than 20 million adults, adolescents, and children in America experience substance abuse-related problems, and 25% of hospitalized clients have alcohol-related problems. The client who is addicted to one or more substances may develop multiple physical, emotional, and psychosocial complications. If a covertly addicted client is admitted to the general hospital for a related or unrelated problem, and is required to stop drinking or stop taking drugs suddenly, the client will be at risk for withdrawal.

Nursing Assessment of the Client with Chemical Dependence

Alcoholism

- Signs of alcohol withdrawal (generally occur 3–36 hours after last drink was taken): tremors, tachycardia, psychomotor hyperactivity, agitation, anxiety, diaphoresis, malaise, anorexia, nausea, vomiting, diarrhea, hypertension, orthostatic hypertension, insomnia, fever, seizures, delirium, disorientation, memory impairment, hallucinations, delusions, delirium tremens.

- Potential complications include sudden death, aspiration pneumonia, peripheral vascular collapse, hyperthermia (it is especially important to monitor the temperature along with vital signs), infection (after hyperthermia), myocardial infarction, alcoholic hepatitis.

- The immediate treatment for present or impending delirium tremens is pharmacological. Valium and Librium are most commonly used to minimize the progression of withdrawal. Doses are gradually titrated down until client is no longer at risk for serious sequelae. Other problems must be addressed: potential for self-harm, trauma, fluid and electrolyte balance, nutritional status, potential for any other imminent physical crisis.

- While the immediate effects of alcohol withdrawal are subsiding, the treatment plan for alcoholism as the primary disease must be formulated. Alcoholics Anonymous (175 Fifth Ave, New York, New York, 10017, (212) 473-6200) is the most well-known and widely used of the outpatient 12-step programs. But each client's unique needs must be considered, and increasingly, multisystem approaches are being taken. Programs may include individual counseling, group therapy, education meetings, occupational therapy, recreational therapy, family therapy, and vocational rehabilitation.

Stimulants

AMPHETAMINES

- Signs of intoxication: euphoria, hyperalertness, anorexia, increased heart rate, increased blood pressure, insomnia, excessive talkativeness.

- Overdose: headache, dizziness, agitation, hostility, tremor, panic, flushed skin, chest pain, palpitations, diaphoresis, vomiting, abdominal cramps.

- Signs of withdrawal: cravings, rebound depression, irritability, anxiety, fatigue, insomnia or hypersomnia, psychomotor agitation, restlessness, increased appetite.

COCAINE

- Signs of intoxication: increased heart rate, blood pressure, intense euphoria, extreme restlessness, followed by depression. Runny nose, needle marks, or brown sputum from smoking crack may be present. Client may suffer from chronic nasal congestion, epistaxis, severe headaches, chest pains, heart problems, increased libido followed by impotence, behavior changes.

- Overdose: anxiety-panic, increased heart rate, increased blood pressure, dilated pupils, perspiration, syncope, seizures, delusions, paranoia, hallucinations, mania. Death may result of cardiac or respiratory failure.

- Withdrawal: similar to amphetamines.

Marijuana

- Signs of intoxication: reddened eyes, dry mouth, drowsiness, lack of coordination, lack of concentration, altered perception, euphoria, craving sweets, impulsiveness, talkativeness, disorientation, illusions.

- Complications: panic attacks, impotence, impaired memory, flashbacks, cognitive deficits.

CNS Depressants

BARBITURATES, SEDATIVES, TRANQUILIZERS

- Signs of intoxication: decreased respirations, slowed heart rate, drowsiness, lack of coordination, slurred speech, confused behavior, sleeping more than 10 hr, confused behavior.

- Withdrawal: depression, irritability, anxiety, tremors, increased heart rate and blood pressure, nausea, vomiting, cramping, weakness, increased reflexes, insomnia, rigidity, stiffness.

- Complications: danger of overdose particularly high when combined with alcohol or liver and kidney disease. Withdrawal requires medical attention.

Hallucinogens

ACID, LSD, PCP, MESCALINE

- Signs and symptoms: obsession with detail, mood swings, panic attacks, nausea and vomiting, synesthesia (seeing sounds and smelling colors), altered perceptions, increased pulse, flushing, cramping, muscle twitching, hallucinations.

- Complications: unpredictable, often dangerous behavior, flashbacks.

Narcotics

OPIUM, HEROIN, CODEINE, MORPHINE, METHADONE

- Signs of use: drowsiness, euphoria, no sensitivity to pain, needle marks, especially on arms, slow and shallow breathing, possible coma.

- Withdrawal: cravings, runny nose, watery eyes, yawning, nausea, panic attacks, tremors, vomiting, constricted or dilated pupils, cold clammy skin, chills, sweating, cramps, insomnia, gooseflesh, decreased appetite, diarrhea.

- Complications: addiction, weight loss, hepatitis, AIDS, overdose.

Nursing Interventions for Client with Chemical Dependency

- Maintain a nonjudgmental attitude when caring for the client with substance abuse problems.

- Provide safety, as client under the influence of a substance is unable to maintain own safety needs.

- Continually monitor the client for negative medical sequelae of intoxication or withdrawal. Death can result from drug-induced respiratory or cardiac failure.

- Assess and monitor the client's mental status, noting fluctuations according to time and amount of drugs taken, or phase of withdrawal.

- Establish a supportive rapport with the client and practice therapeutic communication. Encourage verbalization in order to assist client identify problem areas. Support from health care professionals can help encourage sobriety and increase self-esteem.

- Administer and monitor psychopharmacological medications with caution as directed by a physician, noting efficacy and client behavior.

- Teach relaxation techniques and encourage use to help relieve anxiety.

- Assess family, community resources, and other significant support; explore available options. The most crucial factor in helping substance users become drug-free is motivation. Major lifestyle issues may have to be changed and as many resources that can be enlisted to help will be needed.

- Provide as much information as possible about substance abuse: the physiological, psychological, and social ramifications. Knowledge about options for rehabilitation will help clients and their families identify a treatment plan in order to build on client's strengths.

- Two groups that provide assistance and information to help deal with substance abuse are: Families Anonymous, P.O. Box 3475, Culver City, CA 90231-3475, 1-800-736-9805; and Narcotics Anonymous, World Service Office, P.O. Box 9999, Van Nuys, CA 91409, (818) 780-3951.

12-11   BODY-IMAGE DISTURBANCE

Body-image disturbance occurs when an individual experiences or is at risk of experiencing disruptive feelings and difficulty accepting changes in his or her perception of self. Chronic disease, loss of a body part, loss of body function, severe trauma, surgery, hospitalization, chemotherapy, radiation, pain, obesity, pregnancy, infertility, immobility, and maturational changes may all trigger responses of discomfort or distress at body-image changes.

Nursing Assessment of the Client with Body-Image Disturbance

- Symptoms may include negative verbal statements, not looking at a particular body part, not touching a body part, hiding or overexposing a body part, a change in social involvement, negative feelings about the body, feelings of hopelessness, helplessness, powerlessness, preoccupation with the loss, denial, and depersonalization of the body part. In eating disorders, clients may be overly concerned about their weight.

Nursing Interventions When There Is Body Image Disturbance

- The goal is to have clients share feelings about their view of self, achieve a sense of integration of their altered body image, and to demonstrate adequate ability to function positively.

- Encourage expression of feelings about how client views and feels about self. Listen actively. Answer any questions about the course of treatment, disease, progress, prognosis. Reinforce client teaching to relieve anxiety.

- Clarify any misconceptions the client may have regarding self, care, or caregivers.

- Encourage client to explore the meaning of the loss. Expect the normal grief response: denial, anger, bargaining, depression, acceptance. Support the client through these stages (see Section 12-7). In selected cases, it may be appropriate to explain the normal grief response so that client may more easily accept what is happening.

- Encourage social visits and other contact (letters, phone calls) from family and significant others. Support the family as the client adapts.

- Other persons with a similar body change may help the person adjust more easily to the new situation. Provide opportunities for support people to meet with client. You may wish to refer a clinical nurse specialist, psychologist, or clergyman.

- Explore strengths, resources, and realistic alternatives for the future with the person.

- For a surgically created alteration of body image: replace the lost body part with prosthesis as soon as possible, and encourage the viewing and touching of site.

- For a client undergoing chemotherapy: be aware of body changes such as hair loss and anticipate what can be expected. Discuss what can be done to minimize trauma ahead of time, i.e., the person can be fitted for a wig, can be psychologically prepared for loss of eyebrows, eyelashes, auxiliary hair, pubic and leg hair, etc. Teach the client that avoiding excessive shampooing, using conditioner, patting hair dry gently, and avoiding electric curlers, dryers, and curling irons will help to minimize the amount of hair loss.

REFERENCES

Barker P. The story of the blues. Nursing Times. June 3, Vol. 88, No. 23, 1992.

Carpenito LJ. Handbook of nursing diagnosis. 4th ed., Philadelphia: Lippincott, 1991.

Diagnostic and statistical manual of mental disorders. DSM IV. 4th ed. Washington, DC: American Psychiatric Association, 1994.

Evans C, Kenny P. Postoperative confusion in the elderly. Nurseweek. Vol. 6, No. 14, April, 1993, 30–31.

Herr K, Mobily P. Chronic pain and depression. Psychosocial Nursing. Vol. 30, (9), 7–11, 1992.

Kneisl C, Ames S. Adult health nursing: a biopsychosocial approach. Menlo Park: Addison-Wesley, 1986.

Nadler-Moodie M. Psychiatric aspects of general patient care. La Mesa, CA: Western Publishing, 1991.

Lewis SM, Collier ID. Medical-surgical nursing: assessment and management of clinical problems. 3rd ed. St. Louis: Mosby, 1992.

Liken M, Collins C. Grieving: facilitating the process for dementia caregivers. Psychosocial Nursing. Vol. 31 (1), 21–26, 1993.

US Department of Health and Human Services, Public Health Service, Agency for Health for Health Care Policy and Research. Depression in primary care: detection, diagnosis, and treatment. Psychosocial Nursing. Vol. 31 (6), 1993, 19–28.

Wann M. Alternative therapies enter the mainstream. Nurseweek. Vol. 6 (9), March, 1993, 10–11.

Worden JW. Grief counseling and grief therapy: a handbook for the mental health practitioner, New York: Springer Publishing Co., 1991.

EMERGENCY ASSESSMENT AND INTERVENTION

An emergency is defined by a sudden change in a client's level of consciousness or by an actual or potentially life-threatening trauma or injury that necessitates immediate intensive treatment. Rapid recognition of an emergency through assessment and history-taking are essential so that life-sustaining measures can be employed.

13-1 EMERGENCY ASSESSMENT

In any trauma or medical emergency, the client's **A**irway, **B**reathing, and **C**irculation are first priorities. The primary survey must focus on these critical areas. Also, the cervical spine is always immobilized in trauma situations until cleared by x-ray or physician exam.

Initial Management (Primary Survey)

Cardiopulmonary resuscitation (CPR) is initiated at any point in the primary survey when respirations or pulses are absent (see Section 13-2).

AIRWAY

- Assess the oral and nasal cavities. *Is the airway clear?*

  - Suction as necessary, perform a jaw lift (maintain spinal integrity as necessary) or use head tilt/chin lift maneuver to open the airway, insert oral or nasopharyngeal airway, or assist with endotracheal intubation.

BREATHING

- Assess the quality of the client's respiratory effort.

  - Assess the respiratory rate (too high or too low), assess for peripheral cyanosis or circumoral pallor, look at the chest for paradoxical chest movement (flail chest), auscultate for crackles, gurgles, wheezing, or absence of breath sounds, and obtain a quick pulse oximetry reading if available.

  - Assist client respirations by applying oxygen or bagging with ambu-bag. Anticipate possible medication intervention or chest tube insertion.

  - Evaluate the effectiveness of interventions by client improvement and/or obtaining arterial blood gases.

CIRCULATION

- **Assess circulating blood volume** for effectiveness in supporting blood pressure and tissue perfusion.

  - Assess peripheral pulses, blood pressure, and check the client for hemorrhage. Maintaining spinal precautions, turn the client, and check for bleeding posteriorly.

  - Apply direct pressure to hemorrhage sites or to the pressure point proximal to the wound when an extremity is involved.

  - Support an ineffective blood pressure (systolic <90) with intravenous fluid boluses given through large-bore catheters and by placing the client in the Trendelenburg position (maintain spinal precautions as necessary) or by using vassopressors.

  - Anticipate possible blood transfusions and/or emergency surgery for internal bleeding.

  - Assess for signs and symptoms of hypovolemic, cardiogenic, septic, or neurogenic shock (see Section 13-4, Table 13-3).

History

Obtain a history from the client (if possible), or from family, friends, bystanders or prehospital personnel. Important details include the mechanism of injury, any chronic or current health problems, time elapsed since any accident, medication history, drug/alcohol history, and any allergies. Check client for medic-alert bands.

Physical Examination (Secondary Survey)

- After establishing the basic ABC's of emergency care, the client has a patent Airway, is Breathing, and has Circulation, do a systematic head-to-toe assessment of the emergency victim.

- The chief complaint will likely give clues as to the cause of the crisis.

- **Head, eyes, ears, nose, throat**
  - Level of consciousness
  - Orientation to time, place, person
  - Pupil size and reaction to light
  - Injuries: lacerations, depressions, contusions, pain, foreign bodies, drainage
  - Smell of breath (distinctive in cirrhosis, ketosis, uremia, cyanide poisoning, alcoholism)
- **Neck**
  - Stiffness
  - Pain
  - Distended neck veins
  - Ability to swallow
- **Chest**
  - Symmetry of chest wall, anterior and posterior
  - Respiratory distress
  - External injuries
  - Breath sounds
  - Rib fractures (gentle palpation can reveal)
- **Abdomen and pelvis**
  - Symmetry of external abdominal wall and structures
  - Pain
  - Rigidity or distention of abdomen
  - Bowel sounds
  - External injuries
- **Extremities**
  - Color, temperature
  - Loss of sensation
  - Motor function
  - Peripheral pulses: presence, quality

- Signs of fracture: swelling, pain, limited movement

- Signs of spinal injury: decreased limb movement, decreased sensation, altered reflexes

13-2 CARDIOPULMONARY RESUSCITATION (CPR)

Be prepared to perform CPR at all times. As research continues and data becomes available, yearly updates on skill or recertification are usually required. The levels of CPR are Basic Life Support (BLS) and Advanced Cardiac Life Support (ACLS). The following guidelines are based on recommendations of the 1992 National Conference of the American Medical Association.

I. Basic Life Support

A. The initial steps of CPR are shown in Figure 13-1.

- Determine unresponsiveness.

- Call for help (or activate local **Emergency Medical System**).

- Position client on back, stabilizing neck.

B. Basic Life Support is illustrated in Figure 13-2.

- **Open the airway,** using head tilt/chin lift maneuver, jaw-thrust maneuver and Heimlich maneuver if necessary.

- **Assist breathing** with mouth-to-mouth breathing (or ambu-bag with adjuncts such as oral or nasopharyngeal airways if readily available).

- **Augment circulation** with external heart massage using designated compression and assessment rates.

C. Client with blocked airway (airway obstruction).
  1. Conscious: (Adult and child)

- Recognize a blocked airway (i.e., inability to speak, breathe, or cough, and/or person's hands clutching the neck).

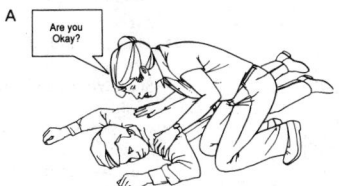

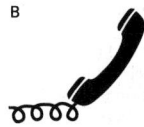

- Activate Emergency Medical System per hospital/ agency protocol.
- Community: Call 911 or local emergency number.
- If not near phone, shout for help and instruct person to phone for emergency services.

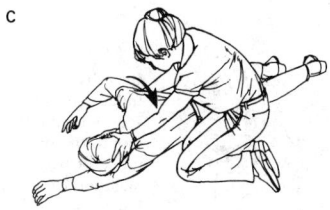

Figure 13–1. Initial steps of cardiopulmonary resuscitation. (A) Determining unresponsiveness. (B) Calling for help (or activate Emergency Medical System). (C) Positioning the victim: Stabilize head and neck, and roll victim onto back as one unit.

- Ask the person, "Are you choking?" If client is able to cough or talk, do not interfere. If choking is not recognized, the client will rapidly become pale, increasingly cyanotic, and unconscious.

- Perform the Heimlich maneuver. Get behind the client and wrap your arms around the waist. This can be done if the client is sitting or standing. A chair back acts as a support and enhances the effectiveness of the maneuver.

- Make a fist with one hand and place the thumb side against the client's abdomen, slightly above

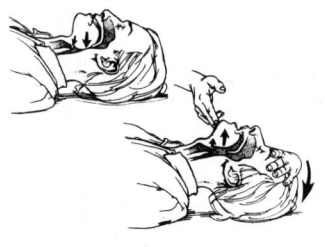

①

IF UNCONSCIOUS (see Figure 13-1 for Initial Steps of Cardio-pulmonary Resuscitation.)

Airway

- Tilt head and lift chin to open airway.
- Stabilize the neck in a neutral position.
- Grasp the angles of the victim's lower jaw, lift with both hands—one on each side of jaw to displace the mandible forward.
- If jaw thrust alone is unsuccessful, the head may be tilted back very slightly.
- Look, listen and feel for breath.
- Perform Heimlich maneuver to relieve obstruction if airway is obstructed (see Figure 13-3, Procedures for Relieving Foreign Body Airway Obstruction).

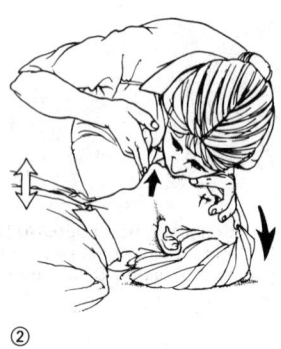

②

IF NOT BREATHING

Breathe

- Inflate lungs twice for 1½ to 2 sec each, mouth to mouth, mouth to nose, mouth to adjunct, or bag to mask.
- Maintain Head Tilt and Chin Lift.
  ...Feel carotid pulse (see Figure 13-5, Pulse Check).
  ...if pulse present, continue lung inflations as follows: Adult: 12/min; Child: 20/min; Infant: 20/min.

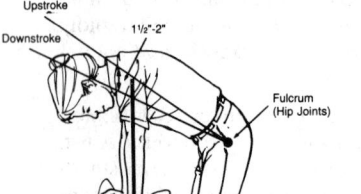

Upstroke
Downstroke
1½"-2"
Fulcrum (Hip Joints)

③

IF PULSE ABSENT

Circulate

ONE RESCUER CPR

- Adult: 80 to 100/min (15 per 9 to 11 sec).
- Alternate 2 lung inflation with 15 chest compressions.
- After 4 cycles check carotid pulse, then give 2 breaths and continue cycles. Child: 100/min, infant: 100/min.
- Alternate lung inflation with 5 chest compressions.
- After 20 cycles, check carotid pulse, ventilate once and continue cycles.

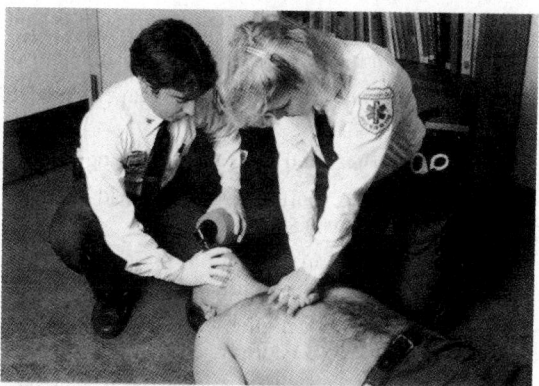

TWO-RESCUER CPR
- Interpose 1 lung inflation after every 5th compression (no pause for ventilation) at following rates:
- Adult: 80 to 100/min;
  Child: 100/min;
  Infant: 100/min.
- Reassess after 20 cycles.

DEPRESS LOWER STERNUM:
Adult: 1½ to 2 in. (4 to 5 cm) (2 hands)
Child: 1½ to 2 in. (4 to 5 cm) (1 hand)
Infant: 1½-1 in. (1 to 2.5 cm) (2 fingers)
(See Figure 13-4 for hand placement)

Figure 13–2. Basic life support.

the navel and below the rib cage, below the tip of the xiphoid process.

- Grasp your fist with the other hand and press into the client's abdomen with repeated quick upward thrusts until the obstruction is expelled or the client becomes unconscious.

2. Conscious pregnant, obese, or ascitic client:

- Chest thrusts are required. Stand behind the client and place your arms under the armpits to encircle the chest.

- Place thumb side of one hand against the middle of the sternum.

- Cover the fist with the other hand and gently press with backward thrusts until the foreign body is expelled or the client becomes unconscious.

3. Unconscious obstructed adult or child:

- Determine unresponsiveness, breathlessness.
- Call for help (or activate local Emergency Medical System).
- Look, listen, and feel for air exchange (3 sec.)
- Attempt to ventilate using the head tilt/chin lift or jaw thrust (See Figure 13-2).
- If ventilation is unsuccessful, resposition client's airway and attempt ventilation again.
- Perform the Heimlich maneuver (as described in Figure 13-3) up to five times.
- Open the client's mouth and remove any visible foreign body with finger sweep or suction.
- Attempt to ventilate client again. Repeat repositioning and successive steps as described. Continue as long as necessary.

4. Unconscious pregnant, obese, or ascitic client

- Determine unresponsivness, breathlessness.
- Call for help (or activate local Emergency Medical System).
- Look, listen and feel for air exchange (3 sec.)
- Attempt to ventilate using the head tilt/chin lift or jaw thrust (see Figure 13-2).
- If ventilation unsuccessful, reposition client's airway and attempt ventilation again.
- With the client lying face up, use the same body position and hand placement as for external chest heart compressions (Figure 13-4). Deliver each thrust slowly and distinctly. Repeat up to five times.
- Open the client's mouth and remove any visible foreign body with finger sweep or suction.
- Attempt to ventilate client again. Repeat repositioning and successive steps as described. Continue as long as necessary.

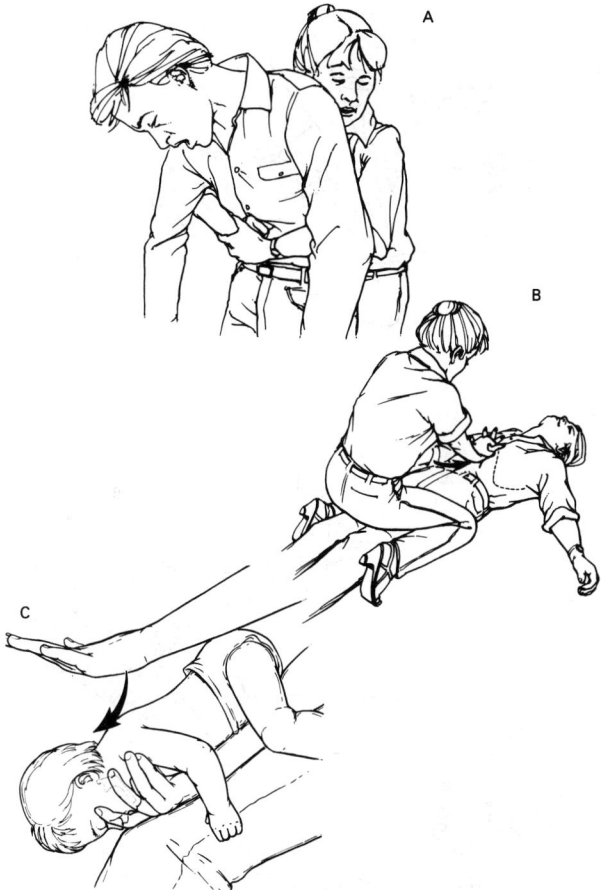

Figure 13–3. Procedures for relieving foreign-body airway obstruction. Use one of these procedures if an attempt to ventilate is unsuccessful. (A) Heimlich maneuver administered to conscious victim of foreign-body airway obstruction. (B) Heimlich maneuver administered to unconscious victim of foreign-body obstruction. (C) Back blow in infant.

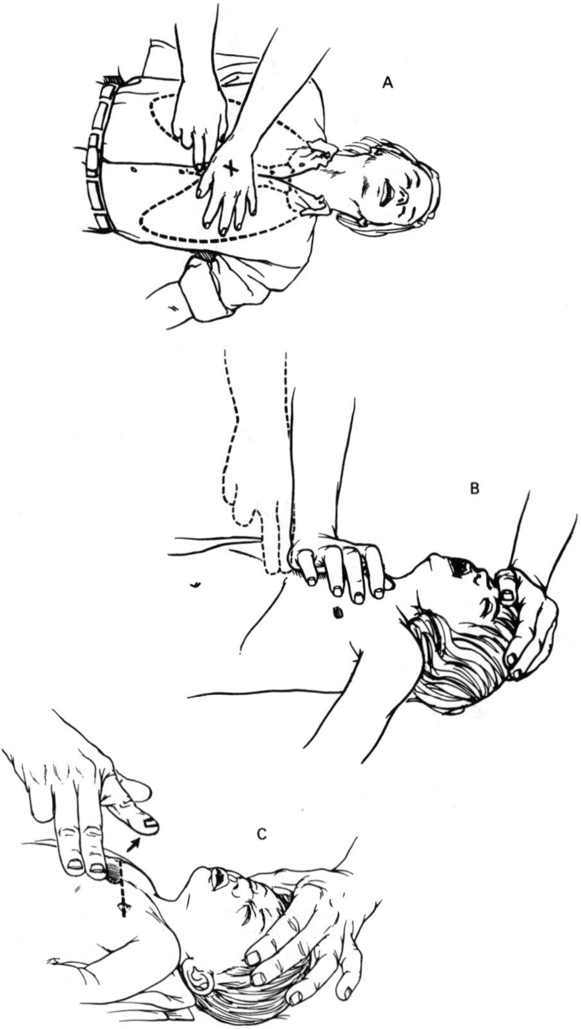

Figure 13–4. Compression hand check. (A) Locating hand position for chest compression in an adult. (B) Locating hand position for chest compression in a child. (C) Locating finger position for chest compression in an infant.

II. Advanced Cardiac Life Support (ACLS). ACLS may be initiated outside the hospital by specially trained medical personnel under the direction of a physician. ACLS may be initiated in the hospital by any certified RN. Contact your education and training department or local emergency medical offices for more information on ACLS certification courses. Usually recertification is required every two years.

ACLS involves:

- Continuous lung ventilation and necessary cardiac compression

- Intubation of the trachea

- Administration of emergency drugs via IV fluid lines, ECG monitoring, and continuation of cardiac arrest management.

A. Airway

- Continue to assess airway; head tilt/chin lift; check for foreign body obstruction.

- Rescue breathing only delivers 16–17% oxygen concentration: administer supplemental oxygen as soon as possible.

- Assist ventilation with oropharyngeal airways when the bag-valve-mask method is used.

- Esophageal obturator airways (EOA's) are used occasionally. They should not be used in clients younger than 16 yr. EOA's block the esophagus with an inflatable cuff, forcing ventilated air into the lungs.

- EOA's should be replaced with endotracheal intubation as soon as possible to improve oxygenation. Intubation is accomplished before the EOA is removed. Removal of the EOA is frequently followed by immediate regurgitation. Take appropriate precautions.

B. Breathing

- If unconsciousness and apnea continue, an endotracheal tube should be inserted to keep the airway open, prevent aspiration and allow a controlled concentration of oxygen to be delivered. Intubation should not interrupt ventilation for more than 30 sec.

- If intubation is unsuccessful, or impossible, the physician may perform a cricothyroidotomy. This is the insertion of a large-bore Teflon IV catheter directly through the cricothyroid membrane and then caudally into the trachea.

C. Circulation

- Continue external compression with the aid of cardiac monitoring, which will guide drug therapy. Evaluate the effectiveness of compressions by palpating femoral pulses.

- Drug therapy treatment will be specific for the particular dysrhythmia the client is experiencing. Electrocardiographic recognition of some dysrhythmias is shown on Table 13-1.

- Figures 13-6 through 13-13 are treatment algorithms for specific dysrhythmias. *Treatment should be individualized for each client, using the algorithms only as guidelines.*

- See Table 13-2 for drugs used in cardiac emergencies.

- One of the more frequently encountered emergency situations is **ventricular fibrillation,** a random, chaotic firing of impulses from the ventricles (see Figure 13-6).

  - Early defibrillation is critically important.

  - Paddle placement is one paddle to the right of the upper sternum below the clavicle and the other in the left anterior axillary line left of the left nipple.

  - In a *witnessed* arrest, a precordial thump is recommended except in children.

- Remember to always, first and last, treat the client—not the monitor.

TABLE 13–1. RECOGNITION OF LIFE-THREATENING DYSRHYTHMIAS

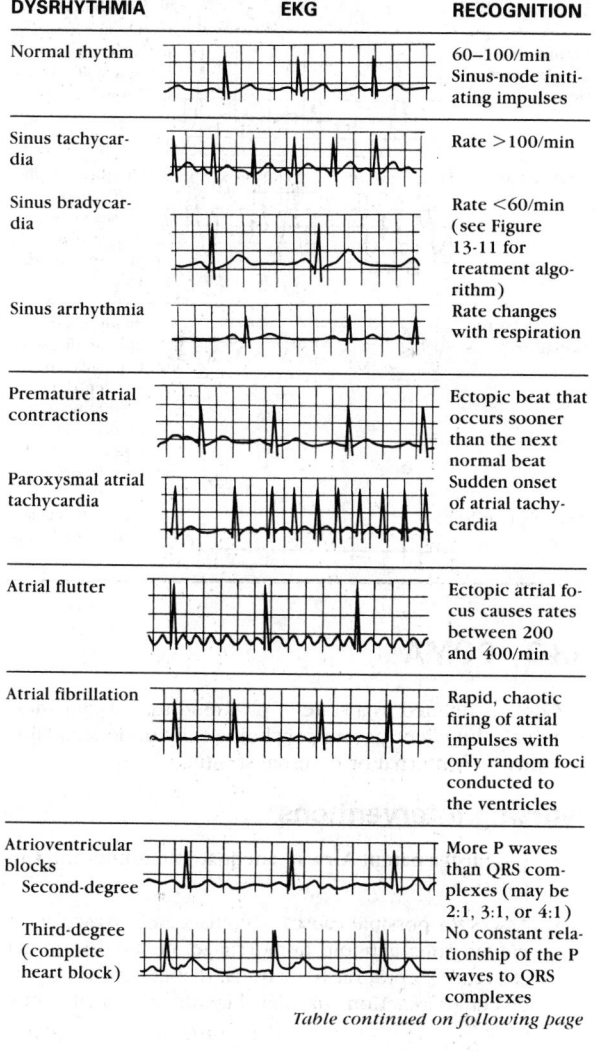

DYSRHYTHMIA	EKG	RECOGNITION
Normal rhythm		60–100/min Sinus-node initiating impulses
Sinus tachycardia		Rate >100/min
Sinus bradycardia		Rate <60/min (see Figure 13-11 for treatment algorithm)
Sinus arrhythmia		Rate changes with respiration
Premature atrial contractions		Ectopic beat that occurs sooner than the next normal beat
Paroxysmal atrial tachycardia		Sudden onset of atrial tachycardia
Atrial flutter		Ectopic atrial focus causes rates between 200 and 400/min
Atrial fibrillation		Rapid, chaotic firing of atrial impulses with only random foci conducted to the ventricles
Atrioventricular blocks Second-degree		More P waves than QRS complexes (may be 2:1, 3:1, or 4:1)
Third-degree (complete heart block)		No constant relationship of the P waves to QRS complexes

Table continued on following page

**TABLE 13–1. RECOGNITION OF
LIFE-THREATENING DYSRHYTHMIAS** *Continued*

DYSRHYTHMIA	EKG	RECOGNITION
Premature ventricular contraction	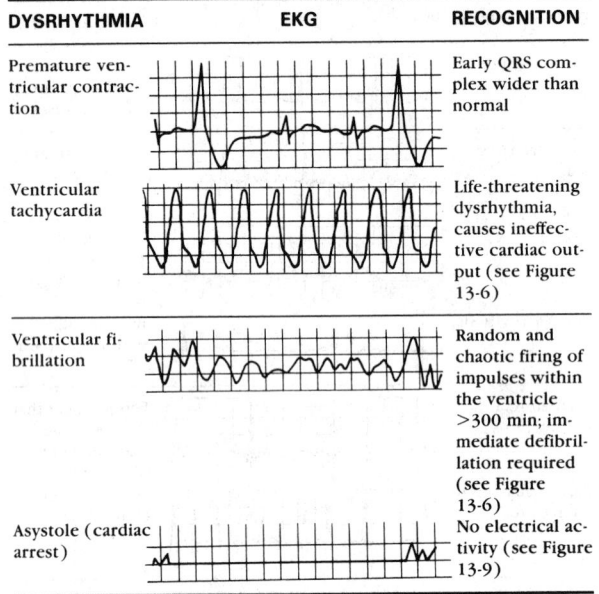	Early QRS complex wider than normal
Ventricular tachycardia		Life-threatening dysrhythmia, causes ineffective cardiac output (see Figure 13-6)
Ventricular fibrillation		Random and chaotic firing of impulses within the ventricle >300 min; immediate defibrillation required (see Figure 13-6)
Asystole (cardiac arrest)		No electrical activity (see Figure 13-9)

13-3 COMA

Coma is defined as a state of profound unconsciousness in which the client has no psychologically understandable responses to internal or external stimuli.

Nursing Interventions

- Establish a patent **A**irway, adequate **B**reathing and **C**irculation.

- Assess for possible causes of coma: cerebrovascular accident, subarachnoid hemorrhage, meningitis, injury (fracture), epidural hematoma, diabetic coma, hypoglycemic reaction, uremia, hepatic encephalopathy,

Text continued on page 605

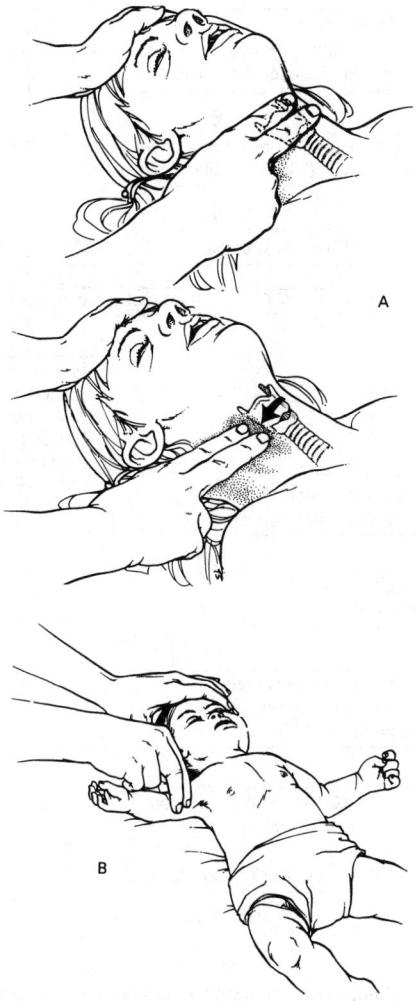

Figure 13–5. Pulse check. (A) Carotid pulse check, adult. (B) Brachial pulse palpation, infant.

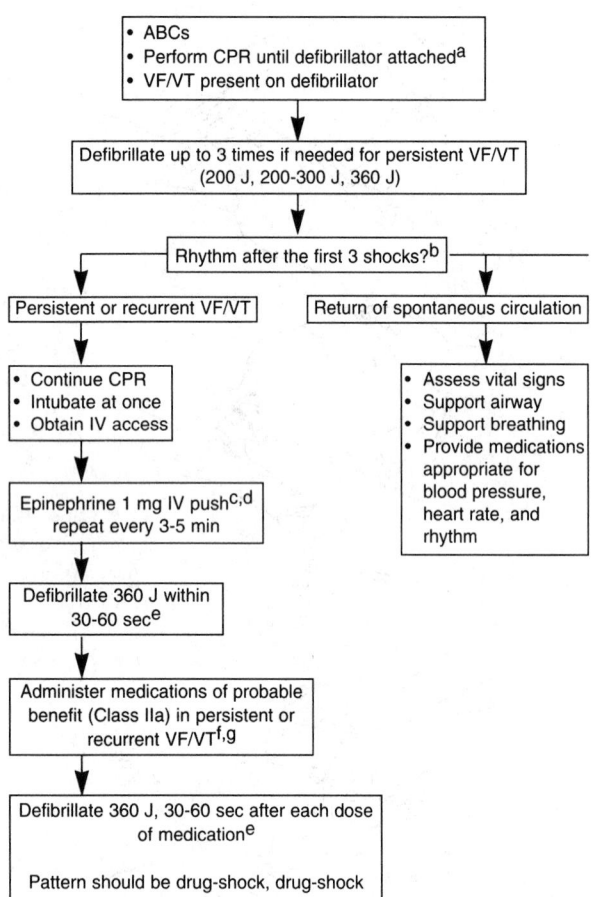

Figure 13–6. Ventricular fibrillation/pulseless ventricular tachycardia algorithm (VF/VT).

Note: Figures 13-6 through 13-12 are treatment algorithms adapted with permission from ACCS Algorithms from *Journal of the American Medical Association,* Oct. 28, 1992, 268:2199–2241. Copyright © 1992, American Medical Association.

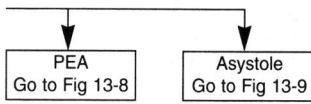

| PEA
Go to Fig 13-8 | Asystole
Go to Fig 13-9 |

Class I:	definitely helpful
Class IIa:	acceptable, probably helpful
Class IIb:	acceptable, possibly helpful
Class III:	not indicated, may be harmful

(a) Precordial thump is a Class IIb action in witnessed arrest, no pulse, and no defibrillator immediately available.

(b) Hypothermic cardiac arrest is treated differently after this point. See section on hypothermia.

(c) The recommended dose of epinephrine is 1 mg IV push every 3-5 min. If this approach fails, several Class IIb dosing regimens can be considered:
• Intermediate: epinephrine 2-5 mg IV push, every 3-5 min
• Escalating: epinephrine 1 mg-3 mg-5 mg IV push, 3 min apart
• High: epinephrine 0.1 mg/kg IV push, every 3-5 min

(d) Sodium bicarbonate (1 mEq/kg) is Class I if patient has known preexisting hyperkalemia.

(e) Multiple sequenced shocks (200, 200-300 J, 360 J) are acceptable here (Class I), especially when medications are delayed.

(f) Medications:
• Lidocaine 1.5 mg/kg IV push. Repeat in 3-5 min to total loading dose of 3 mg/kg; then use
• Bretylium 5 mg/kg IV push. Repeat in 5 min at 10 mg/kg
• Magnesium sulfate 1-2 g IV in torsades de pointes or suspected hypomagnesemic state or severe refractory VF
• Procainamide 30 mg/min in refractory VF (maximum total 17 mg/kg)

(g) Sodium bicarbonate (1 mEq/kg IV):
Class IIa
• if known preexisting bicarbonate-responsive acidosis
• if overddose with tricyclic antidepressants
• to alkalinize the urine in drug overdoses
Class IIb
• if intubated and continued long arrest interval
• upon return of spontaneous circulation after long arrest interval
Class III
• hypoxic lactic acidosis

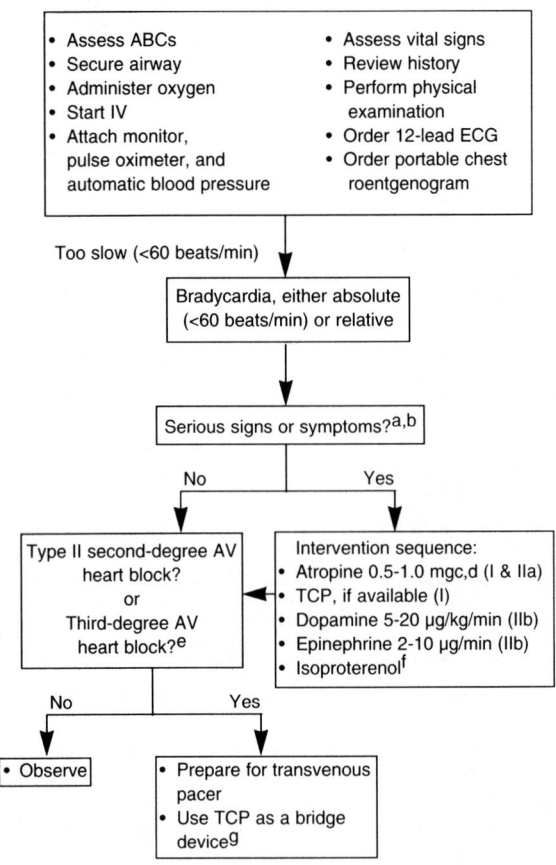

Figure 13-7. Bradycardia algorithm (client is not in cardiac arrest).

(a)Serious signs or symptoms must be related to the slow rate. Clinical manifestations include:
- symptoms (chest pain, shortness of breath, decreased level of consciousness)
- signs (low BP, shock, pulmonary congestion, CHF, acute MI).

(b)Do not delay TCP while awaiting IV access or for atropine to take effect if patient is symptomatic.

(c)Denervated transplanted hearts will not respond to atropine. Go at once to pacing, catecholamine infusion, or both.

(d)Atropine should be given in repeat doses in 3-5 min up to total of 0.04 mg/kg. consider shorter dosing intervals in severe clinical conditions. It has been suggested that atropine should be used with caution in atrioventricular (AV) block at the His-Purkinje level (type II AV block and new third-degree block with wide QRS complexes) (Class IIb).

(e)Never treat third-degree heart block plus ventricular escape beats with lidocaine.

(f)Isoproterenol should be used, if at all, with extreme caution. At low doses it is Class IIb (possibly helpful); at higher doses it is Class III (harmful).

(g)Verify patient tolerance and mechanical capture. Use analgesia and sedation as needed.

TCP = Trans cardiac pacemaker

Figure 13–7. *Continued*

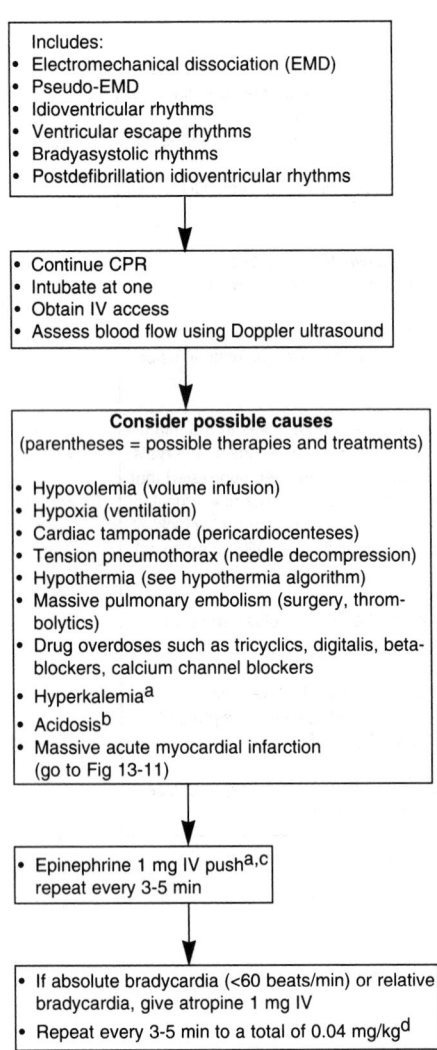

Includes:
- Electromechanical dissociation (EMD)
- Pseudo-EMD
- Idioventricular rhythms
- Ventricular escape rhythms
- Bradyasystolic rhythms
- Postdefibrillation idioventricular rhythms

- Continue CPR
- Intubate at one
- Obtain IV access
- Assess blood flow using Doppler ultrasound

Consider possible causes
(parentheses = possible therapies and treatments)

- Hypovolemia (volume infusion)
- Hypoxia (ventilation)
- Cardiac tamponade (pericardiocenteses)
- Tension pneumothorax (needle decompression)
- Hypothermia (see hypothermia algorithm)
- Massive pulmonary embolism (surgery, thrombolytics)
- Drug overdoses such as tricyclics, digitalis, beta-blockers, calcium channel blockers
- Hyperkalemia[a]
- Acidosis[b]
- Massive acute myocardial infarction (go to Fig 13-11)

- Epinephrine 1 mg IV push[a,c] repeat every 3-5 min

- If absolute bradycardia (<60 beats/min) or relative bradycardia, give atropine 1 mg IV
- Repeat every 3-5 min to a total of 0.04 mg/kg[d]

Figure 13-8. Pulseless electrical activity (PEA) algorithm (electromechanical dissociation [EMD]).

Class I: definitely helpful
Class IIa: acceptable, probably helpful
Class IIb: acceptable, possibly helpful
Class III: not indicated, may be harmful

(a) Sodium bicarbonate 1 mEq/kg is Class I if patient has known preexisting hyperkalemia

(b) Sodium bicarbonate (1 mEq/kg):
Class IIA
- if known preexisting bicarbonate-responsive acidosis
- if overdose with tricyclic antidepressants
- to alkalinize the urine in drug overdoses

Class IIb
- if intubated and long arrest interval
- upon return of spontaneous circulation after long arrest interval

Class III
- hypoxic lactic acidosis

(c) The recommended dose of epinephrine is 1 mg IV push every 3-5 min. If this approach fails, several Class IIb dosing regimens can be considered:
- Intermediate: epinephrine 2-5 mg IV push, every 3-5 min
- Escalating: epinephrine 1 mg-3 mg-5 mg IV push, 3 min apart
- High: epinephrine 0.1 mg/kg IV push every 3-5 min

(d) Shorter atropine dosing intervals are possibly helpful in cardiac arrest (Class IIb).

Figure 13–8. *Continued*

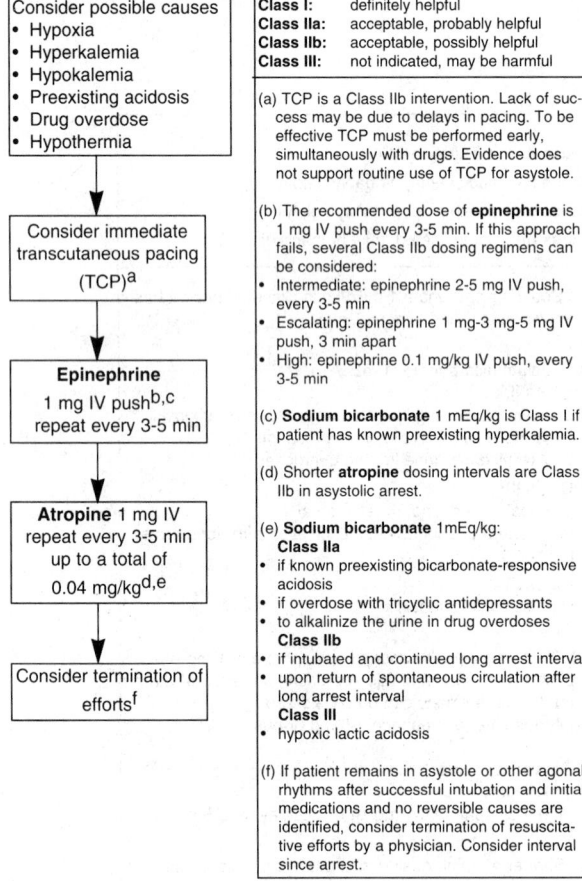

- Continue CPR
- Intubate at one
- Obtain IV access
- Confirm asystole in more than one lead

Consider possible causes
- Hypoxia
- Hyperkalemia
- Hypokalemia
- Preexisting acidosis
- Drug overdose
- Hypothermia

Consider immediate transcutaneous pacing (TCP)[a]

Epinephrine
1 mg IV push[b,c]
repeat every 3-5 min

Atropine 1 mg IV
repeat every 3-5 min
up to a total of
0.04 mg/kg[d,e]

Consider termination of efforts[f]

Class I:	definitely helpful
Class IIa:	acceptable, probably helpful
Class IIb:	acceptable, possibly helpful
Class III:	not indicated, may be harmful

(a) TCP is a Class IIb intervention. Lack of success may be due to delays in pacing. To be effective TCP must be performed early, simultaneously with drugs. Evidence does not support routine use of TCP for asystole.

(b) The recommended dose of **epinephrine** is 1 mg IV push every 3-5 min. If this approach fails, several Class IIb dosing regimens can be considered:
- Intermediate: epinephrine 2-5 mg IV push, every 3-5 min
- Escalating: epinephrine 1 mg-3 mg-5 mg IV push, 3 min apart
- High: epinephrine 0.1 mg/kg IV push, every 3-5 min

(c) **Sodium bicarbonate** 1 mEq/kg is Class I if patient has known preexisting hyperkalemia.

(d) Shorter **atropine** dosing intervals are Class IIb in asystolic arrest.

(e) **Sodium bicarbonate** 1mEq/kg:
Class IIa
- if known preexisting bicarbonate-responsive acidosis
- if overdose with tricyclic antidepressants
- to alkalinize the urine in drug overdoses
Class IIb
- if intubated and continued long arrest interval
- upon return of spontaneous circulation after long arrest interval
Class III
- hypoxic lactic acidosis

(f) If patient remains in asystole or other agonal rhythms after successful intubation and initial medications and no reversible causes are identified, consider termination of resuscitative efforts by a physician. Consider interval since arrest.

Figure 13–9. Asystole treatment algorithm.

alcohol/drug overdose, hypothermia, acid-base disturbances, myxedema, epilepsy, or psychosis.

- Maintain a patent airway. An oral airway or intubation
  may be needed. If trauma is suspected, maintain spinal integrity until a cervical fracture is ruled out.

- Using a flow sheet, obtain vital signs (including tem-
  perature) and level of consciousness (may utilize
  Glasgow Coma Scale—See Section 1-5, Neurological
  Assessment).

- Obtain x-rays as ordered—anticipate Computerized
  Tomography (CT) scanning. Obtain laboratory values
  as necessary and anticipate obtaining arterial blood
  gases.

- *Naloxone (Narcan), 0.4 mg IV* may be given × 3 in
  suspected narcotic overdose, *50 ml of 50% dextrose
  IV* in suspected hypoglycemia may be given, and consider *Flumazenil (Mazicon) 3–5 mg. IV* given 0.5 mg
  per min in suspected benzodiazipine overdoses. The
  recommended doses represent a compromise between desirable slow awakening and the need for
  prompt response and a persistent effect in an overdose situation. If circumstances permit, the physician
  may elect to use 0.2 mg per min titration rate to
  slowly awaken the client over 5–10 min which may
  help to reduce withdrawal symptoms. Most overdoses
  respond to a total dose of 1–3 mg.

- Insert a Foley catheter, obtain urinalysis, consider
  urine toxicology, and monitor output.

- Monitor client response to procedures and treatment.

- Remember that many comatose clients are able to
  hear and understand people around them.

13-4 SHOCK

Shock is a life-threatening state in which tissues are not
perfused with blood. It is always secondary to a cause that
may be cardiac (heart fails to pump properly), hemato-
genic (blood volume is decreased), septic (bacterial endo-

Text continued on page 611

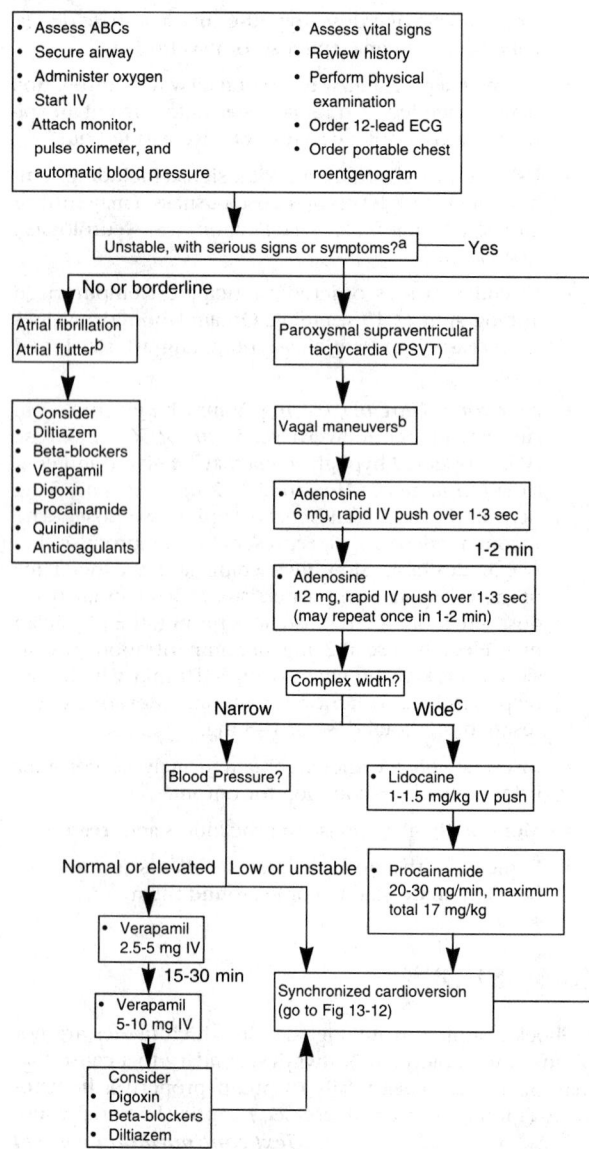

Figure 13–10. Tachycardia algorithm.

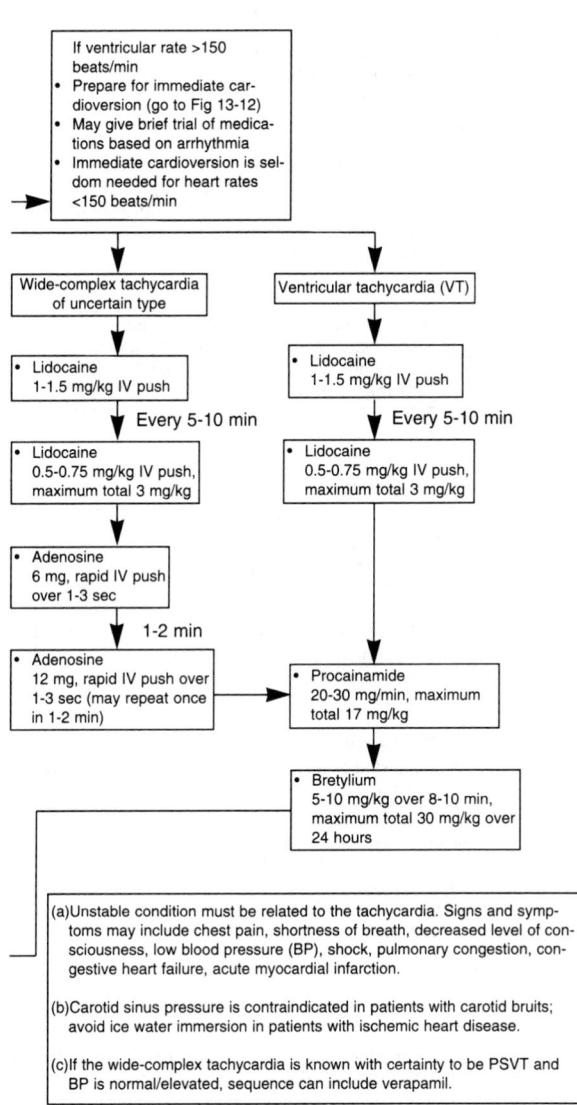

If ventricular rate >150 beats/min
- Prepare for immediate cardioversion (go to Fig 13-12)
- May give brief trial of medications based on arrhythmia
- Immediate cardioversion is seldom needed for heart rates <150 beats/min

Wide-complex tachycardia of uncertain type

Ventricular tachycardia (VT)

- Lidocaine
  1-1.5 mg/kg IV push

- Lidocaine
  1-1.5 mg/kg IV push

Every 5-10 min

Every 5-10 min

- Lidocaine
  0.5-0.75 mg/kg IV push, maximum total 3 mg/kg

- Lidocaine
  0.5-0.75 mg/kg IV push, maximum total 3 mg/kg

- Adenosine
  6 mg, rapid IV push over 1-3 sec

1-2 min

- Adenosine
  12 mg, rapid IV push over 1-3 sec (may repeat once in 1-2 min)

- Procainamide
  20-30 mg/min, maximum total 17 mg/kg

- Bretylium
  5-10 mg/kg over 8-10 min, maximum total 30 mg/kg over 24 hours

(a) Unstable condition must be related to the tachycardia. Signs and symptoms may include chest pain, shortness of breath, decreased level of consciousness, low blood pressure (BP), shock, pulmonary congestion, congestive heart failure, acute myocardial infarction.

(b) Carotid sinus pressure is contraindicated in patients with carotid bruits; avoid ice water immersion in patients with ischemic heart disease.

(c) If the wide-complex tachycardia is known with certainty to be PSVT and BP is normal/elevated, sequence can include verapamil.

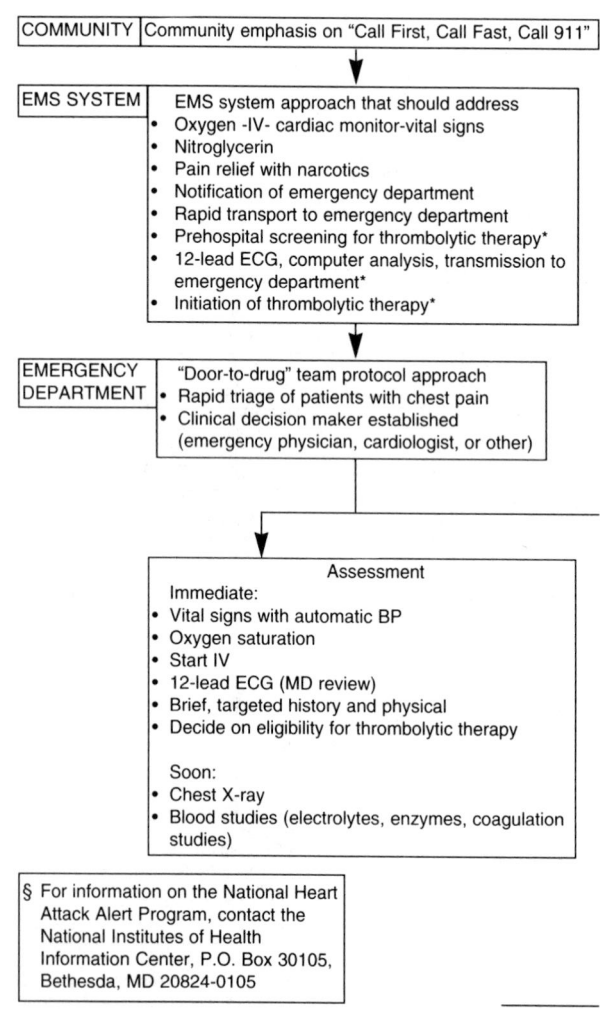

| COMMUNITY | Community emphasis on "Call First, Call Fast, Call 911" |

| EMS SYSTEM | EMS system approach that should address
• Oxygen -IV- cardiac monitor-vital signs
• Nitroglycerin
• Pain relief with narcotics
• Notification of emergency department
• Rapid transport to emergency department
• Prehospital screening for thrombolytic therapy*
• 12-lead ECG, computer analysis, transmission to emergency department*
• Initiation of thrombolytic therapy* |

| EMERGENCY DEPARTMENT | "Door-to-drug" team protocol approach
• Rapid triage of patients with chest pain
• Clinical decision maker established (emergency physician, cardiologist, or other) |

Assessment
Immediate:
• Vital signs with automatic BP
• Oxygen saturation
• Start IV
• 12-lead ECG (MD review)
• Brief, targeted history and physical
• Decide on eligibility for thrombolytic therapy

Soon:
• Chest X-ray
• Blood studies (electrolytes, enzymes, coagulation studies)

§ For information on the National Heart Attack Alert Program, contact the National Institutes of Health Information Center, P.O. Box 30105, Bethesda, MD 20824-0105

*Optional guidelines

Figure 13–11. Acute myocardial infarction algorithm (recommendations for early management of clients with chest pain and possible AMI).

Time interval in emergency department

Treatments to consider if there is evidence of coronary thrombosis plus no reasons for exclusion:
(some but not all may be appropriate)
- Oxygen at 4 L/min
- Nitroglycerin SL paste or spray (if systolic blood pressure >90 mm Hg)
- Morphine IV
- Aspirin PO
- Thrombolytic agents
- Nitroglycerin IV (limit systolic BP drop to 10% if normotensive; 30% drop if hypertensive; never drop below 90 mm Hg systolic)
- Beta-blockers IV
- Heparin IV
- Routine lidocaine administration is NOT recommended for all patients with AMI
- Magnesium sulfate IV
- Percutaneous transluminal coronary angioplasty

30-60 min to thrombolytic therapy

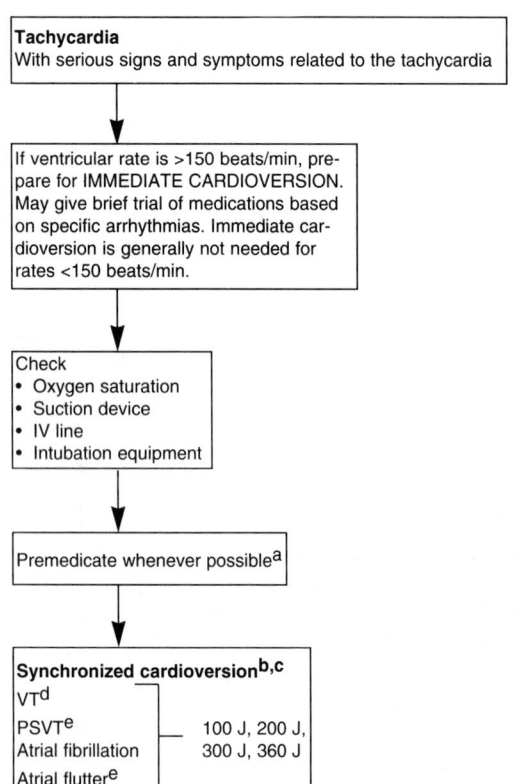

> **Tachycardia**
> With serious signs and symptoms related to the tachycardia

> If ventricular rate is >150 beats/min, prepare for IMMEDIATE CARDIOVERSION. May give brief trial of medications based on specific arrhythmias. Immediate cardioversion is generally not needed for rates <150 beats/min.

> Check
> • Oxygen saturation
> • Suction device
> • IV line
> • Intubation equipment

> Premedicate whenever possible[a]

> **Synchronized cardioversion[b,c]**
> VT[d]
> PSVT[e]   ⎤ 100 J, 200 J,
> Atrial fibrillation ⎥ 300 J, 360 J
> Atrial flutter[e] ⎦

> (a) Effective regimens have included a sedative (eg, diazepam, midazolam, barbiturates, etomidate, ketamine, methohexital) with or without an analgesic agent (eg, fentanyl, morphine, meperidine). Many experts recommend anesthesia if service is readily available.
> (b) Note possible need to resynchronize after each cardioversion.
> (c) If delays in synchronization occur and clinical conditions are critical, go to immediate unsynchronized shocks.
> (d) Treat polymorphic VT (irregular form and rate) like VF: 200 J, 200-300 J, 360 J.
> (e) PSVT and atrial flutter often respond to lower energy levels (start with 50 J).

Figure 13–12. Electrical cardioversion algorithm (client is not in cardiac arrest).

toxins may cause severe fluid volume loss and vasodilation), or neurogenic (a severe shock to the nervous system causes increased size of the vascular bed due to massive vasodilitation).

Signs and symptoms of shock are cool, clammy skin, marked hypotension, restlessness, diaphoresis, rapid shallow breathing, rapid thready pulse, dilated pupils, decreased level of consciousness, and decreased urine output (Table 13-3). Any adult client with a systolic blood pressure of 40–55 mm Hg below his or her usual resting level or below 80–90 mm Hg should be checked thoroughly for other manifestations of shock.

Circulating blood volume must be restored and the underlying cause identified and corrected while keeping the client warm, reassured, and monitored frequently.

Nursing Interventions for Hypovolemic, Cardiogenic, or Septic Shock

- Maintain the airway, administer oxygen at 6–10 liters/min (unless client has COPD–Chronic Obstructive Pulmonary Disease), observe for pulmonary edema

- Control any obvious bleeding by applying pressure to the site and/or pressure points (Figure 13-14).

- Take frequent vital signs to monitor status: check BP, respirations, apical and peripheral pulses every 5–15 min.

- Start at least one IV with a 14–16 gauge needle: 5% dextrose in water to keep vein open

  - For hypovolemic shock, start a second IV with Ringer's Lactate or normal saline

  - For cardiogenic shock, use 5% dextrose in water to keep vein open with microdripper and mechanical controller.

  - For septic shock, Ringer's lactate, normal saline, or other volume expanders as ordered.

- Monitor the heart with heart monitor or 12-lead ECG: ICU monitoring may be required.

Text continued on page 617

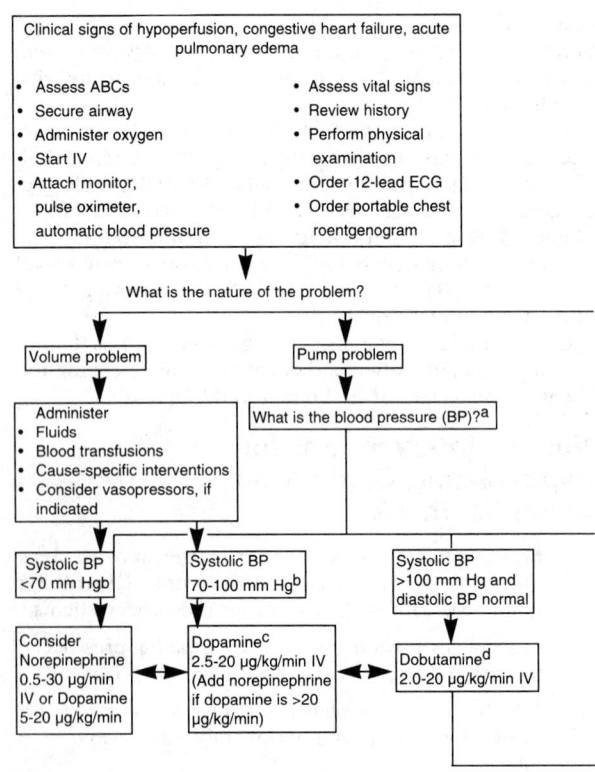

Clinical signs of hypoperfusion, congestive heart failure, acute pulmonary edema

- Assess ABCs
- Secure airway
- Administer oxygen
- Start IV
- Attach monitor, pulse oximeter, automatic blood pressure

- Assess vital signs
- Review history
- Perform physical examination
- Order 12-lead ECG
- Order portable chest roentgenogram

What is the nature of the problem?

Volume problem

Pump problem

Administer
- Fluids
- Blood transfusions
- Cause-specific interventions
- Consider vasopressors, if indicated

What is the blood pressure (BP)?[a]

Systolic BP <70 mm Hg[b]

Systolic BP 70-100 mm Hg[b]

Systolic BP >100 mm Hg and diastolic BP normal

Consider Norepinephrine 0.5-30 μg/min IV or Dopamine 5-20 μg/kg/min

Dopamine[c] 2.5-20 μg/kg/min IV (Add norepinephrine if dopamine is >20 μg/kg/min)

Dobutamine[d] 2.0-20 μg/kg/min IV

(a) Base management after this point on invasive hemodynamic monitoring if possible.
(b) Fluid bolus of 250-500 mL normal saline should be tried. If no response, consider sympathomimetics.
(c) Move to dopamine and stop norepinephrine when BP improves.
(d) Add dopamine when BP improves. Avoid dobutamine when systolic BP <100 mm Hg.

Figure 13–13. Hypotension/shock/acute pulmonary edema algorithm.

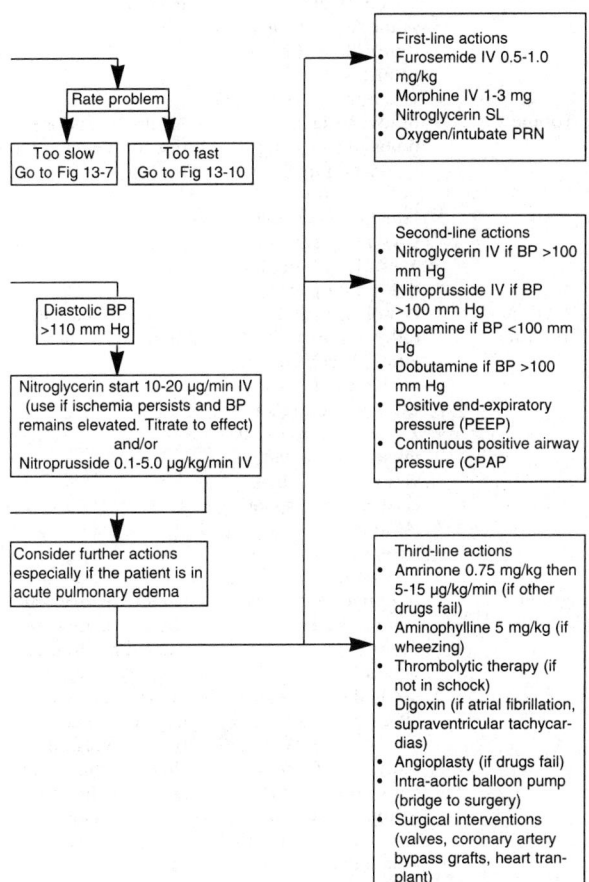

Rate problem

Too slow
Go to Fig 13-7

Too fast
Go to Fig 13-10

Diastolic BP
>110 mm Hg

Nitroglycerin start 10-20 μg/min IV
(use if ischemia persists and BP
remains elevated. Titrate to effect)
and/or
Nitroprusside 0.1-5.0 μg/kg/min IV

Consider further actions
especially if the patient is in
acute pulmonary edema

First-line actions
• Furosemide IV 0.5-1.0
  mg/kg
• Morphine IV 1-3 mg
• Nitroglycerin SL
• Oxygen/intubate PRN

Second-line actions
• Nitroglycerin IV if BP >100
  mm Hg
• Nitroprusside IV if BP
  >100 mm Hg
• Dopamine if BP <100 mm
  Hg
• Dobutamine if BP >100
  mm Hg
• Positive end-expiratory
  pressure (PEEP)
• Continuous positive airway
  pressure (CPAP)

Third-line actions
• Amrinone 0.75 mg/kg then
  5-15 μg/kg/min (if other
  drugs fail)
• Aminophylline 5 mg/kg (if
  wheezing)
• Thrombolytic therapy (if
  not in schock)
• Digoxin (if atrial fibrillation,
  supraventricular tachycar-
  dias)
• Angioplasty (if drugs fail)
• Intra-aortic balloon pump
  (bridge to surgery)
• Surgical interventions
  (valves, coronary artery
  bypass grafts, heart tran-
  plant)

TABLE 13–2. DRUGS USED IN CARDIAC EMERGENCIES (ADULT DOSAGES)

DRUG	SUGGESTED DOSE AND ROUTE	REMARKS
Adenosine	6 mg rapid bolus IV over 1–3 sec followed by 20 ml saline flush. 12 mg repeat dose if no response in 1–2 min	Should not be used in clients on carbamazepine
Atropine	Bradycardia: IV bolus. 0.5–1.0 mg q 3–5 min until pulse is >60 (smaller doses may slow heart rate) Asystole: 1.0 mg IV q 3–5 min prn	Adult: Total dose not to exceed 0.04 mg/kg
Bretylium (Bretylol)	IV bolus, 5 mg/kg, followed by defibrillation. If ventricular fibrillation persists, can give 10 mg/kg q 15–30 min up to 30 mg/kg; for persistent ventricular tachycardia: 5–10 mg/kg in 50 ml 5% dextrose in water over 8–10 min	Use cautiously in digitalized clients
Digoxin (Lanoxin)	In congestive heart failure, digitalizing doses (unless evidence of recent use) tailored to specific need: typically 0.25–0.5 mg IV initially, then 0.25–0.5 mg IV q 4–6 hr IV to total dose of 1 mg, then daily maintenance dose (see	Check history—arrhythmias may be caused by digitalis toxicity instead of congestive heart failure; assess blood levels. Also, slow digitalization (po) may be indicated for elderly or debilitated clients.

TABLE 13–2. DRUGS USED IN CARDIAC EMERGENCIES (ADULT DOSAGES) *Continued*

DRUG	SUGGESTED DOSE AND ROUTE	REMARKS
	also Selected Drug Therapies, Section 7-5)	
Dopamine	IV infusion only— 2–5 µg/kg/min, may increase to 10 µg/kg/min. Using microdrip tubing, 1 drop/min will equal 1 µg/kg/min.	Used after cardiac rhythm has been restored, to stabilize BP.
Epinephrine (Adrenalin)	IV bolus, intratracheally: 1.0 mg of a 1:10,000 solution; repeat q 3–5 min Intracardially: 0.3–0.05 mg of a 1:10,000 solution	For IV drip through central venous line, add 1 mg of epinephrine to 250 ml of fluid, start at 1 µg/min, increase to 4 µg/min as needed; Note dilution; Half dosages are given to children
Inderal	1–3 mg IV q 5 min up to 0.1 mg/kg	
Isoproterenol (Isuprel)	IV drip, 1 mg in 500 ml 5% dextrose in water: 1 mg/500 ml = 2 µg/ml, infuse at 2–10 µg/min	Titrate for desired effect.
Levarterenol (Levophed)	IV bolus, 2–5 mg every 5–10 min IV drip; titrate for desired blood pressure	Don't use in endotoxic shock or renal shutdown.
Lidocaine (Xylocaine)	IV bolus, 1.5 mg/kg, repeat q 2–5 min until ventricular tachycardia resolves. Do not exceed a total of 3 mg/kg.	See Figure 13-6 for ventricular tachycardia algorithm.

Table continued on following page

TABLE 13–2. DRUGS USED IN CARDIAC EMERGENCIES (ADULT DOSAGES) *Continued*

DRUG	SUGGESTED DOSE AND ROUTE	REMARKS
Morphine sulfate	1–3 mg IV doses at 5 min intervals until the desired response is achieved.	Analgesic of choice for pain of acute MI.
Nitroglycerin	IV bolus, 10 μg/min: increase in 5–10 μg/min increments as mandated by the response	A toxic effect is hypotension.
Pronestyl	50 mg IV q 5 min up to 1 g until either dysrhythmia is suppressed, hypotension occurs, or QRS complex widens; 50% maintenance infusion: 1–4 mg/min	Indicated when lidocaine is contraindicated or has failed to suppress ventricular ectopy. Give IV bolus slowly, watch for hypotension.
Sodium bicarbonate*	May vary based on the clinical situation	Do not give intratracheally. Flush tubing after administration. Cannot be given with CA, catecholamines in same line.
Verapamil	5 mg IV initially; if supraventricular tachycardia persists, give 10 mg IV in 10–15 min	Observe for hypotension. Antidote: calcium chloride. See also Figure 13-10.

*To be used after defibrillation, cardiac compression, ventilatory support, and pharmacologic support.

Data from Guidelines for Cardiopulmonary Resuscitation, JAMA, Oct 28, Vol. 268, No. 16, 1992.

TABLE 13–3. SHOCK—INITIAL SIGNS AND SYMPTOMS

	HYPO-VOLEMIC	CARDIO-GENIC	SEPTIC	ANAPHY-LACTIC	NEURO-GENIC
Decreased BP	√	√	√	√	√
Increased, thready pulse	√	√	√	√	Brady-cardia
Cold, clammy skin	√	√	Warm, flushed, diapho-retic	Sweating	Skin warm, dry
Restlessness	√	√	√	√	√
Pallor	Extreme	√	√	√	√
Gross bleed-ing (observed or occult)	√	0	0	0	0
Signs and symptoms of myocardial in-farction or congestive heart failure (distended neck veins, chest pain)	0	√	0	0	0
Heart arrhyth-mias	In ad-vanced stages	√	0	√	0
Fever, infec-tion	0	0	√	0	0
Urticaria (hives)	0	0	0	√	0
Generalized swelling	0	0	0	√	0
Broncho-spasm, short-ness of breath	0	0	0	√	0

- Monitor client response to fluids and treatment. Adjust nursing care plan as indicated.

- Pneumatic Anti-Shock Garments (PASG) markedly redistribute intravascular fluid into the upper circulation and can be valuable in the treatment of shock. However, their use is controversial in cardiogenic shock, absolutely contraindicated in the presence of

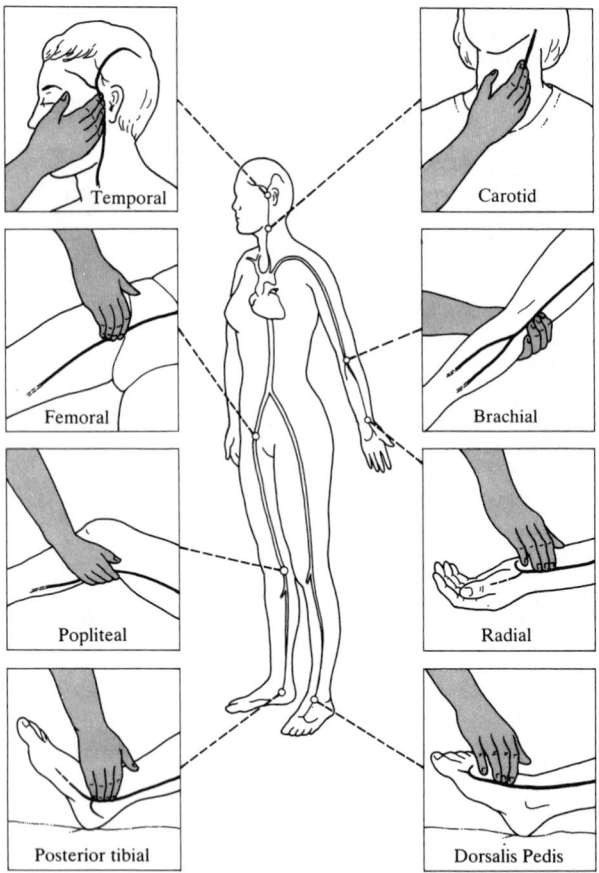

Figure 13–14. Pulse points.

congestive heart failure or pulmonary edema, and highly questionable in cases of head injury, chest injury, or pregnancy.

- Use a modified-shock position, except in cardiogenic shock: supine, legs elevated 45 degrees with knees straight, head and neck level with trunk, slightly raised.

- Keep client warm.

- Obtain laboratory values: complete blood count, electrolytes, blood urea nitrogen, sugar, coagulation, screen, type and crossmatch for blood (if there is blood loss), arterial blood gases, blood cultures q20 min × 3 for septic shock and consider urine and sputum cultures.

- Administer appropriate medications, i.e., vasopressors, antiarrhythmics, digitalis, or antibiotics (after cultures obtained).

- Obtain x-rays.

- Monitor hourly intake and output: report output <30 ml. per hr.

- Lower anxiety by frequent reassurance of client and family.

Neurogenic Shock

Neurogenic shock may be due to psychological trauma, simple faint, or spinal or general anesthesia. The assessment finding that distinguishes this kind of shock from the others is bradycardia.

NURSING INTERVENTIONS

- Many times, elevating the legs is enough to stimulate perfusion (only if spinal fractures have been ruled out).

- If due to psychogenic factors, remove the source of the stimulus, lower the client's head, and have client inhale aromatic spirits of ammonia.

- Pressor agents, e.g., dopamine, aramine, neosynephrine, dobutamine, or norepinephrine may be useful.

- An IV may be started to restore circulating volume if other measures fail.

Anaphylactic Shock

Anaphylaxis is a severe, generalized antigen-antibody reaction resulting from exposure to an allergen. The two most common precipitating agents are penicillin and bee-sting venom. Signs and symptoms are urticaria; respiratory distress, wheezing, stridor, hoarseness, total body swelling, hypotension, sense of impending doom, and respiratory and cardiac arrest.

NURSING INTERVENTIONS

- Maintain airway. Intubation, cricothyroidectomy, or tracheotomy may be necessary.

- Oxygen at 6–10 liters/min by mask (if tolerated).

- If bee sting is the cause, scrape the stinger out of the skin with fingernail or other flat edge (do not use tweezers as squeezing the stinger may release more venom).

- Epinephrine 0.3 to 0.5 mg (0.01 mg/kg) of 1 : 1000 concentration is given subcutaneously or intramuscularly, injected sublingually, or instilled through the endotracheal tube. For extreme reactions: epinephrine 0.5–1.0 ml of 1 : 10,000 solution IV. Or a tourniquet above the sting or injection site may be applied and the arm may be injected with 0.1–0.3 ml of epinephrine: 1 : 1000 solution.

- Start an IV with a large-bore cathlon of Ringer's lactate or normal saline or 5% dextrose in water, depending on condition.

- Apply cardiac monitor.

- Diphenhydramine (Benadryl) 25–50 mg intramuscularly or IV may be ordered, or Aminophylline 250–500 mg IV push, *very slowly,* or IV drip over 20 minutes. Monitor cardiac status continuously during administration.

- Steroids such as methylprednisolone (Solu-Medrol) or dexamethasone may be given IV.

- Provide constant nursing observation with vital signs q5 minutes until client condition stabilizes.

- Apply PASG (Pneumatic Anti-Shock Trousers) as indicated.

- Teach client to wear medic-alert device, about use of a bee sting kit, and to avoid allergens.

- See also Injected Poisons in Section 13-12
- Reassure the client and the family.

13-5   HEMORRHAGE

In hemorrage, bleeding and clinical signs of shock occur: cool, moist skin; falling blood pressure; rapid heart rate, then decreasing heart rate.

Nursing Interventions

- Cut the client's clothing away quickly.

- Apply firm, steady pressure over any obvious bleeding, or at the pulse point above the involved sites (see Figure 13-14). Almost all external bleeding can be stopped by direct pressure. Untreated arterial bleeding results in death.

- Apply a firm pressure dressing. Elevate the injured part to stop venous and capillary bleeding. Immobilize an injured extremity to control blood loss.

- Apply a tourniquet to an extremity only as a last resort, when the hemorrhage cannot be controlled by any other means. If using an inflated blood pressure cuff, inflate above the systolic blood pressure. If tourniquet is applied, loss of the limb is likely.

- Start an IV with a large needle (14–16 gauge) and carry out measures for hypovolemic shock (Section 13-4).

13-6   MYOCARDIAL INFARCTION

Myocardial infarction is a localized ischemic necrosis of an area of the myocardium caused by a narrowing of one or more of the coronary arteries. The narrowing may be caused by any of the following: occlusion of a main coronary artery by embolism, atherosclerotic plaque formation and hemorrhage within coronary artery(s), gradual sclerotic occlusion, post-operative or traumatic shock, or myocardial aneurysm. The severity of an MI depends on the location and extent of the ischemia, adequacy of collateral circulation, and presence of previously infarcted tissue.

Nursing Assessment

- Identify the high risk client:
  - Client with a history of MI, angina, atherosclerosis, hypertension, congestive heart failure (CHF), thromboembolic problems, carditis, aneurysm, or other cardiovascular disease.
  - Obese people, heavy smokers, people with high stress occupations, type A behavior patterns and/or sedentary lifestyles.

- **Signs and Symptoms of MI**
  - Severe, prolonged substernal chest pain/pressure, unchanged with respirations or movement. Pain/pressure may or may not radiate to the jaw, neck, arms, or back. The client may also complain primarily of arm, jaw, or neck pain.
  - Dyspnea
  - Cold, clammy skin with pallor
  - Hypotension or hypertension initially
  - Tachycardia or bradycardia
  - Nausea, possibly vomiting
  - Severe apprehension and anxiety.

Nursing Interventions
ACUTE STAGE ON THE MEDICAL-SURGICAL UNIT

- Notify the physician and nursing supervisor immediately upon recognizing symptoms. Prepare for probable transfer to CCU.
- Maintain strict bedrest in semi-Fowler's position.
- Administer oxygen, usually 4–6 liters by nasal canula or 2 liters for COPD (Chronic Obstructive Pulmonary Disease) clients.

- Obtain 12-lead ECG, and apply cardiac monitor.

- Position crash cart outside room until transferred to CCU. Be prepared to initiate CPR if pulse and respirations cease.

- Establish IV access—usually 5% dextrose in water at a keep open rate.

- Obtain orders for pain medication—may be sublingual nitroglycerin progressing to IV morphine sulfate as necessary.

- Obtain laboratory values to include: CBC, electrolytes, BUN, creatinine, cardiac enzymes (SGOT, LDH, CPK, and CPK iso-enzymes), and consider coagulation studies.

- Obtain portable chest x-ray before transfer to CCU, if possible.

- Treat arrhythmias as necessary, e.g., lidocaine HCL, procainamide HCL, atropine, etc. (see Figures 13-6 through 13-13 for treatment algorithms).

- Provide calm reassurance and a quiet atmosphere. Transfer client to CCU at earliest opportunity. Anticipate treatment based on type of MI, client risk factors and history, and hospital capabilities. For example:

MEDICAL TREATMENT OPTIONS

- Streptokinase and urokinase are clot-dissolving agents effective in reducing tissue damage if given within 4–6 hr of an MI.

- Newer "clot-busters" include t-pa (tissue plasminogen activator) and Eminase. The primary advantage over streptokinase and urokinase is decreased incidence of allergic reactions and faster deactivation of anticoagulation effect after injection.

- Cardiac catheterization, including coronary angioplasty. This method threads a catheter through the groin into the heart, identifies narrowed or occluded arteries with dye and opens the artery by inflating a balloon at the tip of the catheter. Cardiac catheterization may be combined with the use of "clot-busters."

- Coronary Artery Bypass Graft surgery (CABG) may be the follow-up to cardiac catheterization when angioplasty is unsuccessful, where more than one artery is occluded, or both.

POST-ACUTE STAGE ON THE MEDICAL-SURGICAL UNIT

- Assess frequently for complications of MI: CHF, pulmonary embolism, arrhythmias (including ventricular fibrillation), pericarditis, cardiac shock, acute renal failure, cerebral infarction, cardiac arrest.

- Take apical pulse with vital signs: assess for arrhythmias. Monitor with cardiac monitor if available.

- Provide emotional reassurance and confidence in looking toward rehabilitation.

- Allow participation in self-care activities but insist that prescribed activity limitations are adhered to. Provide uninterrupted periods of rest, but prevent complications of bed rest. Encourage range of motion exercises to strengthen upper extremities and prevent shoulder-hand syndrome.

- Make sure dietary restrictions are followed. These usually include avoidance of caffeine, nicotine, alcohol and iced drinks, restriction of sodium and cholesterol.

- Clients post-MI should not use a bedpan or strain at stool. Provide a bedside commode and see that stool softeners are ordered.

- Meet the client's psychosocial needs by listening to fears and anxieties, offering reassurance, and providing information about treatment and medication. Include significant others in the care plan and encourage non-fatiguing socializing. Obtain referral for a psychiatric nurse specialist or other mental health professional if possible.

- Refer the client and family to a cardiac rehabilitation program.

- Client teaching: prepare individualized teaching plan. Consult with the physician as to any limitations. At appropriate time, stress the importance of weight control, medication regime, smoking cessation, diet therapy, stress reduction and relaxation techniques, exercise program, and guidelines for resuming sexual activities.

13-7 HEAD INJURIES

Fracture of the cervical spine frequently accompanies head injury. Suspect it until ruled out (see Section 13-8). Exercise great care in positioning these clients and maintaining a patent airway (Figure 13-15). The brain is particularly vulnerable to anoxia.

Skull Fractures

Skull fractures are usually a result of trauma. There may or may not be brain injuries or hemorrhage with the fracture. Fractures may be simple, depressed, compound, or basilar. Clinical signs of basilar skull fracture (occurring at the base of the brain and frequently accompanied by cervical spine fracture) are ecchymosis at the mastoid process (Battles' sign), periorbital ecchymosis (racoon eyes), and blood behind the tympanic membrane. The main concern is that the skull fracture(s) may have caused one of the following brain injuries.

Types of Brain Injury

CONCUSSION

Concussion is the loss of consciousness associated with a blow to the head that clears within 24 hr. There may be transient amnesia, vertigo, nausea, and weak pulse. When client regains consciousness, there may be a severe headache and blurred vision. If the injury is severe client may lapse into a coma.

CONTUSION

Contusions are similar to a concussion, but there is more severe brain-stem damage and unconsciousness is prolonged beyond 24 hr. There is extravasation of red blood cells into the substance of the brain and cerebral edema.

Extreme care must be taken to fully support the neck of anyone suspected of having a cervical spine injury until a rigid immobilization device is applied.

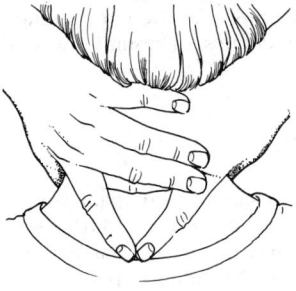

The hand position for supporting the neck is shown at left ● The neck is supported in a neutral position by placing the index fingers just below C7, at the base of the neck ● The thumbs support the mandible (taking care to avoid the area under the mandible, where vessels could be compressed) ● The remaining interlocked fingers cradle the occiput and posterior neck ● By keeping the elbows extended outward, the temptation to support the head laterally with the forearm is minimized. Lateral forearm support of the head is advisable because inadvertent flexion of the neck could occur during lifting.

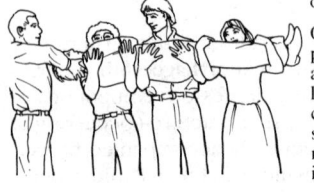

Once the neck is stabilized, assisting personnel can slide their hands and arms under the patient as shown at left. The first arm to go under the client should be nearest the fracture site. Personnel at the shoulders and neck must coordinate closely and act in unison.

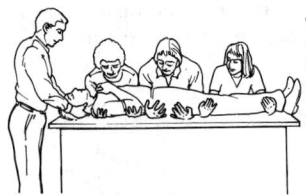

The client can be lifted and rolled as a unit, if necessary, while the person managing at the head directs each action.

Figure 13–15. Moving the client with a possible cervical spine injury.

EPIDURAL HEMATOMA

Epidural hematoma is a rapidly developing accumulation of blood between the skull and the dura mater. It is usually a manifestation of skull fracture with the laceration of the middle meningeal artery. It often occurs after trauma. The classic picture of an epidural is the client with an episode of brief unconsciousness immediately after injury who regains consciousness with complete alertness. Then the client develops headache, rapidly deteriorating neurologic signs (confusion, coma, death), signs of increased intracranial pressure, and loss of motor function of the opposite side of the injury. The mortality for epidural hematomas is 50%. Rapid treatment and surgical intervention are vital.

SUBDURAL HEMATOMA

A subdural hematoma is often caused by venous bleeding, and may develop in the short or long term.

- Acute subdural hematoma may mimic epidural hematoma exactly. The danger in the acute subdural is a mass lesion, which may result in increased intracranial pressure (ICP), brain midline shift, and herniation.

- Subacute subdural hematoma has an onset in symptoms of 48 hr to two weeks.

- Chronic subdural hematoma may develop slowly over time with only subtle behavioral changes as signs. The initial injury may be forgotten and the clinical picture may look like dementia.

Nursing Interventions

- Remember the ABCs of trauma. Suspect cervical spine injury (See section 13-8 and Figure 13-15).

- Maintain airway. Keep passages clear by means of suctioning and positioning the client in a lateral recumbent, prone, or semiprone position, after making certain there is no cervical spine injury. A cricothyroidotomy may be necessary if there is acute respiratory distress.

- Assist with endotracheal intubation if client is comatose.

- Control any hemorrhage and shock. Look for extracranial source of bleeding (thorax, abdomen, long-bone fracture) that may be causing hypovolemic shock or bradycardia, which indicates neurogenic or spinal shock.

- Administer IV fluids at keep-open rate.

- Determine the baseline condition of the client and do frequent assessments comparing client responsiveness to baseline. Take complete vital signs. Marked intracranial pressure produces hypertension in adults and widening pulse pressure.

- Perform neurologic exam at regular intervals which includes: (see also Neurologic Assessment, Section 1-5; use Glasgow Coma Scale):

  - Level of consciousness: alert, lethargic, stuporous, semicomatose, comatose

  - Orientation to person, place, time and event

  - Response to commands or painful stimuli

  - Pupil size and reaction to light

  - Motor activity

  - Restless, combative, or irrational behavior (may indicate increased intracranial pressure)

- Monitor client responsiveness; it is the most sensitive measure of client improvement or deterioration

- Never let the head be lowered in head trauma. Keep the head of the bed at a 30 degree angle.

- Assist with diagnostic procedures: CT scan, skull x-rays, angiography, echoencephalography, arteriograms, laboratory studies (complete blood count, urinalysis, arterial blood gases, electrolytes, glucose, etc).

- Insert Foley catheter and monitor output.

- Consider inserting a nasogastric tube. An NG tube must be ordered by a physician, since in some skull fractures, the tube could enter the fracture site.

- Administer medications as ordered (could include Mannitol (20%) 1.5 gm/kg IV over 30–60 min; dexamethasone (Decadron) 10 mg: IV initially, then maintenance dosage).

- Narcotic pain medications are contraindicated.

- Talk to the unconscious client as if he were awake and maintain a quiet, calm environment.

- Anticipate surgical intervention for head trauma.

13-8 SPINAL-CORD INJURIES

Spinal-cord injuries are usually due to trauma, especially when they occur in clients age 15–35. All unconscious clients and those with head, neck, or back injuries should be suspected of having spinal-cord injury. The severity may vary from a mild cord concussion with transient numbness to permanent quadriplegia. Proper transport is of critical importance, as the injury can very easily be made worse. Figure 13-15 shows proper head positioning and method for transport of the client when there is a possibility of spinal-cord injury. Client should be immobilized as much as possible or carried supine on a flat surface with bolsters at the sides of the head and neck to prevent rotation. Four to five people are required to move the client as one unit to a transfer board.

Nursing Interventions

- Keep head and neck in alignment with the spine. Apply continuous, gentle traction to the head to eliminate any rotation. Carefully apply a cervical collar (if not done already) while keeping head and neck in the neutral position (see Figure 13-15).

- Caution the client not to move head.

- Remember the ABC's of trauma as for head injury (see Section 13-7).

- Apply oxygen by prongs or mask.

- Start an IV with normal saline or Ringer's lactate.

- Take frequent vital signs and neurological assessments. Assess for neurogenic shock: bradycardia, warm, dry extremities.

- Obtain cross-table lateral x-rays of the C-spine before any other films. The physician will evalute the x-rays, and if possible, C-spine x-rays will be completed.

Hopefully the cervical spine will be completely cleared by the physician.

- Assess and treat for other injuries.
- Stabilize fractures under physician direction or prepare for surgical intervention.
- Admit to a spinal-cord injury treatment center if appropriate.

13-9 SEIZURES: STATUS EPILEPTICUS

Most seizures are self-limiting. In the case of status epilepticus, or prolonged, uncontrollable seizures, seizure activity continues longer than 5 min and medical intervention becomes necessary.

Nursing Interventions

- Keep the airway open. Administer high-flow 100% oxygen.
- Establish IV access with normal saline at keep-open rate.
- Administer IV medications—usually diazepam (Valium) 5–10 mg. and/or lorazepam (Ativan), 4–8 mg. over 2 min and phenytoin (Dilantin) 15–18 mg/kg: not to exceed 50 mg/min. Occasionally phenobarbital is given IV to break a seizure cycle.
- Be prepared to intubate client if large doses of sedation are given. Consider continuous pulse oximetry for early warning of hypoxemia.
- Keep airway free of secretions as much as possible.
- Protect client from injury. Position client on side. Provide padding on rails of bed or stretcher.
- Constantly monitor ABC's of trauma, seizure activity.
- Assess for conditions that can precipitate seizures: forgetting to take prescribed anticonvulsant (a loading dose will be needed), infection, high fever, hypoglycemia, toxemia, anoxia, cerebrovascular accident,

acute cerebral edema, tumors, or alcohol/drug ingestion.

- See Potential for Injury Related to Seizures, Section 2–13 for types of seizures, precautionary measures, and care during self-limited incidences (less than 5 min).

13-10 BURNS

Burn clients have multiple, complex problems. It is important to consider the type of burn, it's location and the percentage of the body impacted.

Immediate Nursing Management

- Stop the burning process. Help the client to stop, drop and roll on the floor.

- Use water if available to douse any flames and cool the wound.

- Remove all restrictive items: jewelry, belts, etc., before swelling occurs and to prevent further burning (metal retains heat). Do not attempt to remove adherent clothing.

- Initiate the ABC's of trauma if necessary: **A**irway, **B**reathing, **C**irculation.

- Irrigate chemical burns with copious amounts of water while removing contaminated clothing. Take care not to contaminate yourself. If in the eyes, irrigate with plain water for at least 15 min for acid or 20 min for alkali (see also Section 13-12).

- Apply cool, moist compresses to burns. Never apply grease or ointment of any kind.

- For larger areas: Avoid cold or ice-water immersion as cold may exaggerate vasoconstriction, impair circulation, cause hypothermia, and cause necrosis. Cover with sterile dressings or any clean cloth to prevent further wound contamination and to lessen the pain.

- Maintain life support and transport to the burn center. If the burn center is more than 30 min away, Ringer's lactate should be started en route to the hospital. Morphine is not recommended as it may depress respirations or interfere with evaluation of other injuries.

Management in the Emergency Treatment Center

- Maintain airway, administer humidified oxygen, particularly if facial burns are present, there is soot around the nose or mouth, client history includes smoke inhalation, or nose hairs appear to be singed.

- Find out how the burn occurred and assess the extent of the injuries. Estimate the degree of burn (Table 13-4) and percent of body-surface area (BSA) affected (Figure 13-16). Suspect other injuries, i.e., head trauma.

- Start or maintain an IV line with Ringer's lactate (14–16 gauge needle). Two lines are used with a BSA greater than 40%.

- Apply cardiac monitor and obtain frequent vital signs.

TABLE 13–4. DEPTH-OF-BURN INDEX

	SUPERFICIAL PARTIAL THICKNESS	DEEP PARTIAL THICKNESS	FULL THICKNESS
Appearance	Pink with blisters	White	Brown with thrombosed veins
Hair	Present	Absent	Absent
Sensation	Light touch, pinprick	Pressure	None
Pain	Exquisitely painful	Painful	Painless
Biomechanical Properties	Elevated, soft, and pliable	Elevated, soft, and pliable	Depressed and leathery

Adapted from Tobiasen JM, Hiebert JM, Sacco WJ, Edlich RF. Burn injury severity scoring systems. Curr Concepts Trauma Care 1981; 4:5–8.

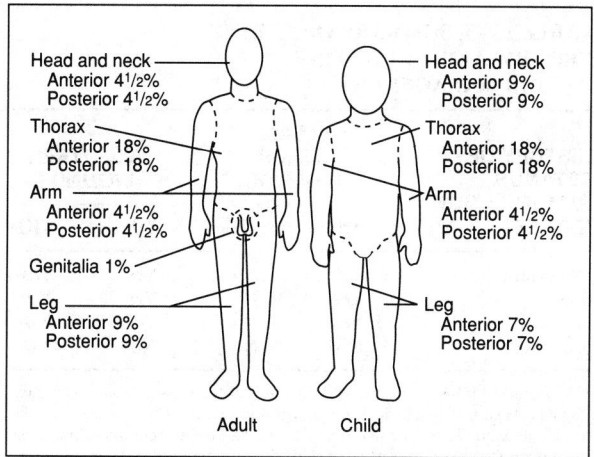

Figure 13-16. Adult and Pediatric "Rule of Nines."

- Relieve pain. Apply moist packs and give small IV doses of Morphine or Meperidine (Demerol). They may also be given intramuscularly for minor burns.

- Consider Foley catheter, urinalysis, and monitor output.

- Obtain laboratory studies: complete blood count, electrolytes, blood urea nitrogen, glucose, creatinine, arterial blood gases, and carbon monoxide levels.

- Obtain chest x-rays.

- Administer tetanus prophylaxis (Table 13-5).

- If client is to be transferred to a burn unit, cover with sterile sheets and blankets.

- Transfer to a burn center or burn unit if client has respiratory-tract burns, has partial thickness burns covering >25% of the total BSA (adult) or >20% total BSA (child), has full-thickness burns covering 10% of the total BSA, is under age 2 or over 65, has burns involving the face, hands, eyes, ears, feet, or perineum, has burns complicated by other injuries, e.g., fractures, or pre-existing conditions, e.g., diabetes or

TABLE 13–5. SUMMARY OF TETANUS PROPHYLAXIS IN ROUTINE WOUND MANAGEMENT

HISTORY OF TETANUS IMMUNIZATION (DOSES)	CLEAN, MINOR WOUNDS		ALL OTHER WOUNDS	
	Td*	TIG	Td*	TIG
Uncertain	Yes	No	Yes	Yes
0–1	Yes	No	Yes	Yes
2	Yes	No	Yes	No†
3 or more	No‡	No	No§	No

*For children less than 7 yr old diphtheria–tetanus–pertussis vaccine (DTP) (DT, if pertussis vaccine is contraindicated) is preferred to tetanus toxoid alone. For persons 7 yr old and older, tetanus–diphtheria (Td) is preferred to tetanus toxoid alone. TIG denotes tetanus immune globulin.

†Yes, if wound more than 24 hr old.

‡Yes, if more than 10 yr since last dose.

§Yes, if more than 5 yr since last dose. (More frequent boosters are not needed and can accentuate side effects.)

Recommendations from the Centers for Disease Control. Atlanta, GA. MMWR 1981; August.

has electrical burns (recommendations of the American Burn Association and the American College of Surgeons). A nurse or physician should accompany the client.

- Burn-wound management is carried out after fluid resuscitation has been initiated and the client is hemodynamically stable.

13-11 FRACTURES

Symptoms of fracture include local pain and tenderness, swelling, deformity, and limited use of the limb. An open or compound fracture occurs when there is direct continuity between the fracture and a break in the skin, with a high risk of infection. Distal parts to the fracture may be evaluated very carefully for circulation and enervation. Figure 13-17 illustrates specific kinds of fractures.

Nursing Interventions

- Remember the ABC's of trauma.

- Check distal pulses.

- Remove any constricting clothes or jewelry.

- Immobilize extremity by splinting above and below the suspected fracture site.

- Do not straighten out joints that are injured.

- Apply ice packs around and on top of injured site.

- Cover a compound fracture with a sterile or clean, dry cloth.

- Frequently assess motor function and neurovascular status (e.g., ask the client with a suspected tibia fracture to move the toes. Check for normal sensation, look for cyanosis and delayed capillary refill time = >2–3 sec).

- Assess for signs of internal injury, e.g., hemoptysis (bloody sputum), which may result from injury to lungs by fractured ribs, or oliguria, anuria, or blood in the urine, which may result from injury to the urethra by a fractured pelvis.

- Elevate extremity unless diminished neurovascularity is suspected (in this case elevation would further decrease blood supply).

- Support the client until medical treatment (reduction, cast, or surgery) is available. Administer pain medication as necessary. Table 13-6 lists specific fractures with management measures and potential complications.

13-12 POISONING

Toxic substances may be absorbed topically, inhaled, ingested orally, or injected. In all cases, the primary concern in treatment is to support vital functions while removing the poison.

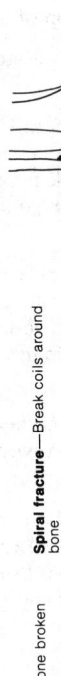

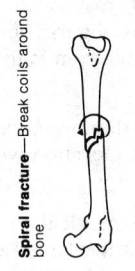

Spiral fracture—Break coils around bone

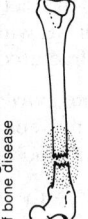

Fracture dislocation—Break complicated by bone out of joint

Depressed fracture—Broken skull bone driven inward

Pathologic fracture—Break is at site of bone disease

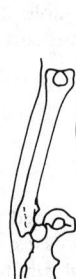

Intracapsular fracture—Bone broken inside joint

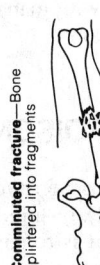

Comminuted fracture—Bone splintered into fragments

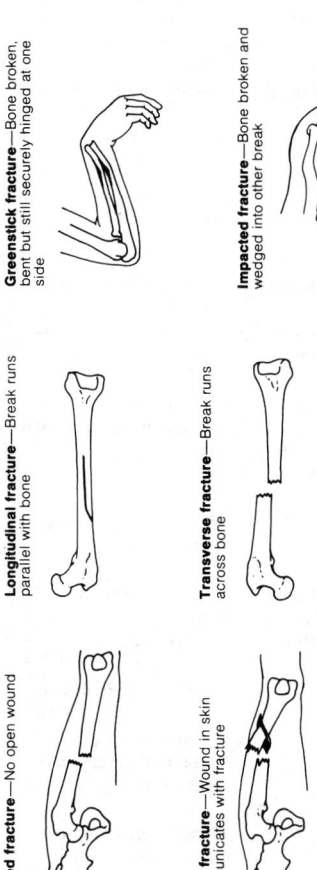
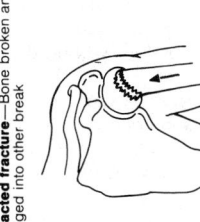
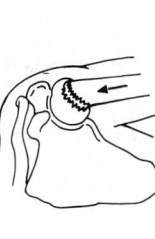
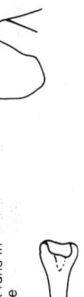

Closed fracture—No open wound

Longitudinal fracture—Break runs parallel with bone

Greenstick fracture—Bone broken, bent but still securely hinged at one side

Open fracture—Wound in skin communicates with fracture

Transverse fracture—Break runs across bone

Impacted fracture—Bone broken and wedged into other break

Extracapsular fracture—Bone broken outside joint

Oblique fracture—Break runs in slanting direction on bone

Figure 13–17. Types of fracture. (From Wolff L, Weitzel NH, Zorhow RA, Zsoher H. *Fundamentals of nursing.* 7th ed. Philadelphia: JB Lippincott, 1983. Reprinted with permission.)

TABLE 13–6. MANAGEMENT AND POTENTIAL COMPLICATIONS OF FRACTURES

SPECIFIC FRACTURE	SPECIFIC MANAGEMENT	POTENTIAL COMPLICATIONS
Pelvis: 3rd leading cause of death in MVA	ABCs of resuscitation Check urethral meatus for blood Do not attempt to insert catheter if blood is present, due to possibility of urethral tear Rectal examination sphincter tone, blood; for males, check location of prostate	Lethal: exsanguinating hemorrhage Other: injury to bladder, urethra, lumbosacral nerves, or lower GI tract Iliac vessel tears
Femur	ABCs of resuscitation Traction splint Analgesia if needed Hospitalization	Femoral nerve impairment Popliteal artery disruption
Hip	ABCs of resuscitation Traction Hospitalization for internal fixation	Shortened extremity Femoral nerve impairment
Tibia and fibula	Reduction Cast	Nerve impairment Vascular disruption
Humerus	Hanging cast for humeral head fracture Sugar-tong splint	Radial nerve impairment Wrist drop Weakness Possible inability to extend fingers and thumb Brachial artery disruptions
Radius and ulna	Closed reduction Cast Elevation	Radial, median, and ulnar nerve impairment

TABLE 13–6. MANAGEMENT AND POTENTIAL COMPLICATIONS OF FRACTURES *Continued*

SPECIFIC FRACTURE	SPECIFIC MANAGEMENT	POTENTIAL COMPLICATIONS
		Radial and ulnar artery disruption
Elbow (fractures and dislocations)	Closed reduction Cast	Median nerve impairment Brachial artery disruption
Shoulder (fractures and dislocations)	Closed reduction Figure-8 or sling Analgesia Early range-of-motion exercises to prevent frozen shoulder	Paralysis of deltoid, possibly triceps Axillary artery injury
Clavicle	Closed reduction Sling	Brachial plexus impairment Subclavian artery disruption

From Hammond BB, Lee G. Quick reference to emergency nursing. Philadelphia: Lippincott, 1984:82. Reprinted with permission.

- Antidotes may be given if the poison is known and there is an antidote available (Table 13-7). Consult your poison control center.

- Keep your local poison control number posted near your telephone at all times (See Table 13-8).

Topically Absorbed Poisons
NURSING INTERVENTIONS

Skin Contamination
- Flood the area continuously with water for 15–30 min while removing contaminated clothes.

Text continued on page 650

TABLE 13–7. SPECIFIC ANTIDOTES FOR TOXIC AGENTS

POISONS	ANTIDOTE
Aspirin	Sodium bicarbonate
Acetaminophen	N-acetylcysteine (Mucomyst) 140 mg/kg initially
Arsenic Mercury*	Dimercaprol (BAL)
Atropine Diphenhydramine (Benadryl) Potato leaves Tricyclic antidepressants	Physostigmine, adult dose usually 2 mg IV, slowly.
Carbon monoxide	Oxygen (100%)
Coumadin (Warfarin)	Vitamin K
Cyanide	Cyanide kit: amyl nitrate, sodium nitrates, sodium thiosulfate
Heparin	Protamine sulfate
Insulin	Glucose
Iron	Deferoxamine, 15 mg/kg, slow IV or intramuscularly
Lead	Calcium disodium edetate (EDTA, Versenate)
Narcotics (morphine, heroin, other opium derivatives)	Naloxone (Narcan) 0.4–0.8 mg IV
Parathion, malathion (pesticides)	Atropine
Phenothiazines	Diphenhydramine (Benadryl), 2.5–5.0 mg/kg

*Contrary to common belief, the metal mercury is inert. In the case of a broken thermometer, one needs to be concerned about the glass rather than the mercury.

TABLE 13–8. POISON CONTROL CENTERS

AMERICAN ASSOCIATION OF POISON CONTROL CENTERS
Certified Regional Poison Centers, February 1994

Alabama
Regional Poison Control Center
The Children's Hospital of Alabama
1600 - 7th Ave. South
Birmingham AL 35233-1711
Emergency Phone: (205) 939-9201, (800) 292-6678 (AL only) or (205) 933-4050

Arizona
Arizona Poison and Drug Information Center
Arizona Health Sciences Center, Rm. #3204-K
1501 N. Campbell Ave.
Tucson AZ 85724
Emergency Phone: (800) 362-0101 (AZ only), (602) 626-6016

Samaritan Regional Poison Center
Teleservices Department
1441 North 12th Street
Phoenix AZ 85006
Emergency Phone: (602) 253-3334

California
Fresno Regional Poison Control Center
of Fresno Community Hospital and Medical Center
2823 Fresno Street
Fresno CA 93721
Emergency Phone: (800) 346-5922 or (209) 445-1222

San Diego Regional Poison Center
UCSD Medical Center; 8925
200 West Arbor Drive
San Diego CA 92103-8925
Emergency Phone: (619) 543-6000, (800) 876-4766 (in 619 area code only)

San Francisco Bay Area Regional Poison Control Center
San Francisco General Hospital
1001 Portrero Ave., Building 80, Room 230
San Francisco CA 94122
Emergency Phone: (800) 523-2222

Table continued on following page

TABLE 13–8. POISON CONTROL CENTERS *Continued*

Santa Clara Valley Medical Center Regional Poison Center
750 South Bascom Ave. Suite 310
San Jose CA 95128
Emergency Phone: (408) 299-5112, (800) 662-9886 (CA only)

University of California, Davis, Medical Center Regional Poison Control Center
2315 Stockton Blvd
Sacramento CA 95817
Emergency Phone: (916) 734-3692; (800) 342-9293
  (Northern California only)

Colorado
Rocky Mountain Poison and Drug Center
645 Bannock St.
Denver CO 80204
Emergency Phone: (303) 629-1123

D.C.
National Capital Poison Center
Georgetown University Hospital
3800 Reservoir Rd., NW
Washington, DC 20007
Emergency Numbers: (202) 625-3333; (202) 784-4660 (TTY)

Florida
The Florida Poison Information Center at Tampa General Hospital
Post Office Box 1289
Tampa FL 33601
Emergency Phone: (813) 253-4444 (Tampa) (800) 282-3171
  (Florida)

Georgia
Georgia Poison Center
Grady Memorial Hospital
80 Butler Street S.E.
P.O. Box 26066
Atlanta GA 30335-3801
Emergency Phone: (800) 282-5846 GA only; (404) 616-9000

TABLE 13–8. POISON CONTROL CENTERS *Continued*

Indiana
Indiana Poison Center
Methodist Hospital of Indiana
1701 N. Senate Boulevard
P.O. Box 1367
Indianapolis IN 46206-1367
Emergency Phone: (800) 382-9097 (IN only), (317) 929-2323

Maryland
Maryland Poison Center
20 N. Pine St.
Baltimore MD 21201
Emergency Phone: (410) 528-7701, (800) 492-2414
  (MD only)

National Capital Poison Center (D.C. suburbs only)
Georgetown University Hospital
3800 Reservoir Rd., NW
Washington, DC 20007
Emergency Numbers: (202) 625-3333; (202) 784-4660 (TTY)

Massachusetts
Massachusetts Poison Control System
300 Longwood Ave.
Boston MA 02115
Emergency Phone: (617) 232-2120, (800) 682-9211

Michigan
Poison Control Center
Children's Hospital of Michigan
3901 Beaubien Blvd.
Detroit MI 48201
Emergency Phone: (313) 745-5711

Minnesota
Hennepin Regional Poison Center
Hennepin County Medical Center
701 Park Ave.
Minneapolis MN 55415
Emergency Phone: (612) 347-3141, Petline: (612) 337-7387,
  TDD (612) 337-7474

Table continued on following page

TABLE 13–8. POISON CONTROL CENTERS *Continued*

Minnesota Regional Poison Center
St. Paul-Ramsey Medical Center
640 Jackson St.
St. Paul MN 55101
Emergency Phone: (612) 221-2113

Missouri
Cardinal Glennon Children's Hospital Regional Poison Center
1465 S. Grand Blvd.
St. Louis MO 63104
Emergency Phone: (314) 772-5200, (800) 366-8888

Montana
Rocky Mountain Poison and Drug Center
645 Bannock St.
Denver CO 80204
Emergency Phone: (303) 629-1123

Nebraska
The Poison Center
8301 Dodge St.
Omaha NE 68114
Emergency Phone: (402) 390-5555 (Omaha), (800) 955-9119 (NE)

New Jersey
New Jersey Poison Information and Education System
201 Lyons Ave.
Newark NJ 07112
Emergency Phone: (800) 962-1253

New Mexico
New Mexico Poison and Drug Information Center
University of New Mexico
Albuquerque NM 87131-1076
Emergency Phone: (505) 843-2551, (800) 432-6866 (NM only)

New York
Hudson Valley Poison Center
Nyack Hospital
160 N. Midland Ave.
Nyack NY 10960
Emergency Phone: (800) 336-6997, (914) 353-1000

TABLE 13–8. POISON CONTROL CENTERS *Continued*

Long Island Regional Poison Control Center
Winthrop University Hospical
259 First Street
Mineola NY 11501
Emergency Phone: (516) 542-2323, 2324, 2325, 3813

New York City Poison Control Center
N.Y.C. Department of Health
455 First Ave., Room 123
New York NY 10016
Emergency Phone: (212) 340-4494, (212) P-O-I-S-O-N-S,
   TDD (212) 689-9014

Ohio
Central Ohio Poison Center
700 Children's Drive
Columbus OH 43205-2696
Emergency Phone: (614) 228-1323, (800) 682-7625,
   (614) 228-2272 (TTY), (614) 461-2012

*Cincinnati Drug & Poison Information Center and
Regional Poison Control System*
231 Bethesda Avenue, M.L. 144
Cincinnati OH 45267-0144
Emergency Phone: (513) 558-5111, 800-872-5111 (OH only)

Oregon
Oregon Poison Center
Oregon Health Sciences University
3181 S.W. Sam Jackson Park Road
Portland OR 97201
Emergency Phone: (503) 494-8968, (800) 452-7165
   (OR only)

Pennsylvania
Central Pennsylvania Poison Center
University Hospital
Milton S. Hershey Medical Center
Hershey PA 17033
Emergency Phone: (800) 521-6110

Table continued on following page

TABLE 13–8. POISON CONTROL CENTERS *Continued*

*The Poison Control Center serving the greater
Philadelphia metropolitan area*
One Children's Center
Philadelphia PA 19104-4303
Emergency Phone: (215) 386-2100

Pittsburgh Poison Center
3705 Fifth Avenue
Pittsburgh PA 15213
Emergency Phone: (412) 681-6669

Rhode Island
Rhode Island Poison Center
593 Eddy St.
Providence RI 02903
Emergency Phone: (401) 277-5727

Texas
North Texas Poison Center
5201 Harry Hines Blvd.
P.O. Box 35926
Dallas TX 75235
Emergency Phone: (214) 590-5000, Texas Watts
   (800) 441-0040

Texas State Poison Center
The University of Texas Medical Branch
Galveston TX 77550-2780
Emergency Phone: (409) 765-1420 (Galveston),
   (713) 654-1701 (Houston)

Utah
Utah Poison Control Center
410 Chipeta Way, Suite 230
Salt Lake City UT 84108
Emergency Phone: (801) 581-2151, (800) 456-7707 (UT only)

Virginia
Blue Ridge Poison Center
Box 67
Blue Ridge Hospital
Charlottesville VA 22901
Emergency Phone: (804) 924-5543, (800) 451-1428

TABLE 13–8. POISON CONTROL CENTERS *Continued*

National Capital Poison Center (Northern VA only)
Georgetown University Hospital
3800 Reservoir Rd., NW
Washington, DC 20007
Emergency Numbers: (202) 625-3333; (202) 784-4660 (TTY)

West Virginia
West Virginia Poison Center
3110 MacCorkle Ave. S.E.
Charleston WV 25304
Emergency Phone: (800) 642-3625 (WV only),
 (304) 348-4211

Wyoming
The Poison Center
8301 Dodge St.
Omaha NE 68114
Emergency Phone: (402) 390-5555 (Omaha), (800) 955-9119
 (NE)

MAJOR CANADIAN POISON CONTROL CENTRES

Newfoundland & Labrador
Emergency Department
The Dr. Charles A. Janeway Child Health Centre,
710 Janeway Place,
St. John's, NF A1A 1R8
(709) 722-1110 local
(709) 726-0830 fax

Nova Scotia & P.E.I.
Poison Control Centre
The Izaak Walton Killam Hospital For Children
P.O. Box 3070
Halifax, NS B3J 3G9
(902) 428-8161 local
(902) 428-3213 fax

Table continued on following page

TABLE 13–8. POISON CONTROL CENTERS *Continued*

New Brunswick
Poison Control Centre
The Moncton Hospital
135 McBeath Ave
Moncton NB E1C 6Z8
1-800-pending
(506) 857-5555 local
(506) 857-5353 business
(506) 857-5360 fax

Emergency Department
Saint John General Hospital
P.O. Box 2100
Saint John NB E2L 4L2
(506) 648-6222
(606) 648-6901 fax

Quebec
Centre antipoison du Québec
Le Centre Hospitalier de l'Université Laval
2705, boul. Laurier
Sainte-Foy, PQ G1V 4G2
1-800-463-5060 Toll-free
(418) 656-8090 local
(418) 654-2747 fax

Ontario
Ontario Regional Poison Information Centre
Children's Hospital of Eastern Ontario
401 Smyth Road
Ottawa, ON K1V 8L1
1-800-267-1373 toll-free
(613) 737-1100 local
(613) 738-4862 fax
(613) 737-2320 business

Ontario Regional Poison Information Centre
The Hospital for Sick Children
555 University Avenue
Toronto, ON M5G 1X8
1-800-268-9017 toll-free
(416) 598-5900 local
(416) 813-7498 fax

TABLE 13–8. POISON CONTROL CENTERS *Continued*

Manitoba
Provincial Poison Information Centre,
Children's Hospital Health Sciences Centre
840 Sherbrooke St.,
Winnipieg, MB R3A 1S1
(204) 787-2591 local
(204) 787-4807 fax
(204) 787-2444 Business

Saskatchewan
Emergency Department
Regina General Hospital
1440 14th Avenue
Regina, SK S4P 0W5
1-800-667-4545 toll-free Southern Saskatchewan
(306) 359-4545 local
(306) 359-4357 fax

Emergency Department
Royal University Hospital
Saskatoon, SK S7N 0X0
1-800-363-7474 toll-free
(306) 966-1010 local
(306) 966-1011 Fax

Alberta
P.A.D.I.S.
Foothills General Hospital
1403 29th Street N.W.
Calgary, AB T2N 2T9
1-800-332-1414 toll-free
(403) 270-1414 local
(403) 670-1472 fax

British Columbia
British Columbia Drug and Poison Information Centre
St. Paul's Hospital
1081 Burrard Street
Vancouver, B.C. V6Z 1Y6
1-800-567-8911 toll-free
(604) 682-5050 Greater Vancouver & lower mainland
(604) 631-5262 fax

Table continued on following page

TABLE 13–8. POISON CONTROL CENTERS *Continued*

Northwest Territories
Emergency Department
Stanton Yellowknife Hospital
P.O.B. 10
Yellowknife NT X1A 2N1
(403) 920-4111 local
(403) 920-2805 fax

Yukon
Emergency Department
Whitehorse General Hospital
5 Hospital Road
Whitehorse YK Y1A 3H7
(403) 667-8726 local
(403) 667-2471 fax

- Take care not to absorb toxic material yourself.
- Call Poison Control or 911 for assistance.

Eye Contamination
- Treat the same as for skin.
- Hold the eyelids open as you flush the eye with water, away from the other eye. If it is an acid substance, wash for at least 15 min; at least 20 min for an alkali substance.
- Transport to an Emergency Department for continued care. A contaminated eye will be irrigated there until the ph is neutral. The eye should be visualized by a physician to evaluate for scarring scleral burns.

Inhaled Poisons

Inhaled poisoning is exposure to substances in the air toxic to lung tissues and systemically such as smoke, some industrial gases and chemical fumes.

NURSING INTERVENTIONS

- Remove client from the toxic environment.
- Establish ABC's of trauma.

- Administer oxygen.
- Observe for respiratory distress. Intubate if necessary.
- Obtain emergency assessment and history, determine the poison if possible and duration of exposure.
- Call poison control for specific instructions (see Table 13-8).
- Observe for chemical pneumonitis. Arterial blood gases may be obtained.

Ingested Poisons

Ingested poisons include drugs, industrial toxins, toxic plants, and food contamination. The most common poisonings today are due to drug overdosages of hypnotics, tranquilizers, antidepressants, and salicylates. In many cases, a mixture of drugs is taken, including alcohol. A nonjudgmental attitude is essential in the treatment of self-induced poisoning.

Many times the toxic substance is uncertain (histories are reliable about 50% of the time).

NURSING INTERVENTIONS

- Establish ABC's of trauma.
- Identify the poison if possible. Establish:
  - Time of exposure
  - Type of substance. Instruct client or family to bring to the hospital, if possible, a sample of the ingested material or the bottle it came in.
  - Amount ingested.
- Call poison control center and obtain specific treatment and side effects to be aware of (see Table 13-8).
- Treatment will depend on the specific poison, the degree of toxicity, and concentration, the amount ingested, and the condition of the client. Be prepared to administer ipecac or lavage the client to clear gastric contents with saline, administer activated charcoal mixed with sorbitol (actidose) 50 gms (adult) or 25 gms (child). The client may require IV intervention with antidotes for narcotics and benzodiazipines.

If respirations become depressed, the client may require intubation.

Injected Poisons

INSECT BITES

Venom injected by yellow jackets, bees, wasps, or hornets can cause local symptoms, e.g., itching, wheals and rash, edema, mildly increased BP, or anaphylactic reaction in a hypersensitive individual.

NURSING INTERVENTIONS IN TREATMENT OF INSECT BITES

- Remove the stinger with a scraping motion with a fingernail, knife, or needle. Do not use tweezers or forceps, as squeezing the stinger may release more venom. If left in, it can continue to release venom.
- Treat the site locally by applying ice and sodium bicarbonate or meat tenderizer to counteract the acid in the venom. An ice pack will help with swelling and localized pain.
- Give Diphenhydramine (Benadryl) 50 mg IV and observe for 2–3 hr for local reactions.
- If there are systemic symptoms, e.g., urticaria, dyspnea, weakness, nausea, muscle cramps, hypotension, tachycardia, etc., maintain the ABC's of resuscitation and treat for anaphylactic shock (see Section 13-4).
- Teach client known to be allergic to insect bites to wear an ID band and to carry a kit containing epinephrine.

SNAKE BITE

Poisonous snakes in the United States include rattlesnakes, moccasins, coral snakes, and copperheads. Other poisonous reptiles include cobras, gila monsters, vipers, and adders. Become familiar with the identifying characteristics of poisonous reptiles in the area where you live. The signs and symptoms of pit viper envenomation are pain, puncture marks, edema, and erythema. The severity of symptoms will depend on the client's size and health, the amount of venom delivered by the snake, the location and depth of the bite, the presence of bacteria in the snake's mouth, and how long it takes the client to receive medical treatment.

NURSING INTERVENTIONS IN TREATMENT OF SNAKE BITES

In the Field

- Immobilize the client and bitten part immediately. Immobilize the affected extremity below heart level to reduce the absorption of venom. Do not apply ice. Transport to the nearest emergency care center.

- Determine the reptile involved. Bring it to the emergency department if possible if it can be accomplished safely.

- Prehospital care should include application of a venous occlusion tourniquet 2–4 in proximal to the bite. Make it tight enough to occlude venous and lymphatic return, but loose enough to allow arterial flow (a finger should be able to slip under easily). Ideally the tourniquet should be loosened every 20–30 min and advanced to keep above the swelling.

In the Emergency Department

- Assess ABC's of trauma.

- Place client at rest in recumbent position. Immobilize affected body part at or just below level of heart. Avoid a completely dependent position.

- Obtain vital signs and monitor every 15 min for the first hour then every 30 min until stable.

- Start an IV with normal saline, using opposite extremity injured.

- Assess for symptoms: swelling, ecchymosis, pain, hypotension, vomiting, weakness, paresthesia. Measure circumference of extremity at the site of the bite every 15–30 min. Prepare to administer supplemental oxygen and resuscitative measures if necessary.

- Administer skin test for hypersensitivity and appropriate antivenin serum according to manufacturer's directions. Serum may be given IV or subcutaneously. Amount of antivenin may be based on severity of symptoms.

- Wash the bite area with antiseptic solution.

- Obtain blood and urine samples—type and cross match, complete blood count, blood urea nitrogen, creatinine, electrolyte levels, prothrombin and partial thromboplastin times.

- Administer pain medication and tetanus prophylaxis as necessary.

- Intensive-care monitoring may be indicated.

13-13 THERMAL EMERGENCIES

Hypothermia (Cold Exposure)

Hypothermia is considered a core temperature of less than 35 degrees centigrade (95F.) resulting from environmental influences. The client is mildly symptomatic at body temperatures between 32 and 35°C (89.6–95°F) and more significantly affected when the core temperature drops below 32°C (90°F). Body temperature below 30C (86°F) is considered profoundly hypothermic and is frequently associated with a high rate of mortality.

Clients with mild hypothermia may initially appear drunk, confused, or disoriented. Symptoms of progressively worsening hypothermia include uncontrollable shivering, slow, slurred speech, amnesia, loss of muscle coordination, drowsiness, and coma. Suspect hypothermia in anyone found ill or injured in cold weather or who has been immersed in water (divers, near-drowning victims). Other groups at risk are alcoholics, street people, the elderly, and newborns.

Treatment in this condition is aimed at:

- Rewarming the core
- Preventing arrhythmias
- Maintaining adequate cardiovascular and pulmonary status

- Managing pH and electrolyte imbalances
- Treating underlying factors, i.e. frostbite.

NURSING INTERVENTIONS

- Maintain airway, breathing, circulation. Initiate CPR if necessary.
- Assist with intubation if necessary.

In the Field

- Move the victim to a warm, dry environment as quickly as possible.
- Remove wet clothing and replace with dry clothing or blankets or lay the victim next to a warm, healthy person.
- If conscious, give warmed fluids by mouth. Transport to hospital.

In the Hospital

- Remove all clothing and apply warm blankets or use warming blanket if possible.
- Apply cardiac monitor. Monitor for dysrhythmias such as atrial fibrillation, bradycardia, premature ventricular contractions. Notify physician if present.
- Apply oxygen, consider heated oxygen (not to exceed 40°C (104°F).
- Consider heated IV fluids.
- Obtain laboratory values. May include CBC, electrolytes, glucose, cardiac enzymes, BUN, Creatinine, coagulation studies, amylase, arterial blood gases.
- Obtain 12-lead ECG.
- Obtain x-rays as ordered including chest x-ray.
- Monitor vital signs, especially rectal temperature, every 15–30 min until client temperature stabilizes at greater than 95°F.
- *Note:* Rewarming shock may occur when the peripheral areas are rewarmed faster than the core. Hyperthermic clients should be rewarmed slowly, espe-

cially if elderly. Body temperature should not rise more than 2 degrees (F) per hour.

- Consider gastric and bladder lavage with warm fluid. In severe hypothermia, peritoneal lavage, or hemodialysis may be used.

- Apply warm packs to trunk, groin, and axillae. Use in conjunction with core rewarming when hypothermia is severe or not responding to passive warming methods.

- Once stable, protect skin integrity by repositioning, applying lotion and massaging bony skin prominences every 30–60 min.

- *Note:* Often resuscitation efforts are not successful until adequate rewarming is achieved. Efforts should not be abandoned until core rewarming has been accomplished. Sometimes revival requires hours of effort.

Frostbite

Frostbite occurs under the same conditions as hypothermia. Freezing temperatures cause vasospasm in a portion of the body and circulation ceases. Manifestation progresses from numbness to total anesthesia of the affected extremity to evidence of necrotic tissue.

NURSING INTERVENTIONS

- Check extremities for:
  - Reddened, white, or cyanotic appearance
  - A temperature anywhere from normal to cold, hard, and nonpliable
  - Blisters (may be serous or blood-filled)
  - Edema or obvious tissue breakdown
  - Presence or absence of distal pulses

- Handle the affected part gently, do not rub or massage. Do not thaw unless injured area will stay thawed.

- Acomplish thawing by immersion in hot water between 37.8–43.3°C (100–110°F). Do not exceed

44.4°C (111.2°F). Monitor water temperature continuously.

- Remove any constrictive clothing, leave blisters intact and encourage gentle exercise to increase the blood flow.

- Smoking, caffeine, and alcohol decrease peripheral circulation and should not be allowed. Untreated, frostbite may result in amputation of the affected part.

- Teach client that the affected part will be hypersensitive to cold in the future and additional protective clothing will be needed.

- Administer tetanus prophylaxis if needed.

Heat Cramps, Heat Exhaustion, and Heat Stroke

Heat cramps and heat exhaustion are due to excessive loss of sodium and are common after profuse sweating. Heat stroke occurs when the body receives more heat externally than it can dissipate.

People at risk are those who engage in sports, people with chronic renal, pulmonary, or cardiac illnesses, the elderly, and people taking phenothiazines, thiazides, antihistamines, tolbutamide (Orinase), or chlorpropamide (Diabenese). After appropriate treatment, client teaching should be aimed at preventing recurrence.

- Symptoms and the three common emergencies that occur in hot weather are outlined in Table 13-9.

Electrical Injury

Electrical burns are caused by contact with an electrical source such as malfunctioning electrical wiring, flash electrical arcs from high-voltage power lines or machines, or even from lightning. Electrical injuries frequently appear minor or localized, but may conceal significant damage internally. Vascular and muscle damage occur similar to those seen with crush injuries.

TABLE 13–9. HEAT CRAMPS, HEAT EXHAUSTION, HEAT STROKE

THERMAL EMERGENCY	SYMPTOMS	NURSING INTERVENTIONS
Heat cramps	Muscle spasms, severe pain in arms, legs, and occasionally in abdomen, faintness, dizziness	Remove client from hot environment and give oral fluids containing sodium, e.g., 1 t of salt per quart of water.
Heat exhaustion	Headache, dizziness, faintness, loss of appetite, nausea, skin may be cool and clammy. There may be profuse sweating, pale skin and decreased BP and increased pulse.	Remove client from source of heat and place in cool environment. Administer oral or IV fluids.
Heat stroke	Profound hyperpyrexia, which could result in brain damage or death; extremely elevated temperature, warm, dry skin, depressed level of consciousness, possible coma, hypertension followed by hypotension or shock.	Cool client rapidly (immerse in or sponge with cool water); hypothermia blanket. Start IV, provide other cardiovascular support. Cardiac monitor, frequent vital signs. Foley catheter unless recovery is prompt.

NURSING INTERVENTIONS

In the Field

- Turn off the source of the electricity immediately. If this is not possible, separate the client from the electrical current by using nonconductive equipment, e.g., dry wood, rope.

- Once the environment is safe for the rescuer, begin assessment and CPR if necessary.

- Apply cool, moist, dressings to the wound, remove when the wound is cooled. Do not apply ice.

- Cover extensive surface burns with sterile dressings or clean, dry cloth to conserve body heat and to minimize bacterial contamination.

- Transport to the emergency department.

In the Emergency Department

- Assess the wounds. Try to identify both the entrance and exit wound. The area between the entrance and exit may be the source of significant vascular and muscle damage.

- Establish IV access with a large-bore catheter and Ringer's Lactate in the large area injuries.

- Assess pulses distal to the injury.

- Client will remain NPO. Nausea and vomiting can occur due to paralytic ileus secondary to the stress of the injury.

- Apply cardiac monitor. Obtain 12-lead ECG if necessary.

- Consider inserting Foley catheter for significant injuries. The urine may appear port-wine or reddish-black due to massive muscle damage.

- Assist with wound exploration. May need to be done in surgery for debridement of necrotic tissue or possible fasciotomy.

- Administer tetanus prophylaxis as necessary. (see Table 13-5).

REFERENCES

Arendt DL, Arendt DB. Rescue operations for snakebite. Am J of Nursing 1992 July: 26–30.

Bayley EW, Smith GA. The three degrees of burn care. Nursing '87 1987; 17:34–41.

Campbell C, Newsome J. Detecting life-threatening arrhythmias. Nursing '90, 1990; December: 34–39.

Centers for Disease Control. Recommendations for tetanus prophylaxis. MMWR 1981; August 28.

Guidelines for cardiopulmonary resuscitation and emergency cardiac care: recommendations of the 1992 national conference on cardiopulmonary resuscitation and emergency cardiac care. JAMA, Vol. 268, No. 16, Oct. 28, 1992; p. 2216–2230.

Huston CJ. Action stat! hypothermia. How to respond quickly to a cold weather emergency. Nursing '90, Vol. 20 (12) December: 33.

Ignativicius D, Bayne M. Medical-surgical nursing: a nursing process approach. Philadelphia: W.B. Saunders, 1991.

Kurecky BA III, Browlee HJ. Venomous snake bites in the United States. J Family Practice, 1987, 25:386–392.

Niemann J. Current concepts, cardiopulmonary resuscitation. New England J Medicine, Vol. 327, (15), October 8, 1992; 1075–1079.

O'Niell S. Dealing with seizures. RN. September, 1984; 39–41.

Rea R, Bourg P, Parker J, Rushing D. Emergency nursing core curriculum. 3rd. ed. Philadelphia: W.B. Saunders Co., 1987.

Sheehy SB. Manual of emergency care. 3rd ed. St. Louis: C.V. Mosby Co., 1990.

Stewart-Amidei. What to do until neurosurgeon arrives. J Emergency Nursing. Vol. 14 (5). Sept./Oct. 1988; 296–301.

Tobiesen SW, Hiebert JM, Sacco WJ, Edlich RF. Burn injury severity scoring systems. Current Concepts Trauma Care 1981; 4:5–8.

NANDA-APPROVED NURSING DIAGNOSES

Activity Intolerance
Activity Intolerance, High Risk for
Adjustment, Impaired
Airway Clearance, Ineffective
*Alcohol Drinking Patterns, Dysfunctional
Anxiety
Aspiration, High Risk for
Body Image Disturbance
Body Temperature, High Risk for Altered
Breastfeeding, Effective
Breastfeeding, Ineffective
Breastfeeding, Interrupted
Breathing Pattern, Ineffective
Caregiver Role Strain
Caregiver Role Strain, High Risk for
Communication, Impaired Verbal
*Community Coping, Ineffective
*Community Coping, Potential for Enhanced
*Confusion, Acute
Constipation
Constipation, Colonic
Constipation, Perceived
Decisional Conflict (Specify)
Decreased Cardiac Output
Defensive Coping

*1994 Diagnoses in Progress

Denial, Ineffective

Diarrhea

Disuse Syndrome, High Risk for

Diversional Activity Deficit

Dysfunctional Ventilatory Weaning Response

Dysreflexia

*Environmental Interpretation Syndrome, Impaired

Family Coping: Compromised, Ineffective

Family Coping: Disabling, Ineffective

Family Coping: Potential for Growth

Family Processes, Altered

*Family Processes: Addictive Behavior (Individual and Family),
   Altered

Fatigue

Fear

Fluid Volume Deficit

Fluid Volume Deficit, High Risk for

Fluid Volume Excess

Gas Exchange, Impaired

Grieving, Anticipatory

Grieving, Dysfunctional

Growth and Development, Altered

Health Maintenance, Altered

Health Seeking Behaviors (Specify)

Home Maintenance Management, Impaired

Hopelessness

Hyperthermia

Hypothermia

Incontinence, Bowel

Incontinence, Functional

*Incontinence, Idiopathic Fecal

Incontinence, Reflex

Incontinence, Stress

Incontinence, Total

Incontinence, Urge

Individual Coping, Ineffective

*Infant Behavior, Disorganized

*Infant Behavior, High Risk for Disorganized

*Infant Behavior, Potential for Enhanced Organized
Infant Feeding Pattern, Ineffective
Infection, High Risk for
Injury, High Risk for
Knowledge Deficit (Specify)
*Loneliness, High Risk for
Management of Therapeutic Regimen (Individuals), Ineffective
*Management of Therapeutic Regimen (Families), Ineffective
Noncompliance (Specify)
Nutrition: Less Than Body Requirements, Altered
Nutrition: More Than Body Requirements, Altered
Nutrition: Potential for More Than Body Requirements, Altered
Oral Mucous Membrane, Altered
Pain
Pain, Chronic
*Pain, Labor
Parental Role Conflict
*Parent/Infant Attachment, Altered
Parenting, Altered
Parenting, High Risk for Altered
Peripheral Neurovascular Dysfunction, High Risk for
Personal Identity Disturbance
Physical Mobility, Impaired
Poisoning, High Risk for
Post-Trauma Response
Powerlessness
*Preservation/Quality of Life, Alteration in
Protection, Altered
Rape-Trauma Syndrome
Rape-Trauma Syndrome: Compound Reaction
Rape-Trauma Syndrome: Silent Reaction
Relocation Stress Syndrome
Role Performance, Altered
Self Care Deficit
   Bathing/Hygiene
   Dressing/Grooming
   Feeding
   *Medication Administration

Toileting

Self Esteem, Chronic Low

Self Esteem, Situational Low

Self Esteem Disturbance

Sensory/Perceptual Alterations (Specify) (Visual, Auditory, Kinesthetic, Gustatory, Tactile, Olfactory)

Self-Mutilation, High Risk for

Sexual Dysfunction

Sexuality Patterns, Altered

Skin Integrity, Impaired

Skin Integrity, High Risk for Impaired

*Skin Integrity: Pressure Ulcer, High Risk for Impaired

Sleep Pattern Disturbance

Social Interaction, Impaired

Social Isolation

*Spasticity

Spiritual Distress

*Spiritual Well Being, Opportunity for Enhanced

Suffocation, High Risk for

Sustain Sponaneous Ventilation, Inability to

Swallowing, Impaired

*Terminal Illness Response

Thermoregulation, Ineffective

Thought Processes, Altered

Tissue Integrity, Impaired

Tissue Perfusion, Altered (Specify Type) (Renal, Cerebral, Cardiopulmonary, Gastrointestinal, Peripheral)

Trauma, High Risk for

Unilateral Neglect

Urinary Elimination, Altered

*Urinary Filtration Syndrome, Impaired

Urinary Retention

Violence, High Risk for: Self-Directed or Directed at Others

CHECKLIST FOR ORIENTING TO THE UNIT

I have familiarized myself with and checked the proper functioning of the following:

Emergency Items

☐ Crash cart, emergency drugs

☐ Fire extinguishers

☐ Emergency exits

☐ Disaster plan

Unit Features

☐ Medication cart or room, controlled substances

☐ IV supplies

☐ Linen closet

☐ Utility room

☐ Extra supply cabinet

☐ Bathrooms, showers

☐ Client rooms, numbering system

☐ Bedside equipment, call lights

☐ Monitoring systems, equipment, oximeters

Nursing Station

☐ Client medical records

☐ Computer system

☐ Essential telephone numbers

☐ Policy and procedures manual

- ☐ Requisition forms
- ☐ Valuables deposit
- ☐ Paging/intercom system

GUIDELINES FOR CLIENT EDUCATION

Teaching clients health principles and about their particular illness is a primary nursing responsibility. To be effective the nurse must have thorough knowledge of the subject matter, understand the mechanisms of learning, and use good communication skills. The nursing process will help you fill your client's learning needs.

ASSESS

- What does the client desire to know?
  Perhaps client is particularly anxious about something.

- What does the client need to know?
  Perhaps knowledge would effect a behavior change that would ameliorate a health problem.

- Are there barriers that might impede the learning process?
  Some of these are:

  - Anxiety

  - Pain

  - Poor environment for learning (i.e. lack of privacy, noise)

  - Mental handicaps, (i.e., short attention span, memory impairment)

  - Physical handicaps, (i.e. impaired hearing, eyesight, coordination)

  - Cultural or language barriers

- Lack of literacy or other educational training
- Unwilling attitude
- Lack of social support

DIAGNOSE

Example: Knowledge deficit regarding disease process and importance of taking prescribed medication.

PLAN

- Establish goals based on your assessment.
  Example: Client will verbalize rationale for taking prescribed medication.

- If there are barriers to learning, remove as many as are within your control.

- Teach at an appropriate time (the acute phase of illness is usually a poor time).

- Plan only short (15 min) learning sessions to prevent client's being overloaded with more information than can be absorbed.

- Arrange for significant others to attend when teaching.

TEACH

- Use more than one method of communication to reinforce the others: verbal, written, audio-visual, three-dimensional models, etc.

- Present the information the client is most anxious about or desires to know first. This will clear the way for other material.

- Use language the client will understand. Keep explanations simple.

- Explain the rationale behind the facts to reinforce understanding.

- Encourage questions. Allow plenty of time. If you don't know the answer to a question, tell the client you will get back to him or her with the information.

- Restate information in different words if necessary, with kindness and gentleness.

- Use additional resource people such as dieticians, pharmacists, and health agency personnel to help educate client. Provide referrals as appropriate to health organizations and support groups.

EVALUATE

Determine if goals have been met by observing client's demonstration of understanding. Realize also that behavior may not change immediately although client has knowledge of the consequences of their actions. Positively reinforce when behavioral goals are met.

MANAGING TIME EFFECTIVELY

Use the nursing process to enhance your organizational skills and maximize work time.

ASSESS

- Arrive before report time to go over care plans, surgery schedules, diagnostic tests, etc.

- Keep to essential information in report; start and end on time.

- Gather information from the Kardex report and initial rounds for making a plan for the shift. The client with a more serious condition, special treatments ordered, or who is recently postoperative will require more nursing time than those who are relatively stable.

PLAN

- Anticipate client needs as much as possible and plan accordingly.

- Use a time chart such as the one in Table D-1 to help organize activities for the shift.

- High priority times are times for surgery, medications, IV's, treatments, vital signs and other ordered activities.

IMPLEMENT

- Stay within alloted time limits as much as possible. Cross off when completed.

TABLE D–1.

	GENERAL	RM 381	382	384	385	386
7:00	report, rounds	7:30 insulin		NPO(sips)	to OR 7:30	TCDB
8:00	VS, brkfst.		tube feeding	enemas till clear		OOB
9:00	am meds	discharge teaching		to x-ray		TCDB bath
10:00		order meds	bath		post op	
11:00		home			VS × 4 prn pain?	TCDB
12:00	VS, lunch		tube feeding		VS × 2	
1:00	meds		IV up	laxative?		TCDB drsg Δ
2:00					IV up	up to w/c
3:00	report					TCDB

- Gather equipment for procedures ahead of time and have ready.

- Group like activities together to save time, i.e., at the desk do charting for several clients at once, make needed phone calls and monitor lab results. While in with client, take vital signs, do assessment, monitor the IV and administer medication.

- Unexpected events will always arise and must be handled with flexibility. Determine priorities and adjust schedule accordingly.

- Ask for assistance when needed. If you know ahead that you will be needing help, i.e., with turning a client q 2 hrs., agree with another staff member at the beginning of the shift on what time the turning will be done.

- Use remaining time between tasks for care planning, charting, helping co-workers, client education, and if possible giving that "extra touch."

EVALUATE

- Evaluate yourself on effective time management often. Establish routines that work best for you. Revise methods as needed. The rewards of increased effectiveness through developed organizational skills are many.

STANDARD ABBREVIATIONS

These are generally accepted abbreviations; however, every hospital may have slight variations that must be used for legal reasons when charting (correct in the margins with pencil if desired).

@	at
AB	abortion
ABG	arterial blood gases
abd	abdominal, abdomen
a.c.	before meals
AD	right ear
ADA	American Diabetes Association
ad lib	as desired
AI	aortic insufficiency
a.m.	before noon
AMA	against medical advice
amp	ampule
amt	amount
ant	anterior
AO	aorta
AP	anterior posterior
APC	aspirin, phenacetin, and caffeine citrate
approx	approximate
ARDS	adult respiratory distress syndrome
AROM	artificial rupture of membranes
AS	left ear
ASA	aspirin
ASAP	as soon as possible
ASHD	arteriosclerotic heart disease

AU	both ears
ax	axillary
Ba	barium
BE	barium enema
bid	twice a day
BM	bowel movement
BP	blood pressure
BPH	benign prostatic hypertrophy
BR	bed rest
br	bathroom
BRP	bathroom privileges
BUN	blood urea nitrogen
BX	biopsy
c̄	with
ca	carcinoma
CABG	coronary artery bypass graft surgery
CAD	coronary artery disease
cal	calorie
caps	capsules
CAT, CT	computerized axial tomography
cath	catheter
C/B	complete bath
CBC	complete blood count
CBG	capillary blood gas
cc	cubic centimeter
c/o	complains of
CHF	congestive heart failure
Circ	circumcision
Cl	chloride
cm	centimeter
CNS	central nervous system
COPD	chronic obstructive pulmonary disease
cpd	compound
CPR	cardiopulmonary resuscitation
C & S	culture and sensitivity
CSF	cerebrospinal fluid
CVA	cerebrovascular accident
Cx	cervix
D.A.T.	diet as tolerated

dc'd, DC'd	discontinued
DOA	dead on arrival
dr	dram
drsg	dressing
DSD	dry sterile dressing
DT's	delirium tremens
D/W,D5W,5%DW	dextrose and water or glucose and water
Dx	diagnosis
EBL	estimated blood loss
ECG,EKG	electrocardiogram
EEG	electroencephalogram
EMG	electromyogram
EOA's	esophageal obturator airways
EPS	electrophysiological study
est	estimate
ext	external, extremity
f	respiratory frequency for 1 min
FIO$_2$	fractional inspired O_2 concentration
FB	foreign body
FBS	fasting blood sugar
FEV	forced expiratory volume in 1 sec
freq	frequent
ft	foot
fx	fracture
gal	gallon
GB	gallbladder
GI	gastrointestinal
g	gram
gr	grain
gtts	drops
HB	heart block
hr	hour
Hbg	hemoglobin
Hb O$_2$ Sat	percentage of hemoglobin saturated by oxygen
HCO$_3$	bicarbonate
Hct	hematocrit
hs	at hour of sleep
ht	height

Hx	history
H₂O	water
H₂O₂	hydrogen peroxide
I & D	incision and drainage
IM	intramuscular
inj	injection
IOL	intraocular lens
IPPB	intermittent positive-pressure breathing
IV	intravenous
IVC	inferior vena cava
IVP	intravenous pyelogram
IVPB	intravenous piggyback
K	potassium
kg	kilogram
KO	keep open
KUB	kidneys, ureters, and bladder
KVO	keep vein open
L, lt	left
L	liter
lab	laboratory
LAD	left anterior descending
lap	laparotomy
LAS	local with anesthesia standby
lat	lateral
lb.,#	pound
LBBB	left bundle branch block
liq	liquid
LLE	left lower extremity
LLL	left lower lobe
LLQ	left lower quadrant
LA	left atrium
LMP	last menstrual period
LP	lumbar puncture
LUE	left upper extremity
LUL	left upper lobe
LUOQ	left upper outer quadrant
LUQ	left upper quadrant
LV	left ventricle
MBC	maximum breathing capacity

MEFR	maximum expiratory flow rate
mEq	milliequivalent
μg	microgram
mg, mgm	milligrams
MI	myocardial infarction
MIFR	maximum inspiratory flow rate
min	minute
ML	midline
ml	milliliter
mm	millimeter
mm Hg	millimeters of mercury
MMFR	mid-maximal expiratory flow rate
M.N.	midnight
mo	month
mod	moderate
MR × 1	may repeat one time
M.S.	morphine sulfate
MVA	motor vehicle accidents
MVV	maximum voluntary ventilation
NA	not applicable
Na	sodium
NaCl	sodium chloride
neg	negative
ng	nanogram
NGT	nasogastric tube
No.,#	number
noc	night
NPO	nothing by mouth
N/S	normal saline
NSR	normal sinus rhythm
N/V	nausea and vomiting
NWB	non-weight-bearing
NKA	no known allergies
O_2	oxygen
occ	occasional
OD	right eye
Od	overdose
ONC	oncology
OR	operating room

ortho	orthopedics
OS	left eye
OU	both eyes
oz	ounce
OOB	out of bed
P̲	pulse
p	after
Para	parity
PA	pulmonary artery
PAR	postanesthesia recovery
PAC	premature atrial contractions
PACU	postanesthesia care unit
PASG	pneumatic anti-shock garments
PAT	paroxysmal atrial tachycardia
P/B	partial bath
pc	after meal
PCN, Pen	penicillin
pCO$_2$	partial pressure of carbon dioxide
PCW	pulmonary capillary wedge
PE	pressure equalization
pH	degree of acidity or alkalinity of a solution
PID	pelvic inflammatory disease
PIP	proximal interphalangeal (joint)
PJC	premature junctional contractions
p.m.	afternoon
PMD	private medical doctor
PO	postoperative
po	by mouth
POD	postoperative day
pO$_2$	partial pressure of oxygen
pp	postpartum
PPBS	postprandial blood sugar
PRE	progressive resistant exercise
prep	preparation
prn	as required
PT	physical therapy
pt	patient
PVC	premature ventricular contractions
q	every

qd	every day
qh	every hour
qid	four times a day
qn, qnoc	every night
qns	quantity not sufficient
R	respiratory
RA	right atrium
RBBB	right bundle branch block
RBC	red blood cells
RV	right ventricle
reg	regular
req	requires
RCA	right coronary artery
REUE	resistive exercise upper extremity
Resp.	respiration
RLE	right lower extremity
RLL	right lower lobe
RLQ	right lower quadrant
RML	right middle lobe
R/O	rule out
ROM	range of motion
R,rt	right
R/I	reverse isolation
RUE	right upper extremity
RUL	right upper lobe
RUOQ	right upper outer quadrant
R.T.O.	return to office
Rx	treatment
s̄	without
SCD	sequential compression device
sec	second
sg	specific gravity
S.G.	Swan-Ganz
S/I	strict isolation
sl	slight
S.L.R.	straight leg raising
S.O.	significant other
SOB	shortness of breath
sol.	solution

S/P	secretion precautions or status post
spec	specimen
S/R	side rails
s̅s̅, ss	half
SSKI	saturated solution of potassium iodide
STAT	immediately
SVC	superior vena cava
S/W	sterile water
Sx,sym	symptom
Syr	syrup
T,Temp	temperature
T & A	tonsils and adenoids, tonsillectomy and adenoidectomy
TAB	therapeutic abortion
tab	tablet
TAH	total abdominal hysterectomy
TAT	tetanus antitoxin
TB,Tce	tuberculosis
TBA	to be absorbed
tbsp, T	tablespoon
tid	three times a day
tinc	tincture
TMJ	temporomandibular joint
TO,PO	telephone order
TPN	total parenteral nutrition
TPR	temperature, pulse and respiration
trans	transfer
tsp,t	teaspoon
TURB	transuretheral resection of the bladder
TUR	transuretheral resection
TURP	transuretheral resection of the prostate
TX	traction, treatment
U,u	unit
ung	ointment
URI	upper respiratory infection
V & P	vagotomy and pyloroplasty
vag	vaginal
VC	vital capacity
VCG	vectorcardiogram

VD	venereal disease
Ve	minute ventilation
VE	vaginal exam
vg	ventral gluteal (injection site)
Vit	vitamin
VO	verbal order
vol	volume
V.S.	vital signs
vs	versus
Vt	tidal volume
vtx	vertex
WBC	white blood cells
w/c	wheelchair
wh	white
WNL	within normal limits
W/S	wound and skin
wt	weight
×	times
yr	year
Δ	change

HELPFUL EXPRESSIONS IN SPANISH

(Mr.)(Mrs.) _____, my name is _____. I am your nurse.
(Senor)(Senora) _____, mi nombre es _____, soy su enfermera.
(Sen-*yor*)(Sen-*yor*-uh), (me *nome*-bray es _____, soy su en-*fair*-mair-uh.

I don't speak Spanish.
Yo no hablo Espanol. (Yo no *ab*-lo *es*-pan-yole).

Point to where it hurts.
Indique donde le duele (in-*dee*-kay *done*-deh leh *dwel*-leh).

Does it hurt mildly, moderately, or severely?
Es el dolor debil, moderdado, o intenso? (Es el doe-*lore deh*-bil, mode-air-*ah*-doh, o een-*ten*-so)?

I will be right back.
Ahora regreso (ah-*or*-rah reh-*gre*-so).

This is a pain pill.
Esta es una píldora para el dolor (*es*-tah es oo-nah *pil*-do-rah pa-rah el doe-*lor*).

I am going to give you an injection.
Voy a ponerle una inyeccion (voy ah poh-*nair*-lay oo-nah een-*yeck*-see-*ohn*).

I'm going to give you medicine.
Le voy a dar medicina (Leh *voy* a dar med-ee-*see*-na)

Are you feeling better?
Se siente mejor? (say see-*yen*-tay may-*hor*)?

Push the button if you need anything.
Oprima el botón si necesita cualquier cosa (Op-*ree*-mah el bo-*tohn* see ness-eh-*see*-tah *qwal*-key-air *ko*-sah).

You need to drink a lot of fluids to help you get better.
Necesita tomar muchos liquidos para que se sienta mejor (Neh-seh-*see*-tah toe-*mar moo*-chos *ee*-quee-dos pah-rah kay seh see-*en*-tah meh-*hor*).

You must not drink.
Usted no debe beber (oo-*stead* no *deh*-beh beh-*bair*).

You must not eat.
Usted no debe comer (oo-*stead* no *deh*-beh coh-*mair*).

You must not smoke.
Usted no debe fumar (oo-*stead* no *deh*-beh fumar).

Try to eat.
Trate de comer (*trah*-teh deh coh-*mair*).

Stand up.
Levantese (leh-*vahn*-teh-seh).

Sit up.
Incorporese (in-cor-*por*-eh-seh).

Lie down.
Acuestese (ah-*kwess*-teh-say).

Relax.
Descanse (des-*cahn*-say).

Breathe deeply.
Respire profundamente (reh-*spee*-reh pro-*foon*-deh-menteh).

Cough.
Tosa (*toe*-sah).

Roll over on your side.
Voltéese de lado (Vol-*teh-eh*-seh deh *lah*-doe).

Try to sleep.
Trate de dormir (trah-tay day dor-meer).

Have you urinated?
Ha orinado? (ah oh-ree-*nah*-doe)?

Please leave urine in the container.
Por favor deje orina en el frasco (pore-fah-*or deh*-hey o *reen*-ah en el *frahs*-ko).

Have you had a bowel movement?
Ha evacuado? (ah eh-vah-*cooah*-doe)?

Are you constipated?
Tiene enstrenimiento? (tee-*eh*-neh ess-treh-nee-*meeyen*-toe)?

Do you have diarrhea?
Tiene diarrhea? (teh-*yeh*-nay dee-ah-*reh*-ah)?

You are going to x-ray.
Van a llevarlo a la sala de radiografia (vahn ah yea-*vahr*-loh ah lah *sah*-lah deh rah-deeoh-grah-*fee*-ah).

You are going to the operating room.
Van a llevarlo a la sala de operaciones (vahn a yeh-*var*-lo a la *sah*-lah deh oh-pay-rah-*seeoh*-nais).

HELPFUL EXPRESSIONS IN FRENCH

(Mr.)(Mrs.) _____, **my name is** _____, **I am your nurse.**
(Monsieur)(Madame) _____, Je m'appelle _____, je suis votre infirmière.
Muh-*syuh,* Ma-*dam,* zhuh-ma-*pel* zhuh-*swee vo*-tra an-feer-myehr.

I don't speak French.
Je ne parle pas français.
Zhuh nuh *par*-lay pa fron-*seh.*

Point to where it hurts.
Indiquez où se trouve la douleur.
An-dee-kay oo suh troov la doo-lur.

Does it hurt mildly, moderately, or severely?
La douleur est-elle légère, moyenne ou sévère?
La doo-lur eh-*tel* lay-*jair, mwah*-yen, oo say-*ver?*

I will be right back.
Je reviens dans un instant.
Zhuh ruh-*vyan* donz un an-*ston.*

This is a pain pill.
C'est une pilule contre la douleur.
Suh-see eh tōōn pee-*l ōōl cont*-ra la doo-lur.

I am going to give you an injection.
Je vais vous faire une injection.
Zhu vay voo fair ōōn en-*jek*-cee-un.

Are you feeling better?
Vous sentez-vous mieux?
Voo son-tay voo myuh?

Push the button if you need anything.
Appuyez sur le bouton si vous avez besoin de quleque chose.
A-*pwee*-yay sōōr luh boo-*ton* see voo za-vay buh-*zwan* duh *kel*-kuh shōz.

You need to drink a lot of fluids to help you get better.
Vous devez boire beaucoup d'eau pour aller mieux.
Voo deh-vay *bwahr* bō-koo dō poor al-lay *myūh*.

You must not drink.
Vous ne devez pas boire.
Voo nuh *deh*-vay pa bwahr.

You must not eat.
Vous ne devez pas manger.
Voo nuh deh-vay pa mon-*zhay*.

You must not smoke.
Vou ne devez pas fumer.
Voo nuh deh-vay pa fu mehr.

Try to eat.
Essayez de manger.
Eh-say-yay duh mon-*zhay*.

Sit up.
Asseyez-vous or voulez vous bien vous assoir.
A-say-yay voo or voo-lay voo bee-en voo zass-*swar*.

Lie down.
Se coucher.
Seh cooh-cheh.

Relax.
Se délasser.
Seh déh-la-sehr.

Breathe deeply.
Respirez profondement.
Res-pee-ray pro-*fon*-day-*mon*.

Cough.
Toussez.
Too-say.

Roll over on your side.
Roulez sur le côté.
Roo-lay sōōr luh kō-*tay.*

Try to sleep.
Essayez de dormir.
Eh-say-yay duh dor-meer.

Have you urinated?
Avez-vous uriné?
A-vay voo ōō-ree-nay?

Please leave urine in the container.
S'il-vous-plait laissez l'urine dans le bocal.
Seel voo pleh leh-*say* lōōr-een don le buk-*al.*

Have you had a bowel movement?
Êtes vous allé aux celles?
Et voos a-lay ō sel?

Are you constipated?
Êtes-vous constipé?
Et voo kon-stee-pay?

Do you have diarrhea?
Avez-vous la diarrhée?
Ah-vay voo la dee-a-ray?

You are going to x-ray.
Vous allez à la radiographie.
Voo za-lay a la *ra*-dee-ō-gra-*fee.*

You are going to the operating room.
Vous allez à la salle d'opération.
Voo za-lay a la *sal* dō-pay-ra-*syon.*

APOTHECARY AND METRIC VOLUME EQUIVALENTS (APPROXIMATE)

Apothecary		Metric	
½ minim	=	0.03 ml	
¾ minim	=	0.05 ml	
1 minim	=	0.06 ml	
1½ minims	=	0.1 ml	
3 minims	=	0.2 ml	
4 minims	=	0.25 ml	
5 minims	=	0.3 ml	
8 minims	=	0.5 ml	
10 minims	=	0.6 ml	
12 minims	=	0.75 ml	
15 minims	=	1 ml	= 1 cc
30 minims	=	2 ml	
45 minims	=	3 ml	
60 minims	=	3.697 ml	= 1 fluid dram
1 fl. dram (1℥)	=	4 ml	= 1 teaspoon = 60 gtts
1¼ drams	=	5 ml	
2 fl drams	=	8 ml	= 1 dessert spoonful
2½ fl drams	=	10 ml	
½ fl oz	=	15 ml	= 3 teaspoons = 1 tablespoon
1 fl oz (1℥)	=	30 ml	= 8 fl drams
1½ fl oz.	=	45 ml	= 1 jigger
2 fl oz	=	60 ml	= 1 wineglass
4 fl oz	=	120 ml	= 1 teacup
8 fl oz	=	240 ml	= 1 glassful
16 fl oz	=	473.2 ml	= 1 pint
32 fl oz	=	946.3 ml	= 1 quart
33.8 fl oz	=	1000 ml	= 1 liter

APOTHECARY AND METRIC WEIGHT EQUIVALENTS

Grains		Milligrams		Grams
1/1000	=	0.06	=	0.00006
1/600	=	0.1	=	0.0001
1/500	=	0.12	=	0.00012
1/250	=	0.25	=	0.00025
1/200	=	0.3	=	0.0003
1/150	=	0.4	=	0.0004
1/120	=	0.5	=	0.0005
1/100	=	0.6	=	0.0006
1/60	=	1	=	0.0001
1/40	=	1.5	=	0.0015
1/30	=	2	=	0.002
1/20	=	3	=	0.003
1/15	=	4	=	0.004
1/10	=	6	=	0.006
1/8	=	8	=	0.008
1/6	=	10	=	0.01
1/4	=	15	=	0.015
1/3	=	20	=	0.02
3/8	=	25	=	0.025
1/2	=	30	=	0.03
3/4	=	50	=	0.05
1	=	60 or 65	=	0.60 or 0.65
1 1/2	=	100	=	0.01
2	=	120	=	0.12
2 1/2	=	150	=	0.15
3	=	200	=	0.2
4	=	250	=	0.25
5	=	300	=	0.3
7 1/2	=	500	=	0.5
10	=	600	=	0.6
15	=	1000	=	1
30	=	2000	=	2

Grains	Milligrams	Grams
437.5 =	28,350	= 28.35 = 1 oz.
7000	= 453,590	= 453.59 = 1 lb. = 2.2 kilograms

AVOIRDUPOIS AND METRIC WEIGHT EQUIALVENTS

lb	kg	kg	lb
1	0.5	1	2.2
2	0.9	2	4.4
4	1.8	3	6.6
6	2.7	4	8.8
8	3.6	5	11.0
10	4.5	6	13.2
20	9.1	8	17.6
30	13.6	10	22
40	18.2	20	44
50	22.7	30	66
60	27.3	40	88
70	31.8	50	110
80	36.4	60	132
90	40.9	70	154
100	45.4	80	176
150	68.2	90	198
200	90.8	100	220

1 lb = 0.454 kg   1 kg = 2.204 lb

Metric Equivalents

Weights

1 picogram	=	10^{-12} gm
1 nanogram	=	10^{-9} gm
1 microgram	=	10^{-3} mg = 10^{-6} gm
1 milligram	=	1000 micrograms = 10^{-6} gram
1 centigram	=	10 milligrams = 10^{-1} decigrams = 10^{-2} gram
1 decigram	=	100 milligrams = 10 centigrams = 10^{-1} gram
1 gram	=	1000 milligrams = 100 centigrams = 10 decigrams
1 kilogram	=	1000 grams

Volume

1 milliliter	=	1 gram
1 liter	=	1 kilogram = 1000 grams (milliliters)

TRADITIONAL LINEAR MEASURE AND METRIC EQUIVALENTS

1 inch	= 2.54 centimeters (cm)
1 cm	= 0.3937 inches
1 foot	= 12 inches = 30.48 cm
1 yard	= 36 inches = 0.9144 meters
1 mile	= 5280 feet = 1.609 kilometers
1 kilometer	= 3281 feet (0.62 mile) = 1000 meters

Inches	Centimeters
½	1.27
1	2.54
1½	3.81
2	5.08
2½	6.35
3	7.62
4	10.16
5	12.7
10	25.4
12	30.5
18	45.7
24	61
36	91
48	122

TEMPERATURE CONVERSION

Celsius (Centigrade) 0	Fahrenheit 32
36.0	96.8
36.5	97.7
37.0 ←————————————————→	98.6 Normal
37.5	99.5
38.0	100.4
38.5	101.3
39.0	102.2
39.5	103.1
40.0	104.0
40.5	104.9
41.0	105.8
41.5	106.7
42.0	107.6

Convert Celsius readings to Fahrenheit by multiplying by 1.8 and adding 32. Convert Fahrenheit readings to Celsius by substracting 32 and dividing by 1.8.

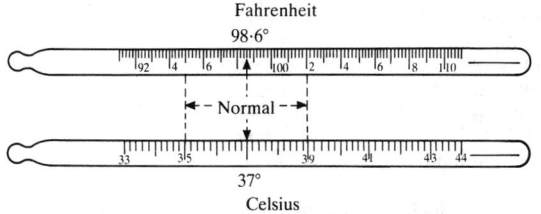

Fahrenheit
98·6°

← - Normal - →

37°
Celsius

24-HOUR CLOCK

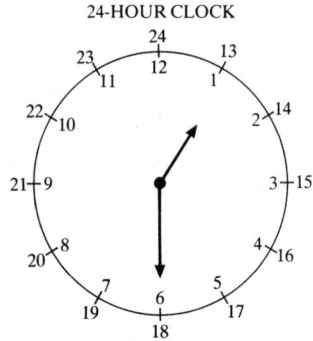

24-HOUR CLOCK

From midnight to noon—12-hr time
                      24-hr time   identical

From noon to midnight—Add 12 to p.m. time = 24-hr time

12-hour time	24-hour Time
12:00 midnight	24:00
12:01 a.m.	00:01
12:59 a.m.	00:59
1:00 a.m.	01:00
12:00 noon	12:00
12:01 p.m.	12:01
1:00 p.m.	13:00
5:30 p.m.	17:30
10:08 p.m.	22:08
12:00 midnight	24:00

**A useful clock for avoiding confusion about a.m. and p.m.
designations**

INDEX

Note: Page numbers followed by the letter i refer to illustrations; page numbers followed by the letter t refer to tables.

KEY TELEPHONE NUMBERS

Admitting_____	Messenger_____
Anesthesia_____	Nuclear medicine_____
Blood bank_____	Nursing office_____
Cardiac care unit_____	OR_____
CT_____	Paging_____
Drug information center____	Pharmacy_____
Dietician_____	Poison control_____
Echocardiology_____	Physical therapy_____
EEG_____	Pulmonary function_____
EKG_____	Recovery room_____
ER_____	Rehabilitation_____
ICU_____	Respiratory therapy_____
Information_____	Security_____
IV team_____	Social service_____
Kitchen_____	Sonography_____
Laboratory_____	Surgery_____
Blood bank_____	Surgical library_____
Blood gases_____	X-ray (diagnostic)_____
Chemistry_____	Angiography_____
Coagulation_____	Cardiac cath_____
Cytology_____	Lymphangiography_____
Drug levels_____	Mammography_____
Hematology_____	Pediatric_____
Pathology_____	Portables_____
Urinalysis_____	Preoperative_____
Maintenance_____	Urologic_____
Medical records_____	X-ray (therapeutic)_____